THYROID
HORMONE
METABOLISM

Thyroid
Hormone
Metabolism

PROCEEDINGS OF AN INTERNATIONAL
SYMPOSIUM HELD IN GLASGOW
7–9 AUGUST 1974

Edited by

W. A. Harland

and

J. S. Orr

Western Infirmary
Glasgow, Scotland

1975

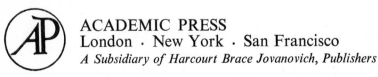
ACADEMIC PRESS
London · New York · San Francisco
A Subsidiary of Harcourt Brace Jovanovich, Publishers

ACADEMIC PRESS INC. (LONDON) LTD.

24–28 Oval Road,

London NW1

U.S. Edition published by

ACADEMIC PRESS INC.

111 Fifth Avenue

New York, New York 10003

Library of Congress Catalog Card Number 75–13622

ISBN: 0–12–325650–X

PRINTED IN GREAT BRITAIN BY

PAGE BROS (NORWICH) LTD, NORWICH

Contributors and Participants

W.D. ALEXANDER, *Gardiner Institute, Western Infirmary, Glasgow, Scotland.*

T.K. BELL, *Royal Victoria Hospital, Belfast, Northern Ireland.*

B. BERNARD, *Department of Internal Medicine III, Medical Faculty, Rotterdam, Holland.*

E.G. BLACK, *Department of Medicine, Queen Elizabeth Hospital, Birmingham, U.K.*

C.C.F. BLAKE, *Laboratory of Molecular Biophysics, South Parks Road, Oxford, U.K.*

A.M.B. BOSS, *Department of Physics, New End Hospital, New End, London, U.K.*

A. BOSSUYT, *Service de Medicine, Hospital Brugmann, Place Van Gehuchten, 1020, Brussels, Belgium.*

A. BURGER, *Laboratoire d'Investigation Clinique, Hopital Cantonal, 1211 Geneve 4, Switzerland.*

C.W. BURKE, *Endocrinology Service, The Radcliffe Infirmary, Oxford, U.K.*

W.A. BURR, *Department of Medicine, Queen Elizabeth Hospital, Birmingham, U.K.*

P.J. CARTER, *Department of Medicine, Queen Elizabeth Hospital, Birmingham, U.K.*

R.R. CAVALIERI, *Veterans Administration Hospital, 4150 Clement Street, San Francisco, California, 94121, U.S.A.*

G.S. CHALLAND, *Radioimmunoassay Unit, Stobhill Hospital, Glasgow, Scotland.*

R. CHAPMAN, *Department of Nuclear Medicine, The Middlesex Hospital Medical School, Nassau Street, London, U.K.*

P. COULOMBE, *Centre Hospitalier Universite Laval, 2705 Blvd. Laurier, Quebec, Canada.*

M. DEMEESTER-MURKINE, *Department des Radioisotopes, Hospital Brugmann, Place Van Gehuchten, 1020, Brussels, Belgium.*

W. DILLMAN, *Endocrine Research Laboratory, Department of Medicine, Montefiore Hospital and Medical Center, Bronx, New York, U.S.A.*

R. DOCTER, *University Hospital Dijkzigt, Erasmus University, Department of Internal Medicine III, Rotterdam, Holland.*

I.P. DRYSDALE, *Division of Clinical Investigation, Clinical Research Centre, Harrow, U.K.*

C.J. EDMONDS, *Medical Unit, University College Hospital Medical School, University Street, London, U.K.*

R.P. EKINS, *Department of Nuclear Medicine, The Middlesex Hospital Medical School, Nassau Street, London, U.K.*

M.J. EVANS, *c/o King's College, Cambridge, U.K.*

D.C. EVERED, *Department of Medicine, Royal Victoria Infirmary, Newcastle upon Tyne, U.K.*

M. FINLAYSON, *Department of Clinical Physics and Bio-Engineering, West Graham Street, Glasgow, Scotland.*

J. FINUCANE, *Department of Medicine, University of Birmingham, Birmingham, U.K.*

N. FISHMAN, *Department of Medicine, Washington University School of Medicine, St. Louis, Missouri, 63110, U.S.A.*

R.D. FRUMESS, *Division of Endocrinology and Metabolism, Department of Medicine, University of Pittsburgh School of Medicine, Pittsburgh, Pennsylvania, U.S.A.*

M.J. GEISOW, *Hatfield Polytechnic, Hatfield, Herts, U.K.*

A.W.G. GOOLDEN, *Radiotherapy Department, Hammersmith Hospital, Ducane Road, London, U.K.*

W. GRAY, *Department of Clinical Physics and Bio-Engineering, West Graham Street, Glasgow, Scotland.*

R.S. GRIFFITHS, *Department of Medicine, University of Birmingham, Birmingham, U.K.*

R.B. GUTTLER, *University of California School of Medicine, 2025 Zonal Avenue, Los Angeles, California 90033, U.S.A.*

D.R. HADDEN, *Metabolic Unit, Royal Victoria Hospital, Belfast, Northern Ireland.*

I. HALES, *Royal North Shore Hospital, St. Leonards, New South Wales, Australia.*

R. HALL, *Royal Victoria Infirmary, Newcastle upon Tyne, U.K.*

K.E. HALNAN, *Glasgow Institute of Radiotherapeutics, Western Infirmary, Glasgow, Scotland.*

S. HAYES, *Department of Chemical Pathology, University College Hospital, London, U.K.*

B.R. HARDING, *The Radiochemical Centre, Amersham, Bucks, U.K.*

W.A. HARLAND, *Department of Forensic Medicine, University of Glasgow, Glasgow, Scotland.*

G. HENNEMANN, *University Hospital Dijkzigt, Erasmus University, Department of Internal Medicine III, Rotterdam, Holland.*

T.E. HILDITCH, *Department of Clinical Physics and Bio-Engineering, West Graham Street, Glasgow, Scotland.*

R. HOFFENBERG, *Department of Medicine, Queen Elizabeth Hospital, Birmingham, U.K.*

M.J. HOOPER, *Gardiner Institute, Western Infirmary, Glasgow, Scotland.*

P.W. HORTON, *Department of Clinical Physics and Bio-Engineering, West Graham Street, Glasgow, Scotland.*

D. HUCKLE, *The Radiochemical Centre, Amersham, Bucks, U.K.*

W.M. HUNTER, *M.R.C. Radioimmunoassay Team, Royal Infirmary, Edinburgh, Scotland.*

W.F. HURST, *10 Oldfield Close, Little Chalfont, Bucks, U.K.*

I.I. IBRAHIM, *Veterans Administration Hospital, Jefferson Barracks and Washington University, St. Louis, Missouri, U.S.A.*

S.H. INGBAR, *Veterans Administration Hospital, 4150 Clement Street, San Francisco, California, 94121, U.S.A.*

M. INTUPRAPA, *Department of Medicine, Royal Victoria Infirmary, Newcastle upon Tyne, U.K.*

T.E. ISLES, *Gardenhurst, Newbigging, Broughty Ferry, Dundee, Scotland.*

C.H.G. IRVINE, *Lincoln College, Canterbury, New Zealand.*

W.J. IRVINE, *Department of Therapeutics, Royal Infirmary, Edinburgh, Scotland.*

D.H. KOERNER, *Endocrine Research Laboratory, Department of Medicine, Montefiore Hospital and Medical Center, Bronx, New York, U.S.A.*

B-A. LAMBERG, *Endocrine Research Unit University of Helsinki, P.O. Box 819, Helsinki 10, Finland.*

J. LAOR, *191 Brickenhall Mansions,Brickenhall Street, London, U.K.*

P.R. LARSEN, *Division of Endocrinology and Metabolism, Department of Medicine, University of Pittsburgh School of Medicine, Pittsburgh, Pennsylvania, U.S.A.*

J.H. LAZARUS, *Department of Medicine, University Hospital of Wales, Heath Park, Cardiff, Wales.*

J.M.A. LENIHAN, *Department of Clinical Physics and Bio-Engineering, West Graham Street, Glasgow, Scotland.*

E.M. McGIRR, *Department of Medicine, Royal Infirmary, Glasgow, Scotland.*

S. McHARDY-YOUNG, *Department of General Medicine and Endo-crinology, Central Middlesex Hospital, London, U.K.*

D.G. McLARTY, *Stobhill Hospital, Glasgow, Scotland.*

A. McMASTER, *Royal Victoria Hospital, Belfast, Northern Ireland.*

M.N. MAISEY, *Department of Nuclear Medicine, Guy's Hospital, St. Thomas Street, London, U.K.*

P.G. MALAN, *Department of Nuclear Medicine, The Middlesex Hospital Medical School, Nassau Street, London, U.K.*

P. MARTIN, *Department of Medicine, University of California, San Fransisco, California, U.S.A.*

P.O. MILCH, *Department of Medicine, Columbia University College of Physicians and Surgeons, New York 10032, and Protein Research Laboratory, Bronx Veterans Adminis-tration Hospital, Bronx, New York, 10468, U.S.A.*

D.A.D. MONTGOMERY, *Royal Victoria Hospital, Belfast, Northern Ireland.*

C. MOSER, *Department of Medicine, University of California, San Francisco, California, U.S.A.*

W. NAEGELE, *Byk-Mallinckrodt Ltd., Germany.*

R. NEWALL, *Miles Laboratories Ltd., Stoke Court, Stoke Poges, Slough, Bucks, U.K.*

J.T. NICOLOFF, *University of Southern California School of Medicine, 2025 Zonal Avenue, Los Angeles, California 90033, U.S.A.*

K. NOBLE, *Mallinckrodt (U.K.) Ltd., Building 521, 59/1 Solent Road, Heathrow Airport, London, U.K.*

L. NYE, *Chemical Pathology Department, St. Bartholomew's Hospital, Bartholomew's Close, London, U.K.*

S.J. OATLEY, *Laboratory of Molecular Biophysics, South Parks Road, Oxford, U.K.*

J.H. OPPENHEIMER, *Montefiore Hospital and Medical Center, Bronx, New York, 10467, U.S.A.*

J.S. ORR, *Department of Clinical Physics and Bio-Engineering, West Graham Street, Glasgow, Scotland.*

C.L. OTIS, *University of Southern California School of Medicine, 2025 Zonal Avenue, Los Angeles, California 90033, U.S.A.*

J.L.W. PARKER, *Department of Medicine, Western Infirmary, Glasgow, Scotland.*

V. PEREZ-MENDEZ, *Department of Radiology, University of California, San Francisco, U.S.A.*

R. PITT-RIVERS, *Department of Zoology, University College London, Gower Street, London, U.K.*

E.E. POCHIN, *MRC Department of Clinical Research, University College Hospital Medical School, University Street, London, U.K.*

B.N. PREMACHANDRA, *Veterans Administration Hospital, Jefferson Barracks, St. Louis, Missouri 63125, U.S.A.*

D.B. RAMSDEN, *Department of Medicine, Queen Elizabeth Hospital, Birmingham, U.K.*

T. RANDALL, *Pathology Department, Western Infirmary, Glasgow, Scotland.*

J.G. RATCLIFFE, *Radioimmunoassay Unit, Stobhill Hospital, Glasgow, Scotland.*

W.A. RATCLIFFE, *Radioimmunoassay Unit, Stobhill Hospital, Glasgow, Scotland.*

L. REES, *Department of Chemical Pathology Research, St. Bartholomew's Hospital, London, U.K.*

T.S. REEVE, *Department of Surgery, The Royal North Shore Hospital of Sydney, St. Leonards, N.S.W. 2065, Australia.*

B. RERAT, *Laboratoire de Cristallographie, C.N.R.S. Laboratoires de Bellevue, Place Aristide Briand, 92-Bellevue, France.*

C. RERAT, *Laboratoire de Cristallographie, C.N.R.S. Laboratoires de Bellevue, Place Aristide Briand, 92-Bellevue, France.*

S.H. RIDGWAY, *Naval Undersea Center, San Diego, California, U.S.A.*

R.S. RIVLIN, *Institute of Human Nutrition, College of Physicians and Surgeons, Columbia University, Black Building 215, 630 West 168th Street, New York, N.Y. 10032, U.S.A.*

J. ROBBINS, *National Institutes of Health, Building 10, Bethesda, Maryland 20017, U.S.A.*

L.L. ROSENBERG, *Department of Physiology-Anatomy, 2549 Life Sciences Building, University of California, Berkeley, California 95720, U.S.A.*

S. ROSENGARD, *The Central Hospital of Middle Ostrobothina, Finland.*

H.L. SCHWARTZ, *Endocrine Research Laboratory, Division of Endocrinology, Department of Medicine, Montefiore Hospital and Medical Center, Bronx, N.Y. 10467, U.S.A.*

J. SETH, *University Department of Clinical Chemistry, Royal Infirmary, Edinburgh, Scotland.*

R.A. SHAKESPEAR, *Department of Clinical Biochemistry, Radcliffe Infirmary, Oxford, U.K.*

D. SHAMES, *Department of Radiology, University of California, San Francisco, U.S.A.*

J.W. SHAW, *University of Southern California School of Medicine, 2025 Zonal Avenue, Los Angeles, California 90033, U.S.A.*

K.J. SHEADER, *Ames Company, P.O. Box 37, Stoke Court, Stoke Poges, Slough, Bucks, U.K.*

J. SMEULERS, *University Hospital Dijkzigt, Erasmus University, Dr. Molewaterplein 40, Rotterdam, Holland.*

D.S. SMITH, *Technicon Methods and Standards Laboratory, 54 St. Bartholomew Close, London, U.K.*

G.F.W. SMITH, *The Radiochemical Centre, White Lion Road, Amersham, Bucks, U.K.*

R.N. SMITH, *Academic Division of Medicine, Section of Therapeutics, Royal Infirmary, Sheffield, U.K.*

C.A. SPENCER, *Radioimmunoassay Unit, Stobhill Hospital, Glasgow, Scotland.*

J.J. STEINBACH, *Nuclear Medicine Service, Veterans Administration Hospital, Buffalo, New York, U.S.A.*

A.V. STEPANAS, *Department of Nuclear Medicine, Guy's Hospital, St. Thomas Street, London, U.K.*

K. STERLING, *Veterans Administration Hospital, 130 West Kingsbridge Road, Bronx, New York 10468, U.S.A.*

J.T. STINIS, *University Hospital Dijkzigt, Erasmus University, Department of Internal Medicine III, Rotterdam, Holland.*

S.B. SUFI, *Department of Nuclear Medicine, The Middlesex Hospital Medical School, Nassau Street, London, U.K.*

M.I. SURKS, *Montefiore Hospital and Medical Center, Bronx, N.Y. 10467, U.S.A.*

I.D. SUTHERLAND, *Mallinckrodt (U.K.) Ltd., Building 521, 59/1 Solent Road, Heathrow Airport, London, U.K.*

R.L. SUTHERLAND, *Department de Chimic Biologique, 78 Avenue General Leclerc, 94 Bicetre, Paris, France.*

I.D.A. SWAN, *Chemistry Department, Glasgow University, Glasgow, Scotland.*

A.I. SWILLER, *1130 Ocean Avenue, Brooklyn, New York, N.Y. 11230, U.S.A.*

H.E. SWILLER, *1130 Ocean Avenue, Brooklyn, New York, N.Y. 11230, U.S.A.*

D. TERGIS, *Institute of Human Nutrition, College of Physicians and Surgeons, Columbia University, New York, U.S.A.*

J.A. THOMSON, *Department of Medicine, Royal Infirmary, Glasgow, Scotland.*

B.D. THOMPSON, *Medical Unit, University College Hospital Medical School, University Street, London, U.K.*

J.M. THORP, *I.C.I. Pharmaceutical Division, Alderley Edge, Macclesfield, Cheshire, U.K.*

A.D. TOFT, *Department of Therapeutics, Royal Infirmary, Edinburgh, Scotland.*

M.B. VALLOTTON, *Endocrine Division, Department of Medicine, University of Geneva, Switzerland.*

P. VICE, *Department of Medicine, Royal Victoria Infirmary, Newcastle upon Tyne, U.K.*

T.J. VISSER, *University Hospital Dijkzigt, Erasmus University, Department of Internal Medicine III, Dr. Molewaterplein 40, Rotterdam, Holland.*

D.W. WARREN, *University of Southern California School of Medicine, 2025 Zonal Avenue, Los Angeles, California 90033, U.S.A.*

J.A. WEAVER, *Metabolic Unit, Royal Victoria Hospital, Grosvenor Road,Belfast, Northern Ireland.*

B. WEINHEIMER, *Medizinische Universitats-Klinik I, 665 Homburg/Saar, Germany.*

K.W. WENZEL, *Klinikum Steglitz, Hindenburgerdamm 30, I Berlin 45, West Germany.*

G.M. WILSON, *Department of Medicine, Western Infirmary, Glasgow, Scotland.*

D. WYPER, *Department of Clinical Physics and Bio-Engineering, West Graham Street, Glasgow, Scotland.*

Foreword

The papers are divided into two sections, which reflect problems uppermost in our interest in the thyroid field at the present time.

In the first section on the specific binding and peripheral action of thyroid hormones, the transport proteins have been reviewed and the precise localisation of thyroxine bound to crystalline prealbumin has been revealed by X-ray analysis. New data are presented concerning hormone binding at the periphery (target organs), a subject of obvious importance in relation to the specific actions of the hormones at a cellular or subcellular level. A number of subcellular targets have been investigated, including the nucleus (the role of thyroid hormones in protein synthesis) and adenyl cyclase (mediator of thyrotrophic activity). It is evident throughout that the role of thyroxine as a prohormone for triiodothyronine is receiving more and more support, although there is no evidence yet to deny thyroxine an intrinsic activity of its own. Indeed, until a test can be devised whereby thyroxine activity is demonstrable in the total absence of deiodination this problem will remain unresolved. Nevertheless, increasingly sensitive methods of analysis of thyroid hormones and their metabolites have revealed a possible role for these in various thyroid states.

In the second section on thyroid hormone function in clinical investigation, a number of new methods or refinements of old ones are described. Radioimmunoassay, which has made such rapid advances in recent years, has been developed to determine the very small amounts of triiodothyronine in various body fluids. The simultaneous estimation of thyroxine and triiodothyronine has also undergone increased precision. Renal turnover of both thyroid hormones has been studied and been shown to correlate with free hormone levels in serum.

Dr. Harland, Dr. Orr and the organising committee are to be congratulated on having arranged a most stimulating programme of papers which has lead to many profitable discussions.

R. Pitt-Rivers.

Preface

Twenty years is a long time for a concept to hold a pre-eminent place in a developing clinical specialty. The concept of the role of free thyroxine has so far maintained its importance both in the teaching and practice of thyroid endocrinology, and in the stimulation of research into thyroid hormone metabolism and into the basis of clinical tests of thyroid function. The studies and the progress which have been inspired are a measure of the insight of Recant, Riggs, Robbins, Rall, and of others, who developed and formulated the concept.

The interest in the plasma binding proteins has led to intensive studies. Valuable clinical correlations with thyroid status have been established, and an extensive range of laboratory tests of thyroid function have been developed, stimulated by the model of free and bound hormone exchanging in plasma. Studies on triiodothyronine have proceeded in parallel with this work and have permeated most aspects of it. In contrast, understanding of the cellular actions of thyroid hormones has not advanced rapidly, and studies in this field have been relatively neglected.

It has, however, been realised for many years that there were numerous observations which could not readily be accounted for in terms of the free thyroxine concept, which, as normally presented, ignores tissue binding. Partly in response to the difficulties encountered in attempting to stretch the concept

to embrace diverse anomalies, interest in the extent and nature
of tissue binding has grown rapidly. This welcome, and fairly
recent trend, has had the effect of bringing together the
clinically motivated studies of cellular binding and the
physiological studies of hormone cellular action.

More recently still, knowledge of the details of the
stereospecific structure of plasma binding proteins has leapt
forward. It may well be that this knowledge will lead to a
further and perhaps quite new understanding of the functions
of the plasma binding proteins in the first instance, and of
tissue binding thereafter.

The organising committee were gratified that the response
to the announcement of this conference brought forward papers
which fitted well together to provide a broad view of the
current status of the whole of this active field, and clearly
illuminated areas in which conflicts of view and of interpretation exist. The discussions showed that thyroid hormone
metabolism is a subject which is marked by a most lively re-
appraisal.

The Editors are grateful to Dr. D. Evered, Mr. W. Gray,
Dr. D. Hadden, Mr. T. Hilditch, Dr. P. Horton and Dr. J.
Thomson for reporting the discussions, but must themselves
accept any blame if the expressions of speakers' views which
fuelled the debate and are recorded here do not always correspond exactly to the actual views held by the speakers at that
time. The Editors are also grateful to Mrs. Norma McCulloch
for her help with the pre-conference organisation, and are
deeply indebted to Mrs. Sheena Lawrence without whose assistance the amorphous mass of documents making up the proceedings

could never have been transformed into the finished volume.

W.A. Harland,

J.S. Orr.

Acknowledgements

Support from the following
is gratefully acknowledged

Abbott Laboratories

Glaxo Ltd.

ICI Pharmaceutical Division

Mallinckrodt (U.K.) Ltd.

Merck, Sharp and Dohme Ltd.

Myles Laboratories Ltd.

The Radiochemical Centre, Amersham

The Royal Society

Contents

Section Two

THYROID HORMONE FUNCTION IN CLINICAL INVESTIGATION

1. Structure and Function of Thyroxine-Transport Proteins

JACOB ROBBINS

Clinical Endocrinology Branch,
National Institute of Arthritis, Metabolism, and Digestive
Diseases, National Institutes of Health,
Bethesda, Maryland, U.S.A.

INTRODUCTION

This is a most appropriate time to discuss the transport
proteins for the thyroid hormones, since we have seen in the
past several years remarkable progress in the chemistry of
these interesting molecules. The thyroxine-binding prealbumin
has become the first hormone-binding protein of any kind to
have its structure fully defined by chemical and physical
studies. The excitement in this advance is not that prealbumin
plays so far-reaching a role in thyroid hormone metabolism,
but rather that we now have a base for further exploration of
thyroxine and triiodothyronine binding sites on other proteins
having specificity for these hormones. In particular, we can
look ahead to a similar definition of the tissue receptor
sites through which the hormones act. As later papers show,
this subject is undergoing a renaissance of major proportions.
I will introduce the topic by describing briefly what we know
about the transport proteins in blood, and will include some
of our own studies of the past few years on the chemistry of

prealbumin (PA).

The first point to make is that there is no evidence
whatever to indicate that any one of them functions as a
transport protein in the sense that it carries the hormone
across the plasma membrane into the cell. The evidence that
the opposite is true, i.e. that the hormone must first dissociate from the protein and then enter the cell, is, however,
entirely indirect. One type of evidence comes from kinetic
studies of thyroxine distribution and metabolism. Table 1 lists
metabolic clearance rates for thyroxine and triiodothyronine
compared to those of the transport proteins. It is obvious
that triiodothyronine is removed from blood at a very much
faster rate than the proteins themselves even though both
thyroxine-binding globulin (TBG) and PA have relatively rapid
disappearance rates. This is also true for thyroxine when one
recognises that only a small portion of the protein is complexed
with hormones. Therefore, the complexes are not metabolized
as hormone-protein units. Further evidence derived from acute
distribution studies is shown in Table 2. Thyroxine clearly
leaves the blood faster than its transport proteins. Oppenheimer *et al.* (7) directly compared the acute loss of thyroxine from blood in the hepatic circulation with that of labeled albumin and prealbumin over a 4-hour period. The clearance of the two proteins was about 10 ml/min, much slower
than that of thyroxine. TBG, having a similar molecular weight,
probably behaves similarly. Since liver capillaries are freely
permeable to protein, the barrier must be at the cell well,
but thyroxine passage into the cells is evidently extremely
rapid. In extrahepatic tissues the barrier to protein is at
the capillary wall, as Irvine and Simpson-Morgan (8) demon-

strated directly by studies of thyroxine and protein kinetics in regional lymph. From a quantitative standpoint, the table shows that the free thyroxine pool must turn over many times per minute to account for the observed rates, especially in the liver.

Table 1.   *Metabolic Clearance Rates*

	Fraction/day	ml Blood/h	Fraction Protein Occupied by T_4
TBG	.14	40	.26
PA	.31	90	.039
ALB	.05	13	.0016
T_4	.10	50	
T_3	.57	1100	

The values are derived from the following sources : TBG, Refetoff *et al.* (1), Cavalieri *et al.* (1a); PA and albumin, Socolow *et al.* (2), Oppenheimer *et al.* (3); T_4 and T_3, Rall *et al.* (4) and Oppenheimer and Surks (5). In the case of the proteins a volume of distribution (V) of 7 liters was assumed. The metabolic clearance rate (MCR) was calculated from the fractional rate (F) or the half time ($t_{\frac{1}{2}}$) by the following equations:

$$\text{MCR (ml h}^{-1}\text{)} = \text{F (day}^{-1}\text{)} \times \text{V (1)} \times \frac{1000}{24}$$

$$\text{F (day}^{-1}\text{)} = \frac{0.693}{t_{\frac{1}{2}}(\text{day})}$$

The question then arises whether thyroxine can dissociate rapidly enough to satisfy these tissue turnover rates. Hillier (9) has measured the off-rates of thyroxine from TBG and PA

(Table 3) and they are indeed rapid enough. Note that the time
scale here is seconds rather than minutes. Therefore, all the
data fit the requirements for free thyroxine transport across
cell barriers and we can assume that triiodothyronine behaves
similarly. Also note that the dissociation rates are such that
TBG and PA contribute equally to free T_4 renewal.

Table 2.   *Acute Thyroxine Clearance*

	Extrahepatic ECF	Hepatic
ml blood/min	5	40
µg/min	0.2	2
Fraction total T_4/min	.002	.03
Fraction free T_4/min	8	100

The clearance rates are from Nicoloff and Dowling (6).
Other values are calculated from the following assumptions :
hepatic blood flow = 1500 ml/min, extrahepatic blood flow =
2500ml/min, total T_4 = 4 µg/100 ml blood, free T_4 = 1 ng/
100ml blood.

On the other hand, Hoch and Lewallen (10) have postulated
that weak binding proteins in plasma could be involved in
intracellular penetration; as they point out, this would still
be compatible with the observation that the hormonal "status"
correlates better with free than with total hormone level since
the hormone-weak binder concentration would parallel the free
hormone concentration. Thus we still cannot reject the possibility that transport into some, or even all, cells requires
the transfer of a hormone-protein complex. In one instance,
however, we can say that the protein TBG is definitely not
required for transport. Cases with totally absent TBG on a

genetic basis can occur with no apparent abnormality in thyroid hormone status of the affected individual (11). Obviously TBG, the protein which carries most of the serum T_4 and T_3, is not essential for thyroid hormone action.

Table 3. T_4 *Dissociation Rates* $(37^{\circ}C)$

	TBG	PA
$t_{\frac{1}{2}}$ (sec)	39	7.4
T_4 equivalents (μg/sec)	0.10	0.19
Free T_4 renewal (times/sec)	48	48

(Adapted from Hillier (9), assuming TBG:PA = 75:15)

If the transport proteins play no specific role in intra-cellular transfer, we can look at them from two points of view. First, they may function as buffers responsible for keeping a large store of thyroid hormone in the extrathyroidal space in a non-diffusable form. In this sense, TBG is the most important since it carries about 75% of the T_4 and T_3 in the blood and much more than is carried by PA (Table 4). The buffer role would prevent wide swings in hormone availability at the target cell and might also avoid excessive hormone action at non-target sites. A second function is their role as donors of hormone from the microcirculation to the cell. Here we can calculate from their dissociation rates, as we have just seen, that TBG and PA contribute equally to the turnover of the free thyroxine pool. If the hormone complexed to albumin and other minor binders has similarly rapid dissociation rates, then these proteins could also contribute to the free hormone pool to an extent which is much greater than their proportional role in thyroid binding. Thus, we have to admit that we cannot estimate how important these transport proteins are, nor can we assert that one is more important than another in all respects.

Table 4.   *Distribution of T_4 and T_3*
                              in serum

	TBG/PA
T_4 bound	5-9
T_3 bound	~10
F T_4 renewal	1

   The values for T_4 and T_3 bound to TBG and PA are derived from the mass action law equations and best estimates of the association constants (12,13,14). The contribution to FT_4 renewal is from Table 3.

   I now turn to the subject of the chemistry and the structure of the two proteins, TBG and PA, which transport most of the circulating thyroid hormones. It is evident from what I have already said that these have the highest affinity for hormone and probably the greatest specificity as well. Therefore, they seem to have the greatest attraction for those interested in thyroid hormone transport. I will not discuss albumin and other weak binders which more properly, perhaps, belong to other disciplines. For completeness, however, I must identify the so-called weak binders, since I have not done so as yet. Serum albumin needs no comment except to say that, despite its far-reaching role as a transport protein for many substances, it does have one strong binding site for T_4 and T_3 in addition to multiple weaker sites. The strong site has an affinity constant for T_4 of 2×10^6 (pH 7.4, .1 M NaCl,

$25^{\circ}C$) (15). This is 2 orders of magnitude lower than the
affinity of PA, and 4 orders lower than TBG, but the high con-
concentration of albumin in blood enables it to carry about
10% of the T_4 and 30% of T_3.

The second category of weak binders is lipoproteins of
the α and β type. Their involvement was indicated some years
ago, mainly from immunoelectrophoretic studies, and more recently was confirmed by Myai *et al.* (16) and Hoch and Lewallen
(10). In fact, there may even be others, and their study may
well be of interest. There is no evidence thus far to indicate whether T_4 is bound to the apoprotein portion of the molecule or is simply dissolved in the lipid. The third category
is γ-globulin, with relatively strong binding of T_4 or T_3 to
antibodies which are developed against thyroglobulin or against
artificial hormone-protein complexes. This occurs not only
when antibodies are produced experimentally (17), but also in
"spontaneous" lymphocytic thyroiditis (18).

Interest in the purification of TBG and PA goes back almost to the first studies on thyroxine transport, when several
laboratories tried unsuccessfully to obtain highly purified
TBG (Table 5). The low concentration of ~15 mg/l made this a
difficult problem. Only recently did the problem meet with
success through the application of affinity chromatography.
Pensky and Marshall (24) used T_4 coupled directly to agarose
to obtain partially purified TBG. They first reported that
DEAE Sephadex chromatography following the affinity column was
sufficient to yield pure TBG, but later indicated (26) that
a third procedure of gel filtration on Sephadex G-150 was
required.

At the same time, Pages and Cahnmann (27) were employing

Table 5.   *Purification of TBG*

	Year	Starting Material	Method
Ingbar *et al.* (19)	1957	Cohn Fr. IV-6,7,9	Anion exchange resin
Tata (20)	1961	Cohn Fr. IV-9	Electrophoresis; DEAE-cellulose
Seal & Doe (21)	1964	Plasma	DEAE-sephadex; Sephadex; hydroxyl-apatite
Andreoli *et al.* (22)	1964	Cohn Fr. IV-4	DEAE-cellulose
Giorgio & Tabachnik (23)	1968	Plasma	$(NH4)_2SO_4$; electro-phoresis; DEAE-cell-ulose; PAGE
Pensky & Marshall (24)	1969	Plasma	T4-sepharose; DEAE-sephadex; gel fil-tration
Sterling *et al.* (25)	1971	Cohn Fr. IV-4	CM-cellulose; Sepha-dex; DEAE-sephadex; PAGE.

aminocaproyl T_4 coupled to agarose on the assumption that this would be superior to T_4-Sepharose. Although the initial purification was somewhat greater, the advantages seemed insufficient to warrant the added synthetic steps. We, therefore, have utilized T_4-Sepharose in our subsequent work (28). One unexpected observation was that the T_4-Sepharose columns retained no prealbumin. Since the T_4 binding site of PA is deep within the molecule we thought that the problem might be that the T_4 residues did not protrude far enough from the gel matrix. However, aminocaproyl T_4 and glycylamino-undecanoyl-T_4 with side arms of 12Å and 23 Å, respectively, also failed to immobilize PA. A possible explanation for this enigma will be apparent shortly.

An additional problem in affinity chromatography was
noted by Marshall and Pensky (29). They found that columns
became contaminated with neuraminidase, leading to the formation of desialylated TBG with slower electrophoretic mobility
than the native protein. This was preventable by adding a
neuraminidase inhibitor or by recycling the T_4-Sepharose with
KOH and $NaHCO_3$.

Purification of PA has been less difficult owing to its
higher concentration in plasma ($\sim$300 mg/l), and was accomplished by conventional separation methods in several laboratories (20,21,30--34). It was also possible to crystallize
PA (31,35), forming the starting point for molecular studies
about which you will hear more later.

I now summarize some of the physical properties of TBG
and PA obtained with these purified preparations. The molecular weights have been the subject of some disagreement
(Table 6), but are now quite well established. The values reported for TBG ranged from 36,000 to 64,000. In our own laboratory, using equilibrium sedimentation, Lord *et al.*(28)
confirmed the value of $\sim$60,000. The available evidence favors
the view that TBG is a single polypeptide chain, although this
is not yet definitive. For PA, reported molecular weights vary
from 50,000 to 73,000. Branch *et al.* (38) using equilibrium
sedimentation, confirmed a molecular weight of 54,000. The
higher values may be due to inclusion of attached retinol
binding protein (mol. wt. 21,000). The tetrameric nature of
PA was first suggested by the genetic polymorphism observed
in the rhesus monkey (39,40) since the homozygous types had
a single PA component whereas the heterozygote showed 5 thy-

Table 6.   *Molecular Weights*

	TBG		PA
Seal & Doe (21)	59,000	Seal & Doe (21)	70,000
Giorgio & Tabachnik (23)	58,000	Schultz *et al.*(30)	61,000
Sterling *et al.* (25)	36,500	Oppenheimer *et al.* (32)	73,000
Marshall & Pensky (36)	64,000	Raz & Goodman (33)	50,000
Lord *et al.* (28)	60,000	Rask *et al.*(37)	62,000
		Branch *et al.* (38)	54,000

roxine-binding components. Although the tetramer is extra-ordinarily stable (38,42) requiring strong denaturing to demonstrate the single subunit, hybridization of the homozygous forms is readily obtained. The rate of hybridization was slower at 25° than in the cold and was reduced when the binding site was occupied by T_4 (39).

Not only does PA not dissociate readily, but its overall shape does not change appreciably between pH 2 and 12 or in 8 M urea, and is only slowly denatured in 6 M guanidine at neutral pH (38,42). Even in 7.3 M guanidine, monkey prealbumin is not totally unfolded until the pH is lowered (41). This remarkable stability may be related to the high degree of β structure, as revealed by circular dichroism (38) and by x-ray diffraction (43). At pH 3.5 a sharp transition in the properties of about half of the tyrosyl and tryptophanyl residues occurs (38), perhaps resulting from the opening up of the binding region to solvent. PA is also highly resistant to enzymatic hydrolysis (44). In our studies on the structure of monkey PA, van Jaarsveld (45) found it impossible to hydrolyze more than

50% of the protein with trypsin even after heating at 100°.
Oxidation with performic acid, however, did permit complete
hydrolysis. Peptide maps showed a great deal of homology between the human and rhesus monkey PA, and the N-terminal 21
amino acids contained only 2 residues which differed in these
species. Interestingly, one of these, residue 5, was the site
of the single amino acid interchange in the PA genetic polymorphism in the monkey.

The amino acid composition of PA (33,37,44-46) is better
known than that of TBG (21,23,25). Until some of the dis-
crepancies between the various TBG preparations are resolved,
I feel that we should retain some reservations about the ex-
act amino acid composition, and also about the carbohydrate
compositions which have been reported (21,23,29). TBG is
notable, however, for its high carbohydrate and sialic acid
content. As with other circulating glycoproteins, the metabolic disappearance rate of TBG is controlled by the terminal
sialic acid residues (1). PA has been referred to as the
tryptophan-rich prealbumin. Although analyses differ, we have
found 3 tryptophans per subunit, or 12 per tetramer, in monkey and human (45). Also, there is only one cysteine per
subunit. Reports that there was only one free sulfhydryl group
per tetramer seemed inconsistent with the ability to dissociate the tetramer with guanidine in the absence of a reducing agent. This must mean that several of the SH groups
are not exposed on the surface of the molecule - another
manifestation of its unusual structure (37,47).

Finally I return to the aspect of TBG and PA structure
which relates to their function - i.e., the nature of their
binding sites.

Table 7.	*Binding relative to* T_4	
	TBG (all at pH 8.6)	PA
L-T_4	100	100
L-T_3	3	10 (pH 7.4)
D-T_4	33	
T_4 Propionic acid	2	
T_4 Acetic acid	38	
T_3 Acetic acid	< 0.1	
T_4 Formic acid	< 0.1	
OMe-D,L-T_4	1	
DIT	< 0.1	1 (pH 7.4)
DIT Propionic acid		200 (pH 8.6)
DIT Benzaldehyde		50 (pH 8.6)

/TBG : Hao & Tabachnik (50)/
/PA : Pages *et al.* (51)- Nilsson & Peterson (52)/

Both proteins show considerable specificity for the thyroid hormones and thyroxine is generally bound more strongly than related molecules. The earlier work (48,49) on this subject employed electrophoretic methods and whole plasma, the complexity of which prevents unequivocal interpretation. Available data with purified proteins are summarised in Table 7. In the case of TBG, a preparation of questionable purity and/or stability was used and the work needs to be repeated with better preparations. The data show a decrease in binding with alteration in the amino acid side chain, in the phenolic group, or in the diphenyl ether structure. On

the other hand certain thyroxyl dipeptides are strongly
bound to TBG (53). In the case of PA, most of these few data
are from our own laboratory. The decreased binding of T_3 must
be due in part to the decreased ionization of the phenolic
group at pH 7.4 since data from a series of halogenated derivatives of T_4 suggested a closer correlation with the pK
of the hydroxyl group than the nature of the substituent *per
se* (54). Titration studies by Nilsson and Peterson (52) showed
that unionized thyroxine, although still bound to PA, inter-
acts much more weakly. In any case, it is evident that the
affinity of T_3 for both TBG and PA at physiologic pH is at
least an order of magnitude lower than that of T_4, a fact of
undoubted importance to the comparative physiology of these
two hormones. The diphenyl ether structure is of less importance in the PA interaction, and deaminated derivatives
of diiodotyrosine exhibit strong binding.

The binding of T_4 by TBG (Table 8) is remarkably strong,
with a constant of 10^{10} at pH 7.4, thus explaining the high
proportion of TBG binding in serum despite the low concentration of the protein, and also accounting for the extremely
high bound/free ratio of > 99/1. From a thermodynamic standpoint, the finding of a small enthalpic change (ΔH^o) and a
large entropic change (ΔS^o) is characteristic of a largely
hydrophobic interaction, and this appears to be more striking
in the case of TBG.

In addition to their binding of the thyroid hormones,
both TBG and PA interact with other small molecules (56).
Some of these are important in pharmacology, since the binding of diphenylhydantoin to TBG, and salicylate especially
to PA, is strong enough to affect thyroid hormone binding

at pharmacologically attained blood levels. Oppenheimer and
Tavernetti (57) pointed out some years ago that the diphenylhydantoin structure is analogous to the diphenyl ether structure of the thyronine derivatives. Even so, less complicated
molecules also interact with the binding sites. One compound
which has been important as a tool for studying hormone binding is the fluorescent probe, 8-anilino-1-naphthalene sul-
fonate (ANS) (Fig. 1), whose fluorescence increases in a non-
polar environment. This property enables it to be used as an
indicator of hormone binding since it has been clearly shown
in our own and other work that ANS and the hormones compete
for the same binding site. When used to study binding to TBG,
as reported by Green *et al.* (55a) the analysis is straight-
forward since there appears to be a single binding site for
both T_4 and ANS. Thus, the affinity constant derived from
the competition reaction is similar to that obtained by conventional methods. Our work with PA, carried out over the
past several years with Drs. Branch, Pages, Ferguson, Edelhoch, Cahnmann and Saroff (54,58) reveals a much more complicated pattern of binding; we found 2 equal binding sites
for ANS per tetramer whereas our own and other work (33,51,
52) identified only one strong site for T_4. Furthermore, we
showed by equilibrium dialysis that certain T_4 analogs (such
as diiodobenzaldehyde) were bound strongly and equally to two
sites whereas others, such as the propionic acid analog of
diiodotyrosine (DIT), seemed to interact with only one site
(51). In our attempts to analyze the T_4-ANS competition, we
could not fit the data to a model for a competitive reaction
between one T_4 and 2 ANS molecules. Finally, we used [³H]
ANS synthesized by Ferguson and Cahnmann (59) as well as

Figure 1.   8-*anilino*-1-*naphthalene Sulfonic Acid (ANS)*

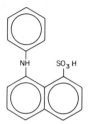

labeled T_4 and studied the binding by the unambiguous dialysis method. This led to the discovery (58) that there was,
in fact, a second binding site for T_4, but its affinity was
about two orders of magnitude lower than the first. We were
then able to show by computer simulation that data for the
binding of ANS and T_4 separately, and data for dialysis of
T_4 in the presence of ANS, fit a single set of parameters.
However, we could not ascertain whether PA had 2 different
binding sites with almost equal affinities for ANS but very
different affinities for T_4 or whether there were two identical binding sites with strongly negative-cooperativity during T_4 occupancy (Table 9).

At this point in our work, we learned that the x-ray
diffraction studies[*] (60) were consistent with 2 identical
binding sites for T_4. Arguing from this and the known stability of the PA molecule, we concluded that the T_4 exhibits
a negative ligand-ligand interaction. We are now in a position to re-evaluate a large accumulation of T_4 analog binding data to map out the properties of the PA binding site.
For example, the finding that the propionic acid analog of
DIT shows the negative cooperativity phenomenon whereas the
* *See also next paper*

Table 8.   *Thermodynamics of T_4 Binding*

TBG (Green *et al.*, 1972) (55)	23°	37°
K (M^{-1})	2.3×10^{10}	1.7×10^{10}
ΔF° (kcal/mole)	-14.0	-14.5
ΔH° (kcal/mole)	$+ 0.21$	$- 0.21$
ΔS° (cal/degree/mole)	$+46.8$	$+46.1$

PA (Nilsson & Peterson, 1971) (52)	4°	37°
K (M^{-1})	2.2×10^{7}	7.8×10^{6}
ΔF° (kcal/mole)	$- 9.3$	$- 9.8$
ΔH° (kcal/mole)		$- 5.3$
ΔS° (cal/degree/mole)		$+14.3$

the aldehyde analog does not (51), suggests that the side
chains of thyroxine interact within the binding site either
by electrostatic or steric hindrance. This orientation is
also consistent with the fact that the phenolic group of
bound T_4 can be titrated (52) and must, therefore, be exposed
to the solvent. This orientation would also explain the
failure of PA to adhere to affinity columns of T_4-Sepharose,
since T_4 is bound to the agarose through its side chain. In
contrast, T_4-Sepharose as well as thyroxyl dipeptides (53)
do bind to TBG.

     In concluding, I turn to another very interesting devel-
opment in our knowledge of the PA molecule which stems from
the work of Goodman and Peterson and their co-workers (34,
47, 61). These groups showed that there exists in serum a
rather tight interaction between PA and another protein,

Table 9.   *Binding of T_4 to PA*

	T_4	ANS
Independent sites		
K_1	$1.0 \times 10^8 \text{ M}^{-1}$	$9.5 \times 10^5 \text{ M}^{-1}$
K_2	$9.5 \times 10^5 \text{ M}^{-1}$	$2.1 \times 10^5 \text{ M}^{-1}$
Interacting sites		
k_1	$5.5 \times 10^7 \text{ M}^{-1}$	$5.5 \times 10^5 \text{ M}^{-1}$
α	0.041	0.62

(interaction energy = $-RT\ln\alpha$)

(from Ferguson *et al.*) (58)

retinol-binding protein (or RBP) which is a specific transport protein for Vitamin A. Furthermore, RBP has a molecular
weight of 21,000, which whould allow its filtration by the
kidney if it were not bound to the larger PA molecule. I
cannot enter into a discussion of this most interesting transport system, which is now under intensive study. We do have
to admit, however, that the physiological implication of this
2-headed transport system for a hormone and a vitamin has
eluded us. One would think that it must hold some significance. To continue my line of thought on protein structure,
however, our studies with van Jaarsveld and Edelhoch (62)
have shown that there are 4 equivalent sites for RBP, although
only one of these is occupied at the concentrations existing
in blood. Dr. Blake in his paper [*] shows where the hormone

molecules are bound in PA, and perhaps he can also identify the location of the RBP molecules. These sites must be separated by some distance since neither T_4 nor RBP interferes with binding of the other ligand (34,47,62).

In this paper, I have simply touched on the high points of our knowledge of these transport proteins. Obviously, I have omitted many details and many interesting ramifications but I want to re-emphasize that, in my view, the studies on PA and its binding sites have achieved a breakthrough in the general field of hormone-binding proteins.

Acknowledgements
   The work reported from my own department has largely been done by the following excellent co-workers : Drs. R. S. Bernstein, W. T. Branch, R. N. Ferguson, R. S. Lord, R. A. Pages and P. P. van Jaarsveld in active collaboration with Drs. H. J. Cahnmann, H. Edelhoch and H. A. Saroff. Their contributions are gratefully acknowledged.

* See next paper

R E F E R E N C E S

1. S. Refetoff, V.S. Fang, N.I. Robin and J.S. Marshall, *Endocrinology,* 92, T8 (1973) abstract.

1a. R.R. Cavalieri, F.A. McMahon and J.N. Castle, *Endocrinology,* 92, T7 (1973) abstract.

2. E.L. Socolow, K.A. Woeber, R.H. Purdy, M.T. Holloway and S.H. Ingbar, *J. Clin. Invest.* 44, 1600-1609 (1965).

3. J.H. Oppenheimer, M.I. Surks, J. Bernstein and J.C. Smith, *Science,* 149, 748-750 (1965).

4. J.E. Rall, J. Robbins and C.G. Lewallen, *In* "The Hormones" (G. Pincus, K.V. Thimann and E.B. Astwood, eds), Vol. 5, pp. 159-439 (1964).

5. J.H. Oppenheimer amd M.I. Surks, *In* "Handbook of Physiology, Section 7: Endocrinology III" (M.A. Greer and D.H. Solomon, eds), Vol. 3, pp. 197-214 (1974).

6. J.T. Nicoloff and J. Dowling, *J. Clin. Invest.* 47, 26-37 (1968).

7. J.H. Oppenheimer, G. Bernstein and J. Hasen, *J. Clin. Invest.* 46, 762-777 (1967).

8. G.H.G. Irvine and M.W. Simpson-Morgan, *J. Clin. Invest.* 54, 156-164 (1974).

9. A.P. Hillier, *J. Physiol.* 217, 625-634 (1971).

10. H. Hoch and C.G. Lewallen, *J. Clin. Endocrinol.* 38, 663-673 (1974).

11. J. Robbins, *Mt. Sinai J. Med.* 60, 511-519, (1973).

12. K.A. Woeber and S.H. Ingbar, *J. Clin. Invest.* 47, 1710-1721 (1968).

13. J. Robbins, *In* "The Thyroid and Biogenic Amines" (J.E. Rall and I. Kopin, eds), pp. 241-254 (1971).

14. R.A. Pages, J. Robbins and H. Edelhoch, *Biochemistry* 12, 2773-2779 (1973).

15. R.F. Steiner, J. Roth and J. Robbins, *J. Biol. Chem.* 241, 560-567 (1966).

16. K. Myai, K.F. Itoh, H. Abe and Y. Kumahara, *Clin. Chim. Acta.* 22, 341-347 (1968).

17. B.N. Premachandra, A.K. Ray, I. Hirata and H.T. Blumenthal, *Endocrinology* 73, 135-154 (1963).

18. B.N. Premachandra and H.T. Blumenthal, *J. Clin. Endocrinol.* 27, 931-936 (1967).

19. S.H. Ingbar, J.T. Dowling and N. Freinkel, *Endocrinology*, 61, 321-326 (1957).

20. J.R. Tata, *Clin. Chim. Acta.* 6, 819-832 (1961).

21. U.S. Seal and R.P. Doe, *In* Proc. Second International Congress of Endocrinology", pp. 325-328 (1964).

22. M. Andreoli, J. Robbins and C. Cassano, *In* "La Thyroide" L'Expansion Scientifique Francaise, Paris, pp. 317-339, (1964).

23. N.A. Giorgio and M. Tabachnik, *J. Biol. Chem.* 243, 2247-2259 (1968).

24. J. Pensky and J.S. Marshall, *Arch. Biochem. Biophys.* 135, 304-310, (1969).

25. K. Sterling, S. Hamada, Y. Takemura, M.A. Brenner, E.S. Newman and M. Inada, *J. Clin. Invest.* 50, 1758, (1971).

26. J.S. Marshall, J. Pensky and S. Williams, *Arch. Biochem. Biophys.* 156, 456-462 (1973).

27. R.A. Pages and H.J. Cahnmann, Abstracts of Fourth International Congress of Endocrinology, Washington, p. 241 (1972).

28. R.S. Lord, H.J. Cahnmann and J. Robbins. Unpublished.

29. J.S. Marshall, J. Pensky and A.M. Green, *J. Clin. Invest.* 51, 3173-3181 (1972).

30. H.E. Schultze, M. Schonenberger and G. Schwick, *Biochem. Z.* 328, 267-284 (1956).

31. R.H. Purdy, K.A. Woeber, M.T. Holloway and S.H. Ingbar, *Biochemistry*, 4, 1888-1895 (1965).

32. J.H. Oppenheimer, M.I. Surks, J.C. Smith and R. Squef, *J. Biol. Chem.* 240, 173-180 (1965).

33. A. Raz and D.S. Goodman, *J. Biol. Chem.* 244, 3230-3237 (1969).

34. P.A. Peterson, *J. Biol. Chem.* 246, 34-43 (1971).

35. H. Haupt and K. Heide, *Experientia,* 22, 449 (1966).

36. J.S. Marshall and J. Pensky, *Arch. Biochem. Biophys.* 146, 76-83 (1971).

37. L. Rask, P.A. Peterson and S.F. Nilsson, *J. Biol. Chem.* 246, 6087-6097 (1971).

38. W.T. Branch, J. Robbins and H. Edelhoch, *J. Biol. Chem.* 246, 6011-6018 (1971).

39. R.S. Bernstein, J. Robbins and J.E. Rall, *Endocrinol.* 86, 383-390 (1970).

40. C.A. Alper, N.I. Robin and S. Refetoff, *Proc. Nat. Acad. Sci. U.S.A.* 63, 775-781 (1969).

41. P.P. Van Jaarsveld, W.T. Branch, H. Edelhoch and J. Robbins, *J. Biol. Chem.* 248, 4706-4712 (1973).

42. W.T. Branch, J. Robbins and H. Edelhoch, *Arch. Biochem. Biophys.* 152, 144-151 (1972).

43. C.C.F. Blake, I.D.A. Swan, C. Rerat, J. Berthou, A. Laurent and B. Rerat, *J. Mol. Biol.* 61, 217-224 (1971).

44. G. Gonzalez and R.E. Offord, *Biochem. J.* 125, 309-317 (1971).

45. P. van Jaarsveld, W.T. Branch, J. Robbins, F.J. Morgan, Y. Kanda and R.E. Canfield, *J. Biol. Chem.* 248, 7898-7903 (1973).

46. Y. Kanda, D.S. Goodman, R.E. Canfield and F.J. Morgan, *J. Biol. Chem. 279, 6796 (1974).*

245, 1903-1912 (1970).

48. J. Robbins and J.E. Rall, *Physiol. Rev.* 40, 415-489 (1960).

49. J.E. Ross and D.F. Tapley, *Endocrinology,* 79, 493-504, (1966).

50. Y.L. Hao and M. Tabachnik, *Endocrinology,* 88, 81-92 (1971).

51. R.A. Pages, J. Robbins and H. Edelhoch, *Biochemistry,* 12, 2773-2779 (1973).

52. S.F. Nilsson and P.A. Peterson, *J. Biol. Chem.* 246, 6098-6105 (1971).

53. M. Tabachnik, Y.L. Hao and L. Korcek, *Endocrinology,* 89, 606-609 (1971).

54. W.T. Branch, R.A. Pages, H.J. Cahnmann, H. Edelhoch and J. Robbins, *Program. Amer. Thyroid Assoc.,* p. 65 (1971).

55. A.M. Green, J.S. Marshall, J. Pensky and J.B. Stanbury, *Biochim.Biophys.Acta.* 278, 117-124 (1972).

55a. A.M. Green, J.S. Marshall, J. Pensky and J.B. Stanbury, *Science,* 175, 1378-1380 (1972).

56. J. Robbins and J.E. Rall, *In* "Hormones in Blood", 2nd ed. (C.H. Gray and A.L. Bacharach, eds), Vol. 1, pp. 383-490 (1967).

57. J.H. Oppenheimer and R.R. Tavernetti, *J. Clin. Invest.* 41, 2213-2220 (1966).

58. R.N. Ferguson, H. Edelhoch, H.A. Saroff and J. Robbins, *Biochemistry,* in press (1974).

59. R.N. Ferguson and H.J. Cahnmann, *Biochemistry* (in press).

60. C.C.F. Blake, M.J. Geisow, I.D.A. Swan, C. Rerat and B. Rerat, *J. Mol. Biol.,* 88, 1-12 (1974).

61. M. Kanai, A. Raz and D.S. Goodman, *J. Clin. Invest.* 47, 2025-2044 (1968).

62. P.P. van Jaarsveld, H. Edelhoch, D.S. Goodman and J. Robbins, *J. Biol. Chem.* 248, 4698-4705 (1973).

2. Crystal Structure of Human Plasma Prealbumin and its Interaction with Thyroxine

C.C.F. BLAKE, I.D.A. SWAN*, M.J. GEISOW** AND S.J. OATLEY

Laboratory of Molecular Biophysics,
South Parks Road, Oxford, England.

C. RERAT AND B. RERAT

Laboratoire de Cristallographie,
C.N.R.S. Laboratoires de Bellevue,
Place Aristide Briand, 92-Bellevue, France.

INTRODUCTION

Prealbumin is a plasma protein that is of considerable biological importance because it transports both a hormone and a vitamin in serum. Thyroxine is bound directly to the prealbumin molecule while retinol (vitamin A alcohol) is bound indirectly through a protein-protein interaction involving its specific carrier molecule, retinol binding protein. Prealbumin has a singly occupied binding site for thyroxine with an association constant of 1.3×10^8 M^{-1} (1) and four binding sites for retinol binding protein with association constants of 1.2×10^6 M^{-1} (2). The complete prealbumin-

* *Present address : Chemistry Department, Glasgow University, Scotland.*
** *Present address : Hatfield Polytechnic, Hatfield, Herts, England.*

retinol binding protein complex can carry one thyroxine molecule and four retinol molecules.

Preliminary X-ray analysis of human prealbumin (3) has
shown that when crystallised from 55% saturated ammonium
sulphate at pH 7.1 (4), the crystals are orthorhombic, space
group $P2_12_12$ with cell dimensions a = 43.2 $\overset{o}{A}$, b = 85.3 $\overset{o}{A}$ and
c = 65.3 $\overset{o}{A}$. The diffraction pattern exhibits marked pseudo-
symmetry, which has been used to show that the molecule is a
tetramer of identical, or nearly identical subunits arranged
tetrahedrally. Two tetrameters each of 54,000 molecular weight
are accommodated in the unit cell. These features have been
confirmed by a 6 $\overset{o}{A}$ resolution electron density map (5) which
shows the four subunits in a compact arrangement around a large
slot that runs through the centre of the molecule. Circular
dichroism studies (6) suggest that about half the residues in
the molecule are in β-conformations. This is in qualitative
agreement with the low-resolution X-ray map, which contains
features consistent with the presence of extensive β-sheet
structures in the molecule. Preliminary results of sequence
studies have been reported by Gonzalez and Offord (7) and
Morgan *et al. (8)*.

E X P E R I M E N T A L

Lyophilised prealbumin, large crystals of native prealbumin and of a mercury derivative, produced by co-crystal-
lisation, with mercuric acetate, were generously provided by
Drs. Heide and Haupt, Behringwerke, A.G. Marburg/Lahn, German
Federal Republic. Unfortunately the native crystals and crystals grown by us from the lyophilised prealbumin showed detailed differences in their medium to high-angle diffraction
patterns and neither was isomorphous with the mercury deri-

vative. A third native form was prepared by removing the mercury (that is probably bound to protein thiol groups)(3) from
the crystals of the mercury derivative by soaking them in
mother liquor containing 10 mM-dithiothreitol and then washing
the crystals in mother liquor. Native crystals produced in
this manner gave diffraction patterns that indicate that the
3 native forms belonged to a single series, with the demercurated crystals most closely isomorphous with the mercury
derivative. The native crystals subsequently used in this
study were all derived from demercuration of mercury-prealbumin
crystals. In addition to the mercury derivative, single and
double uranyl derivations were prepared by soaking the native
and mercury-prealbumin crystals, respectively, in 10 mM UO_2
$(NO_3)_2$.

Diffracted intensities for the native and the 3 derivatives were collected to 2.5 Å resolutions on automatic dif-
fractometers modified to measure 5 reflections quasi-simul-
taneously in the flat cone setting (9). The native, mercury
and mercury-uranyl derivative data were collected on a Hilger
and Watts linear diffractometer and the uranyl derivative on
the prototype Hilger and Watts 5 circle diffractometer. Each
data set, consisting of about 25,000 reflections, was obtained
from two crystals mounted about their b*- and c*-axes. The data
included measurements of Friedel related reflections, reflections from one mounting to fill in the blind region in the
flat cone setting of the other, and overlapping data for
scaling.

The intensities were corrected for Lorentz and polaris-
ation factors, and for absorption by the method of North *et*
al. *(10)*. Duplicate intensity measurements from the b* and c*

crystals were used to obtain the interlevel and intercrystal scaling factors for each data set. The derivative measurements were scaled to those of the native by Kraut's method.

Heavy-atom positions were determined from difference Patterson and difference Fourier syntheses calculated at 2.5 Å resolution. The heavy-atom parameters were refined by the F_{HLE} procedure of Dodson and Vijayan (11), using empirically determined values of the real/imaginary scattering ratio (12). Temperature factors were obtained from refining the site occupancies only in overlapping ranges of $sin^2\theta/\lambda^2$. Difference Fourier syntheses were calculated after refinement of major sites to determine the presence of any minor sites that were then included in further rounds of refinement.

"Best phases" were calculated by the method of Blow and Crick (13) using the 3 derivatives, including measurements of their anomalous dispersion. The mean figure merit for the 8500 unique reflections expected to 2.5 Å resolution was 0.65. The correct enantiomorph was established by the Bijvoet Fourier technique described by Kraut (14).

Protein Fourier sections were produced on a scale of 2 cm/Å and contoured at equal intervals of $0.3e/Å^3$ on a computer-controlled graph plotter. Only positive contours were drawn; the F_{000} term was not included. The contours were transferred to acetate sheets and hung in a Richards comparator (15) modified to take a vertical mirror. The map was interpreted using standard model parts produced by Cambridge Repetition Engineers.

THE PREALBUMIN MOLECULE

The location of the tetrameric prealbumin molecule on a crystallographic 2-fold rotation axis indicates that the subunits are identical in pairs, but does not distinguish between an $\alpha_2\beta_2$ or α_4 tetramer. The two monomers in the asymmetric unit of the crystal (the potential $\alpha\beta$ pair) have been built independently and within experimental error they seem to be identical. The molecule therefore appears to be an α_4 tetramer, and this has been assumed in the following description.

With the exception of the first nine residues that are not marked with any very clear density, we have been able to fit the polypeptide chain throughout its course. Residue 10 is the single -SH group in the chain (7,8) and its position is indicated by the mercury site of the mercury-prealbumin derivative. We have been able to place residues 10 to 126 in the polypeptide chain, with a possible error of one or two residues. A chain of 124 to 128 residues is consistent with the molecular weight of the tetramer of 54,000 (3,6).

The polypeptide chain conformation of the prealbumin monomer is shown schematically in Fig. 1. Much of the chain is organised into eight extended strands that run parallel or antiparallel to one another in two layers. Within each layer the chains exhibit the characteristic pleating and twisting (16) of a β-sheet structure; while the position of the main-chain carbonyl groups and the spacing between the strands indicate that they are extensively hydrogen-bonded together within the sheets. These strands are shown in Fig. 1 by the flat arrows that also indicate the direction of each strand.

The eight extended segments of chain are organised into two β-sheets spaced about 10 Å apart, one composed of strands HGAD and the other of strands FEBC. In addition, it is possible that the rather irregular strand D may be able to form hydro-

C

Blake et al.

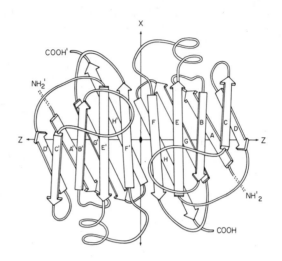

Fig. 1. *A schematic drawing of the main-chain conformation in the prealbumin dimer looking down the molecular Y-axis. The arrows indicate β-sheet strands labelled A to H in one monomer and A' to H' in the other, in the order in which they occur in the polypeptide chain. The molecular X- and Y-axes are indicated.*

gen bonds with strand C as well as strand A, in which case the monomer has the form of an eight-stranded β-sheet folded back on itself. With the exception of the interaction between strands A and G, all strand interactions are antiparallel. Linking the strands together are a number of loops of chain that vary in length between zero or one residue in the GH loop to 12 to 15 residuess in the BC and EF loops. The latter loop contains the single α-helical segment in the monomer, which is composed of about seven residues. A total of 68 residues have been provisionally placed in the β-strands to give the monomer a β-content of 55%; the helix content is about 5%.

The overall shape of the monomer is an elongated cylinder with dimensions 45Å x 25Å x 25Å with the β-strands running approximately parallel to the long axis. However the BC loop forms a pronounced local projection from the surface of the monomer, that can be most clearly seen in Fig. 3. The interior of the monomer is composed almost entirely of side chains projecting from the two β-sheet structures. They appear to be almost exclusively aliphatic residues, while the internal aromatic residues appear to be confined largely to the initial and terminal positions in the β-strands, or to the loops, and are consequently clustered at each end of the cylindrical subunit. It is clear that the internal residues from the β-sheets do not interdigitate but rather tend to be opposed in pairs.

Each monomer makes contacts with its neighbours that differ greatly. One interaction that is very close and extensive, links the monomers into what appears to be stable dimers. These dimers are shown schematically in Fig. 1. The interactions that link the dimers together in the complete molecule appear much more tenuous and are described below. The dimer interactions involve the β-strands H and F, which form a number of β-type hydrogen bonds with the equivalent strands H' and F' respectively, in the second monomer. Both pairs of equivalent strands run antiparallel as a consequence of the molecular 2-fold rotation axis relating the two monomers in the dimer. These interactions extend the two four-stranded β-sheets into eight-stranded β-sheets. DAGHH'G'A'D' (sheet 1) and CBEFF'E'B'C' (sheet 2) in the dimer. The extensive interchain hydrogen bonding in the dimer could account, in part at least, for the extraordinary stability of the molecule to denaturing agents (17).

The dimers are assembled in the tetrameric molecule with sheet 1 in each dimer opposed at the centre of the molecule at a distance of about 10Å. The β-strands in the opposed sheets run nearly at right angles to one another (Fig. 2).

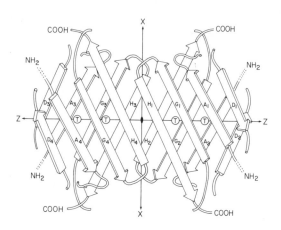

Fig. 2. *A schematic drawing of the opposed β-sheets at the centre of the molecule in the same orientation as Fig. 1. The arrows indicate β-sheet strands, labelled as Fig. 1 with subscripts indicating the monomer in which they occur.*

There is, however, little evidence for direct interaction between the two sheets because the side chains located at the interface appear to be too small to form intersheet contacts. The major contact appears to involve the short AB loop that in each monomer projects through the plain of sheet 1 to contact the opposing dimer near its monomer-monomer interface. These loops, which can be clearly seen in Fig. 3 appear to act as spacers between the sheets. The nature of the interaction of this loop with the opposing dimer is not clear at present but it can only involve four or five residues or an

equivalent length of main-chain. In the tetramer, the four AB
loops are arranged in two close pairs, which together with
the two opposed but separated β-sheets form the surface of a
slot that runs right through the centre of the molecule, which
is clearly visible in Fig. 3.

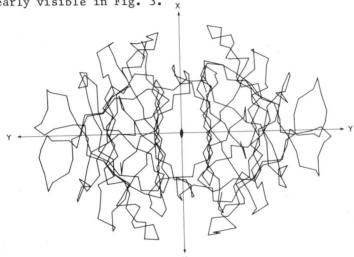

Fig. 3. *A view of the prealbumin tetramer looking down the
molecular Z-axis. The thyroxine binding sites are superim-
posed in the large central slot in the molecule formed by
the opposition of the β-sheets shown in Fig. 2. The long BC
loops can be seen on the outside of the molecule along the
Y-axis.*

The right-hand twist of each β-sheet element, DAGH and D'A'G'H',
in sheet 1, coupled with the 2-fold axis that relates them,
makes the outer, opposed face of sheet 1 markedly convex. The
opposition of the convex faces of these β-sheets gives the
central slot the shape of two funnel-like depressions, each
25Å deep, located in opposite sides of the molecule, which
meet and coalesce at the molecular centre. This can be observed
in Figs 2 and 3.

T H Y R O X I N E   B I N D I N G

Thyroxine and triiodothyronine were bound to the demercurated prealbumin crystals by soaking them in saturated solutions of L-thyroxine and L-3,5,3'-triiodothyronine made up in 55% saturated ammonium sulphate at pH 7.5, for one month in the dark. We suppose that the long soaking time is required because of their extreme insolubility in the mother liquor. Difference maps calculated at 6Å resolution of both derivatives show two symmetry-related peaks of electron density, several times higher than the background features, located deep in the central slot of the prealbumin molecule. The peaks are of an appropriate size and shape to represent the added molecules, and the general location of the di-iodotyrosyl rings of the bound hormone are indicated in Fig. 2. The electron density peaks are located on the crystallographic 2-fold rotation axis that defines the axis of the central slot. The T_4 and T_3 molecules do not have the appropriate symmetry and it is not clear at present whether each site is occupied statistically so that the symmetry is obeyed, or whether the symmetry is broken by the hormone.

Pages *et al.* (1) have shown that prealbumin can bind only one T_4 or T_3 molecule, but in a survey of thyroxine analogues found that di-iodobenzaldehyde has two binding sites. They have proposed that the prealbumin molecule has two binding sites but for steric factors T_4 and T_3 can only occupy one of these in each protein molecule. The X-ray studies clearly show two symmetrically equivalent sites for both T_4 and T_3, although it is not clear from the present difference maps that both sites can be occupied simultaneously. However, Fig. 2 shows that the sites are probably too far apart ($\sim 10\text{\AA}$) for the switching off of one of the sites by T_4 or T_3 bound in the other to be possible in the direct sense. Future high–resolution studies of thyroxine binding may indicate a solution to this problem.

One feature of the thyroxine binding sites that has become evident during the X–ray work is their lack of specificity. During the search for heavy–atom derivatives and during other experiments we have found that a number of diverse molecules can occupy the sites with high occupancy. They include HgI_4^{2-} (or HgI_3^-), $Au\ (CN)_2^-$, ethylmercurithiosalicylate, m–hydroxymercuri–p–toluenesulphonic acid, iodoacetic acid and dithiothreitol. In addition, following the reports of barbiturate inhibition of T_4 binding to prealbumin (18) and the rise in free T_4 in the plasma of patients undergoing aspirin therapy (19) we calculated 6 $\text{\AA}$ difference maps of prealbumin crystals soaked in veronal (5,5'–diethyl–barbituric acid) and sodium salicylate. Both molecules were found to occupy the T_4 binding sites.

Acknowledgements
We are very grateful to Drs. K. Heide and H. Haupt of Behringwerke A. G for their generous gifts of prealbumin and prealbumin crystals, and to Professor D.C. Phillips for his help and encouragement. We acknowledge the financial support of this project by the Medical Research Council who also provided IDAS and SJO with research studentships. We also acknowledge the Science Research Council for providing another of us (MJG) with a research studentship and the European Molecular Biology Organisation for the provision of grants to two of us (CR and BR).

R E F E R E N C E S

1.   R.A. Pages, J. Robbins and H. Edelhoch, *Biochemistry*, 12, 2773–2779 (1973).

2. P.P. Van Jaarsveld, H. Edelhoch, De W.S. Goodman and J. Robbins, *J. Biol. Chem.* 248, 4698-4705 (1973).

3. C.C.F. Blake, I.D.A. Swan, C. Rerat, J. Berthou, A. Laurent and B. Rerat, *J. Mol. Biol.* 61, 217-224 (1971).

4. H. Haupt and K. Heide, *Experientia* 22, 449-451 (1966).

5. C.C.F. Blake, K. Heide, C. Rerat and I.D.A. Swan, *C.R. Acad. Sci.* 272, 195-198 (1971).

6. W.T. Branch, J. Robbins and H. Edelhoch, *J. Biol. Chem.* 246, 6011-6018 (1971).

7. G. Gonzalez and R.E. Offord, *Biochem. J.* 125, 309-317 (1971).

8. F.J. Morgan, R.E. Canfield and De W.S. Goodman, *Biochim. Biophys. Acta.* 236, 798-801 (1971).

9. D.C. Phillips, *J. Sci. Instr.* 41, 123-129 (1964).

10. A.C.T. North, D.C. Phillips and F.S. Mathews, *Acta. Cryst.* 24, 351-359 (1968).

11. E. Dodson and M. Vijayan, *Acta. Cryst.* B27, 2402-2411 (1971).

12. B.W. Matthews, *Acta. Cryst.* 20, 230-239 (1966).

13. D.M. Blow and F.H.C. Crick, *Acta. Cryst.* 13, 794-802 (1959).

14. J. Kraut, *J. Mol. Biol.* 35, 511-513 (1968).

15. F.M. Richards, *J. Mol. Biol.* 37, 225-230 (1968).

16. C. Chothia, *J. Mol. Biol.* 75, 295-302 (1973).

17. P.P. van Jaarsveld, W.T. Branch, H. Edelhoch and J. Robbins, *J. Biol.Chem.* 248, 4706-4712 (1973).

18. S.M. Ingbar, *J. Clin. Invest.* 42, 143-148 (1963).

19. P.R. Larsen, *J. Clin. Invest.* 51, 1125-1134 (1972).

3.   Binding of L-Triiodothyronine to Rat Liver Cytosol and Nuclei

T.J. VISSER, R. DOCTER, J.T. STINIS, B. BERNARD
AND G. HENNEMANN.

Department of Internal Medicine III, Medical Faculty,
Erasmus University, Rotterdam.

INTRODUCTION

Thyroid hormones probably exert their biological activity
by occupying specific binding sites, which are present in
the nuclei from several tissue cells. Samuels and Tsai reported
the interaction of T_3 with nuclei from cultured GH_1 cells (a
rat pituitary tumour cell line) (1), from rat liver (2) and
from human lymphocytes (3).

Oppenheimer *et al* using *in vivo* (4-6) and *in vitro* (7)
techniques also showed that in rat liver nuclei specific T_3
binding sites do exist. Torresani and DeGroot (8) and Thomopoulos *et al* (9) reported the interaction of T_3 with proteins
extracted from rat liver nuclei. A condition, for T_3 and T_4
to reach the nucleus from outside the cell, might be the presence of a mechanism in the plasma membrane facilitating the
entry of the hormone and the presence of a transport protein
in the cytoplasm. Sufi *et al* demonstrated that in the cytosol
from porcine anterior pituitary specific T_3 and T_4 binding
sites are present (10). Spaulding and Davis (11) and Hamada
et al (12), using electrophoretic and gel chromatographic

techniques, provided evidence that specific thyroid hormone
binding proteins are also present in rat liver cytosol.

We have already estimated some parameters of the binding
reaction of T_3 and T_4 with a protein present in rat liver
cytosol (13). The purpose of the present study was to extend
our knowledge concerning the interaction of T_3 with the cytosol
binding protein. In addition the effect of this protein on
the binding of T_3 to rat liver nuclei was investigated.

MATERIALS AND METHODS

Preparation of cytosol

Livers from male Wistar rats (200-250 g) were perfused
in situ with ice cold saline through the portal vein. The
tissue was minced in 50 mM Tris-HCl, 2 mM EDTA, 2 mM 2-mer-
captoethanol, pH 7.4 (TEM) and was homogenised in two volumes
of TEM in a Potter-Elvehjem homogeniser. The cytosol was obtained after centrifugation at 104,000 x g for one hour. For
the preparation of kidney cytosol, kidneys from two rats were
pooled and homogenised in approximately 12 ml of TEM. The cytosol was obtained as described above. All procedures were carried
out at $0^{\circ}C$.

Binding studies with cytosol

All reagents were dissolved in TEM and all determinations
were performed at least in triplicate. Reaction mixtures contained 0.2 ml of cytosol (approximately 30 mg protein per ml),
0.1 ml of ^{125}I-T_3 and 0.1 ml of unlabelled T_3 or other substances to be tested. The mixtures were incubated for at least
30 min at $0^{\circ}C$. Preliminary results demonstrated that equilibrium was reached in this period. Then 0.2 ml of a suspension
of 1.25% acid washed charcoal and 0.125% dextran T70 was added

(14). The resulting suspensions were mixed briefly and left for 15 min at $0^{\circ}C$. The tubes were centrifuged and 0.3 ml aliquots of the supernatants were counted. Under these conditions minimal amounts of $^{125}I\text{-}T_3$ are bound to rat serum proteins which moreover cannot be displaced by high concentrations of cold T_3. Incubations containing TEM instead of cytosol were used as blanks. The data were plotted in a Scatchard diagram (15) and the affinity constant (K_a) and maximal binding capacity (MBC) were calculated according to Rosenthal (16).

Preparation of rat liver nuclei

Nuclei were prepared according to Samuels and Tsai (1) with slight modifications. The whole procedure was carried out at 4° C. After perfusion with ice cold 0.25 M sucrose, 20 mM Tris-HCl, 1.1 mM $MgCl_2$, pH 7.85 (STM), the liver was minced and homogenised in three volumes of STM in a Potter-Elvehjem homogeniser. The homogenate was filtered through nylon cloth and centrifuged at 1,500 x g for 5 min. The pellet was homogenised in 30 ml of STM and centrifuged again. Nuclei were purified by centrifuging the pellet through 15 ml of 2.3 M sucrose, 20 mM Tris-HCl, 1.1 mM $MgCl_2$, pH 7.85 at 40,000 x g for one hour.

The pellet was suspended in 20 ml of STM-Triton buffer (STM, 0.5% Triton X-100) and the nuclei were sedimented at 500 x g for 5 min. This step was repeated once with STM-Triton buffer and a second time with STM. Finally the nuclei were suspended in 10 ml of STM-EDTA buffer (STM, 2.5 mM EDTA). The procedure yielded nuclei with a protein/DNA ratio of approximately 2.5.

Binding studies with rat liver nuclei

0.2 ml aliquots of the nuclei suspension (containing

approximately 150 μg of DNA) were mixed with 0.8 ml of STM-
EDTA-DTT buffer (STM, 2.5 mM EDTA, 5 mM dithiotreitol) containing 3.5 pg of $^{125}I-T_3$ and various amounts of unlabelled
T_3. Some incubations were performed in STM-EDTA-DTT buffer
containing 5.1 mM $MgCl_2$ instead of 1.1 mM $MgCl_2$. After incubation for 30 min at 37° C the mixtures were centrifuged at
1500 x g for 10 min. The pellets were washed with 1 ml of
STM-Triton buffer and counted. The binding parameters were
calculated as described for the cytosol experiments.

Miscellaneous

T_4, T_3, D-T_4, D-T_3, Tetrac, Triac, Tetraprop and Triprop
were purchased from Sigma. MIT and DIT were obtained from
Calbiochem and $^{125}I-T_3$ from Abbott. Triton X-100 is a product
of BDH. Protein content was measured using either the Biuret
method or according to Lowry (17); DNA with the method of
Burton (18).

R E S U L T S

Binding of T_3 to cytosol

Figure 1 shows a Scatchard plot of data from a typical
displacement experiment with liver cytosol. The calculated
K_a in eleven experiments for the reaction of T_3 with the
binding protein averaged 4.8 (± 3.0) x 10^7 M^{-1} (mean ± S.D.).
The MBC of the binding protein for T_3 was 4.3 (± 0.8) pmol/mg
total cytosol protein. The relative affinity of various thyroid
hormone analogues for the binding protein is depicted in
Table 1. The specificity of the binding was assessed by studying the displacement of $^{125}I-T_3$ by various concentrations
of the analogue.

Figure 2 demonstrates that a similar interaction of T_3

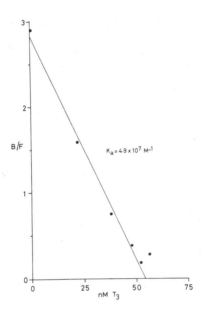

Fig. 1. *Scatchard analysis of T3 binding to rat liver cytosol. The binding at each hormone concentration is the average of three determinations. The line shown is derived from experimental data according to Rosenthal (16).*

with kidney cytosol was observed. The K_a of this reaction was 1.8 ($\pm$ 0.8) x 10^7 M^{-1}, the MBC 33.2 ($\pm$ 8.8) pmol/mg protein (mean $\pm$ S.D. for five experiments).

Binding of T₃ to rat liver nuclei

Figure 3 illustrates an estimation of the K_a for the nuclear binding of T_3 when the experiments were conducted in buffer with an excess of EDTA. The binding parameters are calculated as K_a, 3.5 ($\pm$ 2.5) x 10^{10} M^{-1}; MBC, 2.9 ($\pm$ 1.0) fmol/100 μg DNA (11 experiments).

Figure 3 also demonstrates a Scatchard diagram of data

Visser et al.

Table 1. *Relative displacement potency of thyroid hormone analogues. The crossreactivity was assessed by studying the displacement of ^{125}I-T_3 from the binding protein in rat liver cytosol by various concentrations of analogue.*

Substance	Crossreactivity (on molar basis)
T_3	1.00
T_4	0.35
D-T_3	0.85
D-T_4	0.17
Triac	0.06
Tetrac	0.06
Triprop	0.16
Tetraprop	0.09
T_2	0.09
MIT	<< 0.01
DIT	<< 0.01
Tyr	<< 0.01

obtained from experiments performed in buffer containing an excess of Mg^{2+}. In this case the K_a is 2.5 ($\pm$ 1.0) x 10^8 M^{-1} and the MBC 0.31 ($\pm$ 0.15) pmol/100 μg DNA (three experiments).

Binding of T_3 to nuclei in the presence of cytosol

Considering the results described above it seemed unlikely that T_3 binding to nuclei was dependent on the prior formation of a T_3-cytosol protein complex. To investigate whether the presence of cytosol would alter the mode of interaction of T_3 with the binding sites in the nuclei the following experiments were carried out.

First the effect of various amounts of cytosol on the uptake of ^{125}I-T_3 by the nuclei was investigated. Figure 4

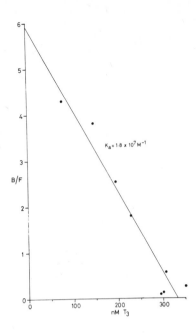

Fig. 2. *Scatchard analysis of T_3 binding to rat kidney cytosol. The diagram is obtained as described in the legend in Fig. 1.*

shows that when the amount of cytosol was increased, the amount of T_3 taken up by the nuclei decreased. Also incubations were performed in which the amount of cytosol and the concentration of ^{125}I-T_3 were kept constant in the presence of varying concentrations of unlabelled T_3. The experiments were carried out as described under Materials and Methods. After incubation and centrifugation aliquots of the supernatant were taken for counting and for determination of the percentage of protein bound ^{125}I-T_3 using dextran coated charcoal.

From these data another Scatchard diagram could be plotted and the calculated binding parameters did not differ

Visser et al.

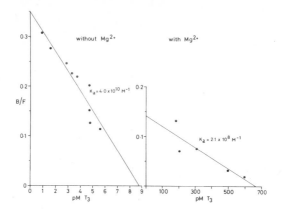

Fig. 3. *Scatchard analysis of T_3 binding to rat liver nuclei. The diagram shown in the left panel is obtained from data of incubations carried out in buffer containing excess EDTA; the diagram in the right panel results from incubations performed in buffer with excess Mg^{2+} as described in the section on Materials and Methods.*

significantly from those measured in the absence of cytosol.

D I S C U S S I O N

One of the early effects of T_3 on intact cells is an increase in the RNA-polymerase activity (19). Studies from other laboratories (1-9) and as described in this paper suggest that this might be a consequence of T_3 binding to high affinity, limited capacity binding sites in the nucleus. This paper demonstrates the presence of specific binding sites for T_3 in rat liver and kidney cytosol. The affinity of T_3 for this high capacity cytosol protein is about three orders of magnitude lower than for the putative receptors located in the nucleus. The present study also shows that T_3 binding to the nucleus is independent of the prior formation of a T_3-cytosol receptor complex as is the case with the steroid hormones (20).

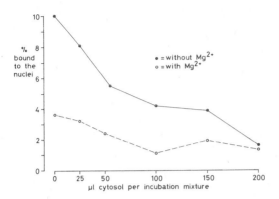

Fig. 4.*Binding of T₃ to rat liver nuclei in the presence of various amounts of cytosol. Rat liver cytosol was prepared by homogenisation in STM as described under Materials and Methods. Closed circles represent binding of T₃ when the medium contains excess EDTA; open circles with excess Mg^{2+}.*

We demonstrated only minimal non-specific binding of T_3 to serum proteins. Since it is not likely that interstitial fluid differs very much from serum in this respect, it is assumed that this so-called cytosol binding protein is indeed derived from intracellular sources. The physiological role of the cytosol binding protein is not yet clear. It might act in a mechanism to transport the thyroid hormones through the cytoplasm, or it might promote T_3 passage through the nuclear membrane or membranes of other subcellular organs, e.g. mitochondria. The present study does not clarify the second point because the Triton X-100 treatment solubilises the outer nuclear membrane.

Of course it cannot be excluded that the function of the cytosol binding protein is a totally different one, e.g. it is not demonstrated that the protein in question is devoid of

any enzymatic activity. The possible relationship to the
tyrosine and thyroxine aminotransferase which is present in
rabbit liver as described by Hechtman *et al.* (21) or to a
thyroxine deiodinase remains also to be elucidated. Anyhow
it is obvious that the presence of the binding protein located
in the cytoplasm will be in favour of the maintenance of a
certain intracellular T_3 concentration necessary for expressing
its biological activity. Little is known about the mechanism
by which thyroid hormone enters the target cell. In our laboratory some experiments have been performed which showed that
the entry of thyroid hormone in lymphocytes, purified from
bovine plasma, is a saturable process (unpublished results).
Samuels and Tsai also demonstrated that the human lymphocyte
is a target cell for thyroid hormones (3).

Concerning the nuclear binding of T_3 the magnesium effect
is intriguing. Also here the physiological implications of
this finding are uncertain. Studies are now being performed
which might clarify some points raised here.

R E F E R E N C E S

1. H.H. Samuels and J.S. Tsai, *Proc.Nat.Acad.Sci.U.S.A.*
    70, 3488 (1973).

2. H.H. Samuels and J.S. Tsai, *J. Clin.Invest.* 53, 656,
    (1974).

3. J.S. Tsai and H.H. Samuels, *J.Clin.Endocrinol.Metab.*
    38, 919 (1974).

4. M.I. Surks, D. Koerner, W. Dillman and J.H. Oppenheimer,
    J. Biol. Chem. 248, 7066 (1973).

5. J.H. Oppenheimer, H.L. Schwartz, W. Dillman and M.I.
    Surks, *Biochem. Biophys. Res. Commun.* 55, 544 (1973).

6. J.H. Oppenheimer, H.L. Schwartz, D. Koerner and M.I.
    Surks, *J. Clin. Invest.* 53, 768 (1974).

7. D. Koerner, M.I. Surks and J.H. Oppenheimer, *J. Clin. Endocrinol. Metab.* 38, 706 (1974).

8. J. Torresani and L.J. DeGroot. Abstr. 6th Ann. Meet. Eur. Thyr.Ass., Prague, June 25-28, 1974. Endocr. Exp. (Bratislava), 8, 202 (1974).

9. P. Thomopoulos, B. Dastugue and N. Defer, *Biochem. Biophys. Res. Commun.* 58, 499 (1974).

10. S.B. Sufi, R.S. Toccafondi, P.G. Malan and R.P. Ekins, *J. Endocr.* 58, 41 (1973).

11. S.W. Spaulding and P.J. Davis, *Biochem. Biophys. Acta.* 229, 279 (1971).

12. S. Hamada, K. Torizuka, T. Miyake and M. Fukase, *Biochim. Biophys. Acta.* 201, 479 (1970).

13. T.J. Visser, B. Bernard, R. Docter and G. Hennemann, Submitted for publication.

14. S.G. Korenman, *Steroids,* 13, 163 (1969).

15. G. Scatchard, *Ann.N.Y. Acad. Sci.* 51, 660 (1949).

16. H.E. Rosenthal, *Anal. Biochem.* 20, 525 (1967).

17. O.H. Lowry, N.J. Rosebrough, A.L. Farr and R.J. Randall, *J. Biol. Chem.* 193, 265 (1951).

18. K. Burton, *Biochem.J.* 62, 315 (1956).

19. J.R. Tata and C.C. Widnell, *Biochem. J.* 98, 604, (1966).

20. E.E. Baulieu *In* Endocrinology; Proc. 4th Int. Congr. of Endocrinology, Washington, D.C. June 18-24, 1972. Ed. R.O. Scow. Excerpta Medica, Amsterdam, 1973. p.30.

21. P. Hechtman, S.D. Schimmel and R.L. Soffer, *Biochem. Biophys. Res. Commun.* 43, 1395 (1971).

4. Subcellular Binding Proteins of Thyroid Hormones

KENNETH STERLING AND PETER O. MILCH

*Department of Medicine, Columbia University College of
Physicians and Surgeons and Protein Research Laboratory,
Bronx Veterans Administration Hospital, Bronx, New York,
U.S.A.*

INTRODUCTION

The subject of subcellular binding proteins of the thyroid hormones has relevance to the primary molecular mechanism of hormone action at the cellular level.

As an introduction to this problem, it is of interest to consider the two classes of hormones as they have been divided regarding transport in the circulation (1). (Table 1). The *Protein and Peptide Hormones* are all water-soluble and exist without any significant binding to the serum proteins. These all have relatively short biologic half-lives of one half hour or less, down to as short as a minute or so if one includes amino acid hormones such as a catecholamines, and the octapeptides vasopressin and Angiotensin II. In contrast, the *Small Molecule Target Hormones* are all more or less hydrophobic, being soluble in whole plasma owing in part to their being bound by serum albumin, as well as to the specific

*This work was supported by Grant AM-10739 from the U.S.
Public Health Service.*

Table 1. *Soluble and Hydrophobic Hormones*

Soluble	Hydrophobic
Protein and peptide hormones	Small-molecule target hormones
Parathyroid	Cortisol
Thyrocalcitonin	Progesterone
Growth Hormone	Oestradiol
FSH, LH, Prolactin	Testosterone
ACTH, MSH	Thyroxine
TSH	
Vasopressin	
Insulin	
Glucagon	

binding proteins, such as *transcortin,* the corticosteroid-binding globulin (CBG) for cortisol, corticosterone, progesterone and aldosterone; the *sex hormone binding globulin* or testosterone and oestrogen binding globulin (TeBG), and, of course, *prealbumin* and the *thyroxine binding alpha-globulin* (TBG). With the exception of aldosterone which is rather weakly bound, the small molecule target hormones have much longer biologic half-lives, ranging from about a week in the case of thyroxine to about an hour in the case of cortisol. The dialysability under conditions of equilibrium dialysis is generally in conformity with expectations: thus, about 95% of cortisol is protein-bound, and about 5% unbound, whereas thyroxine (T_4) is about 99.96% bound, and about 0.04% free.

The currently exploding field of the so-called "second messenger", that is, the hormonal activation of the membrane-

bound enzyme, adenylate cyclase, to increase the formation
of 3'5' cyclic adenosine monophosphate (cAMP) has been shown
most clearly to be crucially important with respect to the
peptide hormones including the action of thyrotropin upon the
thyroid gland, but not convincingly with respect to the primary actions of the thyroid hormones themselves, despite some
suggestions to the contrary.

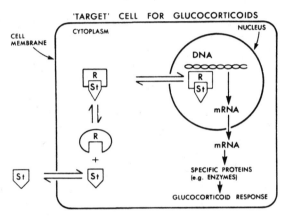

Fig. 1. *Sequence of events in the action of a steroid hormone*
upon a target cell. St=steroid hormone molecule- R=specific
protein receptor for the glucocorticoid hormone. The change
in shape of the receptor, R, is intended to signify a change
in protein conformation, as discussed in the text.

The most extensively studied mechanisms of hormone actions
have been tne sex steroid, progesterone, the glucocorticoids,
and aldosterone. The model for hormone action currently enjoy-
ing widespread enthusiastic support is outlined in Fig. 1
from a recent review article by Baxter and Forsham (2). In
this illustration the steroid is bound by cytoplasmic recept-
or protein, which steroid-receptor complex is then translocated to the nucleus. The alteration depicted from a round to

a square shape suggests an alteration, perhaps, of the protein
conformation. Most recently P.K. Siiteri of the University of
California (personal communication) has observed rather con-
vincing evidence of sequential alteration of the hormone-
receptor complex from 4S to 5S sedimentation characteristics
in the nucleus in pulse-chase experiments with labeled oestra-
dial. Within the nucleus the hormone-receptor complex is
evidently bound to the nuclear chromatin where it influences
transcription of the genetic message of the DNA. Recently,
Schutz, Beato and Feigelson have shown that cortisol increases
the amount of messenger RNA (mRNA) which directs the synthesis
of a specifically inducible hepatic enzyme (tryptophan oxy-
genase) in the livers of cortisol treated rats (3). The many
studies by O'Malley and colleagues (4,5) show similar results
in terms of oestrogen action upon the oviduct.

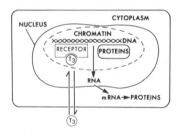

THYROID HORMONE-RESPONSIVE CELL

Fig. 2. *Thyroid hormone-responsive cell.*

The model of thyroid hormone action in Fig. 2. also devised by John D. Baxter (6) is of considerable interest in
that it illustrates the interaction of the thyroid hormone
triiodothyronine (T_3) with nuclear chromatin, which Baxter
has found in studies of "sheared" DNA corresponds to the more

active DNA as opposed to that in the "inactive" chromatin, and also to the DNA fraction possessing more RNA polymerase activity. It will be noted that this illustration lacks any representation of a cytosol receptor or cytosol binding protein (CBP), notwithstanding clear demonstrations of the existence of such a protein not only by our laboratory (7a,7b), but also by Refetoff and co-workers (8), by Davis and Spaulding (9a,9b), by Hamada and co-workers (10), and by Hamada and Ingbar (11a,11b), studies (in press) from Oppenheimer's laboratory, as well as the distinguished investigators from Rotterdam (12).*

The major reason is that this receptor of thyroid hormone may differ from steroid receptor proteins in not being translocated into the nucleus as a prerequisite for hormone action, although this matter is far from settled. An attractive hypothesis has been the so-called "bucket brigade" model of Stephen Spaulding in which CBP functions as an intracellular transport protein, analogous to TBG in the serum with bound hormone in equilibrium with a minute moiety of free hormone which penetrates the nuclear and possible mitochondrial effectors.

Our own experience (7) with cytosol binding protein dates back almost three years when we investigated it in the homogenates of rat kidneys which had been perfused *in situ* with ice cold isotonic saline for 20 to 30 mins until the renal venous effluent was crystal clear and shown to be devoid of serum protein by the Oyama-Eagle modification (13) of the Lowry Folin phenol reaction (14). The cytosol represented the supernatant from ultracentrifugation at 140,000 g for 1.5 hours.

* *See previous paper*

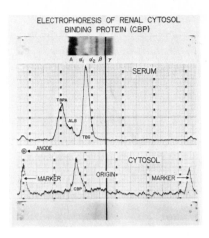

Fig. 3. *Comparison of radioactive scans of the carriers of human serum and rat renal cytosol binding proteins. Electrophoresis in glycine-acetate, pH 8.6. The label is* T_4 ^{125}I.

As shown in Fig. 3, a radioactive scan of a paper strip electrophoretogram revealed a peak with mobility differing from that of simultaneously run human serum proteins, shown in the upper part of the figure. The CBP illustrated represented radioactive T_4 bound to protein and retained after overnight dialysis against a large volume of buffer. The findings were confirmed by other procedures including Pevikon thin layer electrophoresis (10b) and polyacrylamide disc gel electrophoresis. Molecular sieving with Sephadex G-200 suggested a molecular weight of approximately 70,000 daltons.

CBP is not limited to the rodent species, as shown in Fig. 4 which illustrates the scan of the supernate obtained from human renal cells grown in cell culture (14).Similar results have also been found from human hepatic cell cultures (Chang liver). The amount of origin radioactivity was an unexplained variable in many of these studies of human

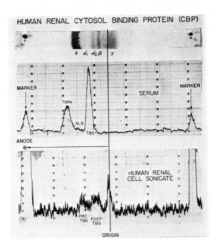

Fig. 4. *Comparison of radioactive scans of human serum and human renal cell binding proteins. Electrophoresis in glycine-acetate, pH 8.6. The label is T_4 ^{125}I.*

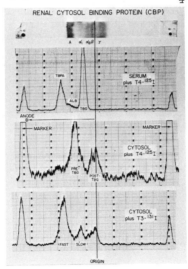

Fig. 5. *Rat renal cytosol binding proteins for T_4 and T_3. Electrophoresis in glycine-acetate, pH 8.6.*

and rodent cytoplasm, and may be due to the thermal instability of the cytosol receptor (7,12).

Different mobilities of cytosol receptors for T_4 ^{125}I and T_3 ^{131}I are suggested in Fig. 5, depicting scans of paper strip electrophoretograms of rat renal cytosol run simultaneously with human serum, shown above for reference.

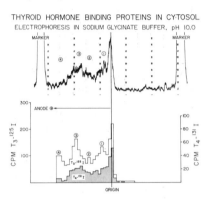

THYROID HORMONE BINDING PROTEINS IN CYTOSOL
ELECTROPHORESIS IN SODIUM GLYCINATE BUFFER, pH 10.0

Fig. 6. *Rat renal cytosol binding proteins for T_4 and T_3. Cytosol was labelled with T_3 ^{125}I and T_4 ^{131}I. Electrophoresis was done in sodium glycinate buffer, pH 10.0. The radioactive scan above reflects mainly ^{131}I, and ^{125}I to a lesser degree. In the histogram below with discrimination between the labels, in addition to origin radioactivity, the labelled T_3 is distributed in four peaks, appropriately numbered, with 4, which has moved furthest towards the anode at the left, clearly showing T_3, but no appreciable T_4 radioactivity. In contrast, the other peaks bound both radioactive hormones. In the run illustrated, the level of T_3 added was 0.16 µg per 100 ml, while the T_4 was 11 µg per 100 ml. Similar results, that is, peak 4 showing T_3 but not T_4 radioactivity were also seen with the same T_3 concentration, but T_4 levels of 1.1, 6.1 and also 21.1 µg per 100 ml.*

Since it could be argued that the different ligands could conceivably cause slightly different electrophoretic mobilities, experiments were carried out in which both labelled hormones as T_3 ^{125}I and T_4 ^{131}I were added to the *same* rat renal cytosol preparation. A peak with greatest anionic mobility was found to bind T_3 but not T_4, even with increments

of non-radioactive T_4 as high as 20 µg/100 ml (2.6 x 10^{-7}M)
as illustrated in Fig. 6. Whereas the glycine-acetate system
at pH 8.6 used in the foregoing studies provided reasonable
separation of peaks, we found that the sodium borate and sodium glycinate buffer systems at pH 10.0 provided more rapid
migration and greater separation of cytosol binding proteins
(although these alkaline buffers are less satisfactory for
study of serum protein carriers). Pevikon thin layer electrophoresis with subsequent autoradiography yielded generally
similar findings, but provided no additional data.

Many studies were carried out in which varying amounts of
thyroid hormones were added to cytosol with findings compatible with the existence of high affinity,low capacity binding
proteins as well as a low affinity, high capacity binder, the
latter presumably a non-specific binding protein (Fig. 7).
In the illustration, an electrophoretogram of human serum
showing both the stained paper strip and its radioactive scan
are shown at the top for orientation. The scan immediately
below it is rat renal cytosol binding protein with added T_4
^{125}I at a T_4 concentration of 5 µg per 100 ml, showing a
single radioactive peak with mobility slightly greater than
that of human serum TBG, hence the designation "Pre-TBG".
Numerous studies in which cytosol was loaded with stepwise
increments of non-radioactive T_4 up to 50 µg per 100 ml revealed an identical scan in every instance. On the other hand,
the addition of lesser amounts of T_4 ^{125}I, down to the limits
of accurate scanning, often revealed additional peaks with
lower electrophoretic mobility, as illustrated, suggesting
binding proteins of limited capacity. These were readily
saturated, hence lost in the background of scans beginning

around a level of 0.5 µg per 100 ml, but certainly quite dis-
tinguishable at lower levels. At 5 µg per 100 ml or above only
a single peak was visible.

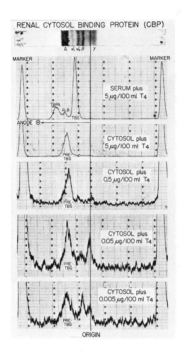

Fig. 7. *The effect of different levels of T_4 addition upon
the peaks visible on scan after electrophoresis of CBP. At
the top the stained paper strip and radioactive scan of human
serum are shown for orientation. Below are aliquots of the
same rat renal cytosol subjected to electrophoresis after
progressively less addition of T_4 as indicated, showing additional peaks visible at the lower levels.*

A more quantitative approach to the evaluation of cytosol
binding proteins was provided by Scatchard plots for measurement of the binding constants (Fig. 8). The Scatchard plot
illustrated represents data obtained for the interaction bet-

ween T_3 and rat renal CBP at $4^\circ C$ for one hour after which
the "bound" and "free" moieties of T_3 were separated rapidly
by dextran-coated charcoal. Similar data could occasionally
be obtained by equilibrium dialysis at $4^\circ C$ for 16 hours, but
more frequently a horizontal line resulted. The latter invariably occurred when undiluted cytosol was used in a dialysis bag; more than 97% of the radioactivity of labelled T_3
would be retained within the bag at all levels. Presumably
this represented some alteration in the protein with standing
overnight in a dialysis bag, even though refrigerated at $4^\circ C$.
This presumed alteration evidently resulted in a vast number
of non-specific binding sites.

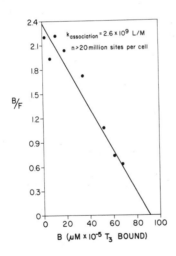

Fig. 8. *Interaction between triiodothyronine (T₃) and rat
renal cytosol binding protein (CBP). Scatchard plot.*

Nevertheless, some equilibrium dialysis studies did
indeed corroborate the binding constants of the rapid charcoal separations, and Fig. 8 typifies the results obtained

with rat renal and also hepatic CBP. As shown, the association constant obtained in a typical study was 2.6×10^9 L/M, a value only slightly below that of about 10^{10} L/M for human TBG. Based on the assumption of 100 million renal cells per gram per weight for rat kidney, the computed number of primary cytosol binding sites exceeds 20 million per cell. It should be observed that the straight line plot of Fig. 8 indicates a predominating primary class of binding sites.

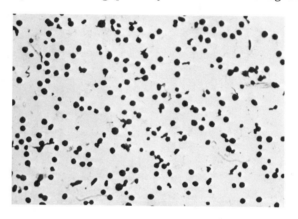

Fig. 9. *Photomicrograph of isolated rat renal cell nuclei.*
3000X

Earlier studies in our laboratory with isolated renal cell nuclei had indicated an appreciable uptake of tracer T_3 *in vitro* at 4°C or 37°C. Fig. 9 is a phase contrast photomicrograph of renal cell nuclei isolated by centrifugation through 2.4 M sucrose solution. Of particular interest has been the finding that the uptake was invariably appreciably greater (usually at least ten times) with nuclei suspended in saline or isotonic potassium phosphate buffer, than with nuclei resuspended in CBP from the very same kidneys, or in human serum albumin at the same protein concentration (about

1%) as the CBP. This finding has suggested that very possibly free hormone rather than receptor-bound hormone may enter the nucleus (or other effectors such as mitochondria), in contrast to the situation with regard to steroid hormone action.

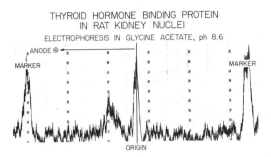

Fig. 10. *Radioactive scan of paper electrophoretic strip of the protein from rat renal nuclei.*

As mentioned earlier, considerable evidence has been accumulated regarding the actions of the steroid hormones in increasing nuclear transcription(1-4). Moreover, as early as 1966 Siegal and Tobias (15) demonstrated the nuclear localisation of thyroid hormone by radioautography of tritium labelled hormone added to cell cultures of human renal epithelial cells, grown in monolayer. The observations of Baxter (6) on T_3 binding by the DNA of active chromatin have been mentioned earlier, and Oppenheimer's group has been reporting the binding of T_3 in comparison with its analogues after injection of the labelled hormone into rats (16,17). They fractionated nuclear chromatin and found binding by the acidic protein (i.e. the non-histone protein), and recently have studied labelling *in vitro* as well (18). Accordingly, we have undertaken study of the nuclear protein which binds thyroid hormone. A radioactive scan of a paper strip electrophoretogram

D

of the protein from isolated rat renal cell nuclei is shown
in Figure 10, which shows a distinct peak which has migrated
toward the anode, in addition to a peak of radioactivity at
the origin. Studies of the nuclear binding constants have
been done by incubation of isolated rat liver nuclei with T_3
^{125}I and graded amounts of non-radioactive hormone for 45 min
at $37^{\circ}C$ in buffer. Counting of the supernate and nuclear pellet
after centrifugation permitted determination of the fraction
bound at each level, and construction of a Scatchard plot
(Fig. 11) which yielded an association constant of 6.6×10^{10}
L/M and approximately 15,000 binding sites per nucleus. Renal
nuclei gave similar data.

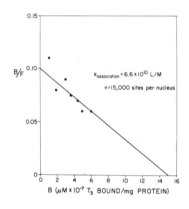

Fig. 11.   *Interaction between triiodothyronine (T_3) and rat
liver nuclei. Scatchard plot.*

In addition to the foregoing, the mitochondria have been
isolated from rat hepatic and renal cells. The rather mono-
tonous granular appearance of the photomicrograph of Fig. 12
is compatible with isolated mitochondria in pure form. When
these mitochondria have been destroyed by sonication, a binding protein may be demonstrated in the supernatant fluid after

centrifugation to remove the membranes. A distinct electrophoretic peak which has migrated toward the anode may be seen
in Fig. 13, which shows the radioactive scan of a paper strip
after electrophoresis in sodium borate buffer at pH 10.0.

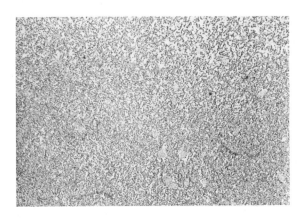

Fig. 12. *Photomicrograph of isolated rat liver mitochondria.*
3000 X

Considerable additional work will be required to eluci-
date fully the molecular mechanism of thyroid hormone action.
For the present it may be justifiable to suggest that more
than a single locus of action may exist within responsive
cells. On general descriptive biological grounds it is reasonable to speak of a duality of thyroid hormone action. The
first action could be an essentially irreversible effect upon
growth and maturation, most strikingly typified by tadpole
metamorphosis, but doubtless having its counterpart in adult
mammalian tissue metabolism. This growth function can most
readily be conceived of as mediated by cell nuclei. A nuclear
locus of action is supported by evidence already cited, including, of course, the analogy to steroid hormone action.

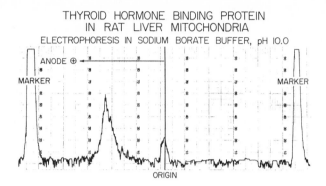

Fig. 13. *Radioactive scan of paper electrophoretic strip of the protein in rat liver mitochondria.*

Attractive though it might appear to some to ascribe all thyroid hormone action to a single pathway, it seems impossible to omit consideration of a direct primary effect upon mitochondria. The mitochondria can readily be conceived of as a locus for a form of reversible thyroid hormone action, including the thermogenic action in homeothermic animals. Working with isolated mitochondria, Tapley's laboratory has shown a number of changes of possible physiologic significance upon addition of thyroid hormone. Most recently this group has observed increased mitochondrial protein synthesis in as short an interval as five minutes after addition of T_4 or T_3 in the physiological range to isolated mitochondria *in vitro* (19). Moreover, Babior, Ingbar, and colleagues have shown increased entry of ^{14}C-labelled adenosine diphosphate (ADP) into mito-chondria after hormone administration (20a). This compound is phosphorylated within the mitochondria to yield the energy-rich phosphate bond of adenosine triphosphate (ATP). Such observations have recently been made after a physiologic replacement dose consisting of daily injections of T_4 in dosage

2 μg/100g body weight to thyroidectomised rats, a finding which affords support for a direct action of thyroid hormone upon mitochondria (20b).

In summary, the evidence presently available suggests a dual action of thyroid hormone: (1) an action upon nuclear transcription, concerned with growth, differentiation, and perhaps certain trophic functions, and (2) an action upon mitochondria concerned with energy and thermogenesis. Our own findings show that upon entering the cell the thyroid hormones are firmly bound by cytosol receptor proteins, and subsequently by proteins of the nucleus and mitochondria which are both considered likely effector loci for hormone action.

R E F E R E N C E S

1. K. Sterling, *In* Radioisotopes in Medicine *In Vitro* Studies, R.L. Hayes, F.A. Goswitz and B.E.P. Murphy, eds. U.S. Atomic Energy Commission, (1968).

2. J.D. Baxter and P.H. Forsham, *Am. J. Med.* 53, 573,(1972).

3. G.Schutz, M. Beato and P. Feigelson, *Proc. Nat. Acad. Sci. U.S.A.* Vol. 70, No. 4, p.p. 1218-1221, (1973).

4. B.W. O'Malley and A.R. Means, *Science,* 183, 610, (1974).

5. B.W. O'Malley, *N.E. J. Med.* 284, 370 (1971).

6. J.D. Baxter, M.A. Charles, G. Ryffel, B.J. McCarthy and K.M. Macleod, Proceedings of the Annual Meeting of the American Society for Clinical Investigation, Inc., Atlantic City, (1974).

7a. K. Sterling, M.A. Brenner, V.F. Saldanha and P.O. Milch, Annual Meeting, American Thyroid Association, Inc. Chicago, III (1972).

7b. K. Sterling, V.F. Saldanha, M.A. Brenner and P.O. Milch, *Nature,* 250, 661 (1974).

8. S. Refetoff, R. Matalon and M. Bigazzi, *Endocrinology,* 91, 934, (1972).

9a. S.W. Spaulding and P.J. Davis, *Biochem. Biophys. Acta.*, <u>229</u>, 279 (1971).

9b. P.J. Davis, B.S. Handwerger and F. Glaser, *J. Biol. Chem.* <u>249</u>, 6268, (1974).

10. S. Hamada, K. Torizuka, T. Miyake and M. Fukase, *Biochem. Biophys. Acta* <u>201</u>, 479 (1970).

11a. S. Hamada and S. Ingbar, Program, Endocrine Society, 53rd Annual Meeting, 1971.

11b. S. Hamada and S. Ingbar, To be published.

12. T.J. Visser, B. Bernard, R. Docter and G. Hennemann, These proceedings.

13. V.I. Oyama and H. Eagle, *Proc. Soc. Exptl. Biol. Med.* <u>91</u>, 305, (1956).

14. O.H. Lowry, N.J. Rosebrough, A.L. Farr and R.J. Randall, *J. Biol. Chem,* <u>193</u>, 265, (1951).

15. E. Siegel and C.A. Tobias, *Science,* <u>153</u>, 763,(1966).

16. J.H. Oppenheimer, H.L. Schwartz, D. Koerner and M.I. Surks, *J. Clin. Invest.* <u>53</u>, 768, (1974).

17. M.I. Surks, D. Koerner, W. Dillman and J.H. Oppenheimer, *J. Biol. Chem.* <u>248</u>, 7066, (1973).

18. D. Koerner, M.I. Surks and J.H. Oppenheimer, *J. Clin. Endocrinol. Metab.* <u>38</u>, 706, (1974).

19. J.L. Buchanan, M.P. Primack and D.F. Tapley, *Endocrinology,* <u>89</u>, 534 (1971).

20a. B.M. Babior, S. Creagan, S.H. Ingbar and R.S. Kipnes, *Proc. Nat. Acad. Sci. U.S.A.* <u>70</u>, 98, (1973).

20b. G.I. Portnay, F.D. McClendon, J.E. Bush, L.E. Braverman and B.M. Babior, *Biochem. Biophys. Res. Commun.* <u>55</u>, 17, (1973).

5. The Effect of Clofibrate on Thyroxine Metabolism

W.A. HARLAND AND J.S. ORR

Department of Pathology, University of Glasgow and West of Scotland Health Boards' Department of Clinical Physics and Bio-Engineering, Glasgow.

INTRODUCTION

Clofibrate /‾ethyl-alpha-(p-chlorophenoxy) isobutyrate‾/ was originally synthesized as one of a series of branched chain acids structurally related to certain synthetic oestrogens. The compound was devoid of oestrogenic activity in the rat, but was found to cause a reduction in cholesterol concentrations in both serum and liver, in doses which were well tolerated over long periods. There is now abundant evidence that the drug has an hypocholesterolaemic effect in man (1-3). The drug has a number of other effects such as reducing serum fibrinogen and uric acid concentrations, and hepatic effects have received special attention (4). Early work demonstrated that clofibrate caused a substantial increase in the liver weight in both rats and monkeys (5). This is associated with a proliferation of smooth-surfaced endoplasmic reticulum and a substantial increase in both size and numbers of mitochondria and microbodies (6). The latter have been shown to contain catalase, urate oxidase and amino acid oxidase and they are now classed as peroxisomes (7). There is also an increase in hepatic glycerol phosphate dehydrogenase (GPD) concentration (8).

Thorp (9) observed a marked seasonal variation in the hypocholesterolaemic effect in rats, and this led him to postulate an endocrine basis for the drug's action. This was though at first to be due to an enhanced effectiveness of adrenal steroids and for this reason the drug was first marketed in combination with androsterone, under the trade name Atromid. Subsequently the steroid was withdrawn and the drug is now sold as Atromid-S.

The possibility that the effectiveness of the drug might depend on thyroid hormones was first suggested by Thorp in 1963 (10) and a number of papers concerning this relationship have now been published (8, 11-13). Of particular interest is the increased hepatic GPD activity because of the known thyroid hormone specificity of this enzyme. It has been claimed that in rats the drug effect is equivalent to administration of 4-8 μg thyroxine /100g body weight/day (13). It was also established that the hypocholesterolaemic effect of the drug is dependent on the presence of thyroid hormone. However, clofibrate was not thyromimetic, and its action was blocked by thyroidectomy and methimazole. It was further noted that clofibrate did not cause an increase in thyroid weight, nor histological evidence of increased activity. Metabolic rate was not increased although oxygen consumption of liver slices was elevated. Westerfield *et al.* (13) as a result of extensive investigations have concluded that clofibrate in some way enhances the effectiveness of thyroid hormones without increasin thyroid gland activity.

One possibility that has been considered is that clofibrate might act by competing with thyroxine for the acidic binding sites on serum albumin (10). This idea led to a number of studie and it was found that clofibrate depressed T_4 binding by TBPA without effect on binding by TBG (14). It was also found that therapeutic doses led to an increased TBG combining capacity together with a slight fall in the dialysable fraction of thyroxine (15,16). However, others found no change in "free thyroxine" concentration after treatment for one month (17). In an experiment designed to see whether the action of clofibrate in relation to T_4 was primarily intrahepatic or whether there was evidence of displacement of thyroxine from plasma binding proteins, Osorio *et al.* (18) examined the effect of a single injection of soluble clofibrate on hepatic uptake and biliary clearance of radiothyroxine. They found that clofibrate caused a fall in the serum/liver thyroxine ratio but was without effect on biliary clearance of thyroxine.

No conclusions as to the relationship of clofibrate to thyroid hormone metabolism emerge from these studies. It seems that these hormones are essential for the drug's action but the mechanism is uncertain. The present paper describes work concerned with these problems. Measurements in rats of T_4 concentrations and flows following acute administration of clofibrate are presented together with experiments designed to study the sequence following chronic drug administration. Some of the methods are novel and the results cast an interesting light on the physiology of thyroid hormone metabolism.

M E T H O D S

General

All experiments were performed on male Charles River rats weighing 220-320 g. Animals were housed in groups of six or twelve and were provided with food and drink in excess.

Tracer techniques

Thyroxine kinetics were studied using L-thyroxine labelled
with ^{131}I or ^{125}I with specific activity of 25-50 mCi/mg
(Radiochemical Centre, Amersham,). The isotope was used within
five days of delivery. Iodide contamination of the tracer was
estimated by thin layer chromatography (19) or by the following
technique. An aliquot of the tracer solution was added to
0.5 g cation exchange resin (Bio-rad Ag 50 WX2, 100-200 mesh,
hydrogen form), suspended in 1 ml distilled water in a plastic
tube. The resin was washed three times with 10 ml distilled
water. Activity washed off the resin, expressed as a fraction
of the total activity, represented the proportion of con-
taminating iodide. Both methods gave equivalent results, with
an average of 7% contamination. Samples with 10% iodide or
more were discarded. At the time of injection, and using the
same syringe, a volume equal to the administered dose was
injected directly into 2N NaOH in a 100 ml flask. Thus the
standard dose was exactly comparable to the doses injected
into the animal, irrespective of any residue left in the
syringe. The NaOH prevents adherence of the label to the
standard flask. Standards of suitable geometry were prepared
from this stock. All activities were measured in an automatic
gamma counter (Nuclear Chicago) and results were expressed
as fractions of dose.

Experiment A.

Six rats on Diet GR 31 (20) were given 10 μCi ^{125}I-T$_4$
intraperitoneally. Blood samples were obtained from the tail
four times in 48 h, and then 100 mg clofibrate and 10 μCi
^{131}I T$_4$ were injected intraperitoneally. Blood samples were
collected for a further 72 h. Activities due to both isotopes

in 0.1 ml serum were measured and expressed as fractions of dose/ml.

Experiment B.

Twelve rats maintained on Diet GR 31 were injected intra-peritoneally with 5 μCi ^{125}I-T$_4$. After 20 h, six of the animals were given 100 mg clofibrate. Four hours later all animals were killed and the activities in plasma and tissue measured as before. In four rats the acute effect of clofibrate on biliary clearance was studied by injecting 100 mg of the sodium salt of clofibrate into the femoral vein 4 hours after radio-thyroxine intraperitoneally and 1 h after the bile duct had been cannulated. The biliary clearance was calculated as described by Myant (21).

Experiment C.

A group of 16 rats was given powdered Diet 41 (22) with clofibrate (2 g/kg) for two weeks prior to and throughout the experiment. A second group of 16 acted as controls. All were injected intraperitoneally with 10 μCi ^{131}I-T$_4$. Four of each group were killed after 24 h and on each subsequent day. Activities in the whole body less thyroid, liver, intestines including contents, and eviscerated carcass including head and pelt, were measured and expressed as a fraction of dose. The animals were killed by exsanguination from the aorta under ether anaesthesia. Serum protein bound iodine (PBI) concentrations were measured on serum from each rat by the Technicon "Auto-analyser" procedure, and plasma T$_4$ concentration was estimated by assuming that PBI was all T$_4$ iodine (Plasma T$_4$ = PBI x 1.53).

Experiment D.

Two groups of six rats were selected. The first was given

powdered Diet GR 31 with clofibrate (2 g/kg) for 20 days
before and throughout the experiment. The second was a control
group.

Rats were given divided intraperitoneal   doses from a
stock of ^{131}I–T$_4$ in saline made up to a concentration of 2
µCi/ml according to the schedule.

Day	Time (h)	Vol. (ml)
1	1600	0.6
2	1600	0.6
3	1600	0.6
4	1600	0.8
5	1000	0.1
5	1400	0.1
5	1600	kill

Animals were killed and radioactivity of plasma and tissue
was measured as in Experiment A. Radioactivity was expressed
as a fraction of the activity in 0.6 ml stock solution, which
was the effective daily dose.

Experiment E.

Biliary clearance of radiothyroxine was measured in six
rats fed for two weeks on clofibrate diet as in Experiment B.
The controls were on Diet GR 31 for six weeks prior to the
experiment.

Calculations.

The methods for T$_4$ secretion rate (T$_4$SR) and tissue T$_4$
concentration depend on the Occupancy Principle (23). This
states that the total flow (F) of any substance in a system
is equal to the ratio of content (C) to Occupancy (θ) in any
part of the system.

i.e. $\qquad F = \dfrac{C_1}{\theta_1} = \dfrac{C_2}{\theta_2} = \dfrac{C_n}{\theta_n}$

where C is the amount of mother substance in the part, and θ for the same part is the total integral with respect to time of the activity-time curve of a radioactive tracer, activity being expressed as a fraction (f) of the activity in the total tracer dose.

i.e. $\qquad \theta = \displaystyle\int_0^\infty f(t) \cdot dt$

Because activity is expressed as a fraction, θ has the dimensions of time. It follows that if θ and C can be measured in any part, F can be calculated, and where θ for another part is known then C for that part can also be calculated.

Since the radioactive tracer in these experiments is administered as the iodine atoms in radiothyroxine, and since both the endogenous T_4 and the radiothyroxine are changed in certain tissues into derivates, C in any part of the system includes, in addition to T_4 itself, all the derivatives of T_4 expressed in terms of the atoms of iodine they contain. The full picture of these metabolic processes is not understood, nor is it known which of the derivatives are metabolically important, nor whether pure T_4 plays an important role other than as a source of the derivatives. It seems reasonable therefore to accept their combination as a useful measure of the effective T_4 content. T_4 content of tissues is used to mean content in this sense.

Single tracer dose. Following single doses of radiothyroxine, it was observed that activity, in all parts measured, diminished in a single exponential manner. These disappearances

were expressed as fractional disappearance rates (k) per day
where

$$k = \frac{\ln 2}{t_{\frac{1}{2}}} = \frac{0.693}{t_{\frac{1}{2}}}$$

and $t_{\frac{1}{2}}$ is the time in days taken for activity to diminish
by half. Curves of this type can be integrated by extrapolating
to zero time and dividing the intercept activity (Ao) by k.
Since there is no exogenous source of thyroid hormone, and
since plasma occupancy (θ_p) and content/g (T_{4p}) were measurable, it follows that

$$T_4 SR = \frac{T_{4p} \times k_p}{Ao_p}$$

and that tissue

$$T_4 = T_4 SR \times \theta_T = T_4 SR \times \frac{Ao_T}{k_T}$$

where the subscript P refers to plasma and T refers to tissue.
Multiple tracer doses. In Experiment D multiple doses of tracer
were administered over a period equal to 5 or 6 half-times
of a single tracer dose. Ideally the tracer should be administered at a constant rate throughout this period, but as
this is not practical in small animals a dose schedule was
chosen to be reasonably equivalent to continuous infusion.
Tracer was given at an average rate of 0.6 ml/day, or 0.1 ml
/4h, the injections being more closely spaced on the final
day. The injection on day 4 includes 0.1 ml to avoid a night
time injection and an addional 0.1 ml of tracer was also
given at this time to compensate for underestimation of θ
which would otherwise result from the intermittent administration of tracer and the slightly curtailed injection schedule.
Activity in any part at death, divided by the activity administered per day is equivalent to θ for that part, the animal

having effectively integrated the tracer activity-time curve.
Calculations for T_4SR and tissue T_4 then follow as above.
Tissue utilisation rates. When tissue T_4 and the fractional
disappearance rates (k_T) are known, then tissue utilisation
rate

$$\text{(TUR)} \quad = \quad \text{Tissue } T_4 \times k_T$$

$$= \quad T_4SR \times \theta_T \times k_T$$

$$= \quad T_4SR \times Ao_T$$

i.e. TUR can be calculated either as the product of the tissue
T_4 content and the fractional disappearance rate, or as the
product of T_4SR and the extrapolated zero time value for
the single exponential tissue disappearance curve. The inclusion of derivatives of T_4 in tissue T_4 in some tissues
implies that the fractional disappearance rates apply to the
sum of T_4 and derivatives. The TUR therefore is the total
outflow of T_4 derivatives from the tissue but this must equal
the inflow of T_4 itself, since the total content is constant.

This method for TUR applies where tracer passes rapidly
into a tissue, and is bound in the same manner as the mother
substance, the molecules of which are being catabolised in
a random fashion. This is not the case in the intestinal tract
where tracer radioactivity increases slowly at first, and
subsequently diminishes at a rate which is dependent on the
rate at which tracer enters the intestines from other sources.
Flow of T_4 through the intestines is therefore calculated as
the quotient of the intestinal T_4 and the faecal transit time,
estimated by faecal markers.

R E S U L T S

Experiment A. This experiment shows the effect of acute clofibrate dosage on radiothyroxine disappearance curves in
plasma. The results are presented in Fig. 1. Two effects are

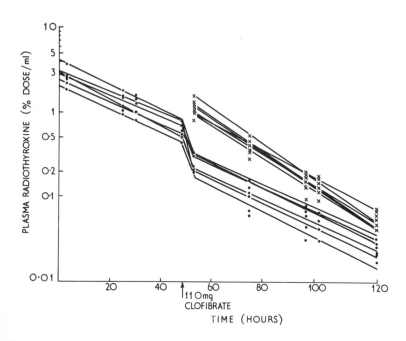

Fig. 1. *The effects of acute clofibrate dosage on radiothyroxine
disappearance curves in plasma.* ^{125}I-T_4 *was given at zero
time and* ^{131}I-T_4 *was given with the clofibrate at 48 h.*

apparent. First, there was an acute drop of approximately
50% in the activity/ml of the tracer given prior to the drug,
and the initial activity/ml of the second tracer was approximately 50% of the initial activity/ml of the first. In
addition the disappearance of the second tracer, given with
the drug, was more rapid than that of the first. The signifi-

cance of this difference was tested by Student's t test in individual rats, and failed to reach significance in only two of the six.

Experiment B. Since acute administration of clofibrate reduced plasma radiothyroxine activity, this experiment was designed to locate the displaced tracer. The results are shown in Table 1 and Fig. 2. The data in the table show that

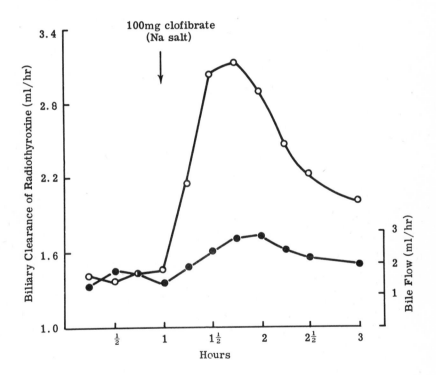

Fig. 2. *The effects of acute clofibrate dosage in bile flow and biliary clearance of radiothyroxine.*

24 h after administration of radiothyroxine and 4 h after clofibrate, there was again a significant reduction in plasma

Table 1.   *Tissue activity (% dose) 24 h after*
    radiothyroxine and 4 hours after 110 mg clofibrate.
    Results represent mean ± S.D. for 6 rats in each group.

	Plasma (1 ml)	Liver	Intestines	Leg	Muscle (1 g)
Control	1.12	4.94	13.0	0.33	0.12
	± 0.15	± 0.94	± 2.1	± 0.01	± 0.02
Clofibrate	0.57	5.84	16.6	0.35	0.14
	± 0.11	± 1.19	± 2.1	± 0.03	± 0.04
p	1.2×10^{-5}	8.7×10^{-2}	1.1×10^{-2}	0.23	0.25

activity/ml, and a rise in activity in muscle and leg. Assuming
that the plasma volume is 4% of the body, total plasma activity
fell by 4.4% of the tracer dose administered, and this was
balanced by a rise of 4.5% of dose in the liver and intestines
taken together. This evidence that all the activity displaced
from the plasma passes to the liver and then into the intestine
is strongly supported by the results in Fig. 2, from which
nearly all the activity lost by plasma could be accounted for
in the acutely raised biliary clearance.

Experiment C. The experiment measured the disappearance
of a pulse of radiothyroxine from plasma and tissues in rats
given clofibrate in the diet for three weeks. The activity
values for all tissues diminished exponentially, and Table 2
shows the extrapolated zero-time values and fractional dis-

Table 2.   *The effect of clofibrate on the distribution and fractional disappearance rates (k) of radiothyroxine in plasma and tissues.*

	Extrapolated zero-time value (% dose)	k (day^{-1})	Extrapolated zero-time value (% dose)	k (day^{-1})
Plasma (1 ml)	2.0	0.846	2.4	0.983
Liver	17.2	0.771	21.8	0.939
Carcass	65.1	0.688	52.8	0.693

appearance rates (day^{-1}). It will be noted that the effect of clofibrate diet was to increase the disappearance rates for plasma and liver substantially but that for the carcass was unchanged. There were small rises in the extrapolated zero-time values for plasma and liver, but that for the carcass was considerably reduced.

Experiment D. This experiment utilised the multiple injection technique and measured the effect of clofibrate diet on T_4SR and T_4 concentration in tissues. The results are shown in Table 3. There was a small but significant reduction in PBI and in the concentration of T_4 in liver, but due to the substantial significant increase in liver weight, T_4 in the whole liver was increased. The small increase in the mean T_4SR and the small decrease in the mean carcass T_4 were not significant.

Table 3.   Effect of clofibrate (0.2% diet) on thyroxine secretion rate and tissue hormone concentration.

	Bd. Wt. (g)	PBI (µg/100ml)	T_4SR (µg/100g Bd. Wt)	Liver Wt. (%Bd.Wt.)	Liver T_4 (µg/g)	Intestine T_4 (µg/g)	Carcass T_4 (µg/g)	Pelt T_4 (µg/g)
Control	327 ±25	3.4 ±0.2	0.87 ±0.10	3.6 ±0.2	0.033 ±0.004	0.046 ±0.007	0.0091 ±0.0010	0.0097 ±0.0018
Clofibrate	322 ±17	3.0 ±0.3	0.94 ±0.24	4.7 ±0.4	0.029 ±0.004	0.051 ±0.007	0.0088 ±0.0017	0.0130 ±0.0023
Significance	0.68	1.3×10^{-2}	0.23	3.9×10^{-6}	0.038	0.088	0.35	0.29

Intestine, Carcass and Pelt weights (g) fell from 24.3 ± 0.7 to 23.9 ± 1.6, 181 ± 16 to 169 ± 12 and 65.8 ± 11.4 to 59.4 ± 10.7 respectively. These changes were not significant.

Experiment E. This experiment measured biliary clearance of radiothyroxine in rats on clofibrate diet. Results are shown in Table 4. There was a marked increase in biliary clearance in clofibrate treated animals, mainly corresponding to an increase in bile flow. Clearance measured immediately after tracer administration was significantly higher than that measured 4 h after administration of tracer, an effect noted in both the clofibrate treated and the control groups.

From Experiments C, D, and E, tissue utilisation rates were calculated, and the results are shown, combined with total tissue T_4's, in Figs 3 and 4, which present the effects of clofibrate diet on the T_4 flow pattern.

DISCUSSION

The results of the experiments reported here confirm that clofibrate has a profound effect on thyroxine economy, although the results are disappointing if considered in the light of the commonly held view that T_4 diffuses rapidly throughout and exchanges within a single "distribution space". The T_4 concentrations in plasma, carcass and liver are all slightly reduced, which would be compatible with the view that clofibrate tends to compete with thyroxine for its binding sites throughout the volume of rapid exchange. However, this notion would contribute little or nothing to an understanding of metabolic mechanisms. Limitation of consideration of the results to T_4 concentrations, and to a hypothetical free and rapid exchange throughout a total distribution space, hides a wealth of information and illumination on physiological mechanisms. It is therefore necessary to consider such physiological mechanisms as those controlling

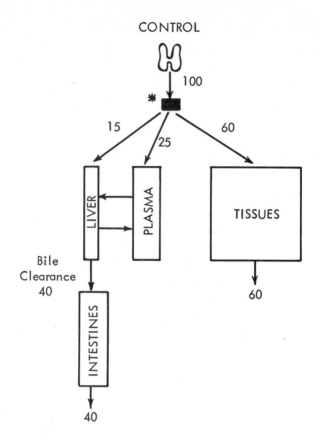

Fig. 3. *Available thyroxine model indicating exchange of protein bound thyroxine in liver and plasma. The area of the compartments is proportional to tissue thyroxine content. Size of the available-thyroxine pool (*) is arbitrary. The numbers indicate the distribution of thyroid output to various tissues in control animals.*

the supply of T_4 to binding sites in the various tissues, and its subsequent utilisation, if the homeostatic reality is to be understood. It is not enough to consider simply an hypothetical model of a completely passive system, even although this model may be all that is required for studies

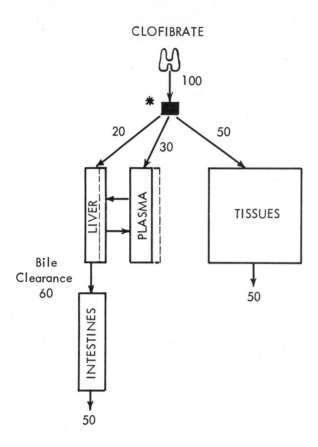

Fig. 4. *The effect of clofibrate on distribution of thyroid hormone in the rat. Note the increased daily flow of thyroxine through the liver.*

of an abnormal thyroid situated in a normal body.

In view of the lack of current knowledge on tissue T_4 mechanisms, it is possible only to draw a general picture of the effects of clofibrate shown by these experiments.

It is clear that a single injection of clofibrate causes radiothyroxine to leave the plasma and enter the liver. This may be by direct displacement in the plasma, from the anionic

Table 4. *Effect of clofibrate on biliary clearance of radiothyroxine (A) immediately after intravenous tracer, (b) four hours after intraperitoneal tracer.*

	Bile Volume (ml/hr)			Clearance (ml/hr)		
	A	B	Significance (p)	A	B	Significance (p)
Control	0.70 ± 0.16 (34)	0.58 ± 0.13 (31)	7.3×10^{-4}	1.57 ± 0.49	0.91 ± 0.24	7.3×10^{-4}
Clofibrate	1.91 ± 0.60 (46)	0.98 ± 0.37 (49)	0.095	2.46 ± 1.14	1.61 ± 0.80	2.4×10^{-2}
Significance	1.14×10^{-6}	5.6×10^{-10}		4.8×10^{-6}	9.0×10^{-8}	

plasma protein binding sites, as suggested by Thorp (10). It
should be noted that if this is the case then the radiothyroxine displaced does not enter the carcass at all but goes
exclusively to the liver and thence by the bile to the intestine. The concept of free and rapid exchange is not compatible with this finding. Another possible mechanism for
the loss of plasma radiothyroxine caused by acute administration of clofibrate is that the drug causes the liver to
strip T_4 from the plasma binding proteins. If this were the
case it should be noted that despite the lowered plasma
radiothyroxine concentration, no radiothyroxine was found
to leave the tissues to balance the plasma loss. The concept
of free and rapid exchange is therefore not compatible with
this mechanism either.

Although in the acute clofibrate situation the fraction
of administered tracer dose held in the plasma is drastically
reduced, by contrast, the fraction of dose initially held in
the plasma in the chronically clofibrate fed rats is slightly
increased. This apparently anomalous finding can be considered
in the light of physiological responses to clofibrate which
do not have time to operate in the acute situation. Experiments A and C show similar increases in disappearance rate
of radiothyroxine from plasma and liver for both acute and
chronic clofibrate administration. The body appears to be
unable to counteract this effect of clofibrate. It can, however, restore the plasma and liver T_4 concentrations almost
to normal, presumably by a considerably increased production
of available binding proteins. This restoration of concentration, in the face of an inexorably increased turnover rate,
necessitates an increase in flow. The net result is that with

chronic dosage of clofibrate, liver and plasma T_4 concentrations
are slightly down and flows per g slightly up. It is not
possible to say whether it is flow, or concentration, or both,
which controls the physiological response.

The experiments suggest a small reduction in carcass T_4
concentration and T_4 flow per g, and there may overall be a
small but insignificant increase in T_4SR. The increase in
liver weight by over 25% has led to a substantial increase in
the total T_4 through the liver. These complex relative changes
are illustrated in Figs. 3 and 4.

In situations where abnormal function is not exclusively
confined to the thyroid gland, we suggest that the complex
relationship between supply and demand for each individual
tissue underlying a euthyroid state, and the complex causes
and effects which must go to the maintenance of such a state,
cannot be expected to be reducible to a simple mechanism such
as suggested by the "free thyroxine" hypothesis (24,25). This
frequently quoted hypothesis claims that the quotient of the
total plasma bound T_4 to the unfilled plasma protein binding
sites is the determinant of thyroid function and a euthyroid
state of the whole body. We have elsewhere presented some
evidence against this hypothesis (26-30), and the data in
this paper are also seen to be incompatible with this sim-
plistic approach.

The third possibility relating thyroxine to the hypocholesterolaemic action of clofibrate is that thyroxine is
essential to the change in hepatic function. A low T_4 disappearance rate is observed in hypothyroidism, consistent with
reduced hepatic function. Since it is generally agreed that
clofibrate acts chiefly on the liver, any reduction of T_4

might be expected to reduce the effect of clofibrate on cholesterol, and complete absence of T_4 would probably abolish
the effect. The results of these experiments show that clofibrate interferes with T_4 economy, and that physiological
responses occur to maintain adequate supplies of T_4 to the
liver and plasma. In such a biological homeostatic situation
it is not surprising both that a physiological response is
required to maintain the T_4 supply, and that the maintenance
of T_4 supply is required for the physiological response. We
suggest that the maintenance of T_4 supply in the face of
interference by clofibrate is also required for the effect of
clofibrate on cholesterol.

R E F E R E N C E S

1. J.M. Thorp, *Lancet*, i, 1323-1326 (1962).

2. R.C. Cotton and E.G. Wade, *J. Atheroscler. Res.*, 6,
    98-102 (1966).

3. M.J. Oliver, *Bull. N.Y. Acad. Med.* 44, 1021-1027 (1967).

4. D.S. Platt and B.L. Cockrill, *Biochem. Pharmacol.*
    15, 927-935 (1966).

5. M.M. Best and C.H. Duncan, *J. Lab. Clin. Med.* 64, 634-
    642 (1964).

6. R. Hess, W. Staubli and W. Riess, *Nature*, 208, 856-858
    (1965).

7. D.J. Svoboda and D.L. Azarnoff, *Fed. Proc.* 30, 841-847
    (1971).

8. D.A. Richert and W.W. Westerfeld, *Endocrinol.* 87,
    1274-1281 (1970).

9. J.M. Thorp and W.S. Waring, *Nature*, 194, 948 (1962).

10. J.M. Thorp, *J. Atheroscler. Res.* 3, 351 (1963).

11. D.S. Platt and J.M. Thorp, *Biochem. Pharmacol.* 15,
    915-925 (1966).

12. J.M. Thorp, R.C. Cotton and M.F. Oliver, *Prog. Biochem.*

Pharmacol. 4, 611-617 (1968).

13. W.W. Westerfeld, D.A. Richert and W.R. Ruegamer, *Biochem. Pharmacol.* 17, 1003 - 1016 (1968).

14. Y. Chang, R.J. Pison and M.H. Malone, *Biochem. Pharmacol.* 16, 2053-2055 (1967).

15. M.T. Harrison and R.McG. Harden, *Scot. Med. J.* 11, 213-217 (1966).

16. C.G. McKerrow, R.L. Scott, S.P. Asper and R.I. Levy, *J. Clin. Endocrinol.* 29, 957-961 (1969).

17. J. Barbosa and L. Oliver, *Metabol.* 18, 141-147 (1969).

18. C. Osorio, K.W. Walton, C.H.W. Browne, D. West and P. Whystock, *Biochem. Pharmacol.* 14, 1479-1481 (1965).

19. P. England, J. Webb, T.W. Randall, W.A. Harland and K. Whaley, *Acta Endocrinol.* 73, 681-688 (1973).

20. P. England, W.A. Harland, J.S. Orr and T.W. Randall, *J. Physiol.* 229, 33-40 (1973).

21. N.B. Myant, *J. Physiol.* 135, 426-441 (1957).

22. H.M. Bruce and A.S. Parkes, *J. Hyg. Camb.* 47, 202-208 (1949).

23. J.S. Orr and F.C. Gillespie, *Science,* 162, 138-139 (1968).

24. J. Robbins and J.E. Rall, *Recent Prog. Hormone Res.* 13, 161-208 (1957).

25. J.E. Rall, J. Robbins and C.G. Lewallen, Chapter III *in* The Hormones, Vol. V, Eds. G. Pincus, K.V. Thimann and E.B. Astwood, Academic Press, New York and London, 159-439 (1964).

26. W.A. Harland and J.S. Orr, *Scot. Med. J.* 14, 375-380 (1969).

27. W.A. Harland and J.S. Orr, *J. Physiol.* 200, 297-310 (1969).

28. W.A. Harland and J.S. Orr, *J. Physiol.* 207, 557-561 (1970).

29. W.A. Harland and J.S. Orr, *in* Further Advances in Thyroid Research, eds. K. Fellinger and R. Hoter, Verlag der Weiner Medizinischen Akademie, 1127-1135 (1971).

30. W.A. Harland, J.S. Orr and J.R. Richards, *Scot. Med.*

J. <u>17</u>, 92-97 (1972).

6. Cytosol Binding Proteins for Thyroid Hormones in Bovine Anterior Pituitary

JEHUDA J. STEINBACH, M.D.

*Nuclear Medicine Service, Veterans Administration Hospital,
Buffalo, New York, and
Departments of Nuclear Medicine and Medicine,
State University of New York at Buffalo,
Buffalo, New York, U.S.A.*

INTRODUCTION

Current views of the mechanism of TSH secretion by the thyrotrophic cells of the anterior pituitary suggest that secretion is stimulated by TRF and inhibited by thyroid hormones (1). Since the initial description of the feedback inhibition loop of thyroid hormones (2), it has been assumed that the site of action of thyroid hormones is in the anterior pituitary. Recent observations utilising synthetic TRF and sensitive measurements of TSH lend experimental support to these assumptions (3,4). It is now recognised, however, that ancillary sites of thyroid hormone action probably are located also at the level of the hypothalamus (5,6). Preferential accumulation of thyroid hormones within the anterior pituitary has been shown (7,8,9), complementing these physiological observations.

The concept that specific receptors mediated by recognition of the appropriate hormones is the initial step of

hormonal function has gained wide acceptance. The existence
of specific binding sites for oestrogens in the cytosol of
the anterior pituitary has been shown by several investigators (10).

In vivo experiments measuring the kinetics of radioiodinated T_3 and T_4 interchange at the anterior pituitary level
have suggested the presence of low capacity, high affinity
binding sites for T_3 (11).

The *in vitro* demonstration of such specific binding sites
has long been delayed because low affinity, high capacity
sites for thyroid hormones are present in almost all tissues
including the anterior pituitary.

The present study describes the chromatographic and
electrophoretic fractionation of thyroid binding proteins in
the cytosol of the anterior pituitary.

M A T E R I A L S   A N D   M E T H O D S
*Preparation and Labeling of Soluble Anterior Pituitary
Fraction*

Bovine anterior pituitaries were obtained in the frozen
state from a commercial supplier (Pel-Freez Corp.) and utilised within three months of receipt. Tissues were thawed and
blotted from all blood and washed repeatedly in 0.9% saline
to remove as much as possible of the residual blood traces.
Anterior pituitaries were then pooled and homogenised in the
cold, using a Waring blender with miniblender attachment, in
0.25 M sucrose at a ratio of 1:3 wt./vol. The homogenate was
then subjected to differential centrifugation at 4°C according to the method of Henninger *et al.* (12). The supernatant
obtained from the final stage of the differential centrifug-

ation (1 hr at 105,000 x g) was incubated overnight at $4^\circ C$ with radioiodinated T_3 and T_4. The amount of carrier T_3 or T_4 added to 250 μl of cytosol (containing 7.5 mg of proteins) was 5 ng, which was calculated on the basis of the specific activity of the tracer supplied. The above incubation time was chosen since a minimum of 4 hours was required to obtain maximal uptake.

$^{131}I\text{-}T_4$, in specific activity range of 40–80 mCi/mg, was obtained from Amersham/Searle Corporation. $^{125}I\text{-}T_4$, in specific activity range of 80–220 mCi/mg, and $^{131}I\text{-}T_3$, in specific activity range of 17–60 mCi, was obtained from Mallinckrodt/ Nuclear Corporation. $^{125}I\text{-}T_3$, in specific activity range of 50–85 mCi/mg, was obtained from Abbot Laboratories.

Excluded from the study were all hormone preparations containing less than 90% of the labelled hormone.

Column Chromatography

The radiolabeled supernatant was subjected to gel chromatography using Sephadex G-200, 15 x 1 cm columns (Pharmacia K-9). Columns were eluted at $4^\circ C$ with tris buffer, pH 7.8. Fractions were collected in a volume of 0.6 ml/tube using an automatic fraction collector (Gilson Micro-Fraction Collector).

The radioactivity of the samples was measured by counting with an automatic gamma spectrometer (Searle Radiographics). In addition, protein concentration in each tube was determined using the Lowry method (13) or by measuring absorption at 280 nm.

The tubes containing the highest protein concentration were then pooled and labelled as fractions 1,2 and 3. Each fraction was rechromatographed, again using Sephadex G-200.

E

Repeat counting and determination of protein concentrations
in the individual fractions was performed as described above.

Control chromatography of bovine serum was performed
following 105,000 x g centrifugation of the serum. 1.5 mg of
serum proteins were added to the incubation mixture with radioiodinated T_3 and T_4. This quantity of serum was chosen to sim-
ulate approximately 20% contamination of the cytosol by serum
proteins. The column chromatography was processed in the same
manner as described above for the anterior pituitary cytosol.

Acrylamide Electrophoresis

Electrophoresis on 5.6% acrylamide gel containing 1%
sodium dodecyl sulfate (SDS) was done using the method of
Fairbanks *et al.* (14). Migration of the pyronine-y dye to a
distance of 60 mm required a running time of about 55 mins.
The gels were scanned at 550 nm with a Gilford Spectrophoto-
meter. Whole pituitary extract and fractions 1, 2 and 3 were
studied separately. Comparison with bovine serum was performed
using whole serum and aliquots eluted from a Sephadex G-200
column corresponding to fractions , 2 and 3 of the cytosol.

R E S U L T S

Sephadex G-200 Chromatography

Sephadex G-200 column chromatography of the anterior
pituitary extract incubated with radioiodinated T_4 consistently revealed four activity peaks. (Fig. 1). The first peak
centred around tube No. 6. This peak is in the void volume
as indicated by a blue dextran marker (15). The second peak
was centred around tube No. 9, the third peak centred around
tube No. 16, and the fourth peak centred around cube No. 26.
Determination of the relative protein concentration (Lowry

method) of tubes 1-30 (Fig. 1) reveals three protein peaks
corresponding to the three radioactivity peaks. The fourth
radioactivity peak represents the free labeled T_4 as confirmed in a control study. Rechromatography of fractions 1, 2
and 3 resulted in activity peaks corresponding to their original location (Figs. 2,3,4). Protein determination, either
by the Lowry method or by light absorbance at 280 nm, confirmed that the major radioactivity peaks were associated with
protein peaks (Figs. 2,3,4). Only slight dissociation of the
radioiodinated T_4 into the free hormone peak could be seen.

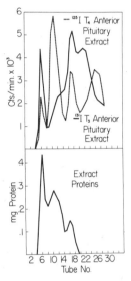

Fig. 1. *Sephadex G-200 column chromatography of the anterior
pituitary extract following simultaneous incubation with* ^{125}I-
T_4 *and* ^{131}I-T_3. *The peak of the void volume as determined with
blue dextran is at tube No. 6 (not shown).*

*The upper frame demonstrates the radioactivity associated
with each of the protein fractions. The last two peaks to the
right are the free hormone peaks. Free T_3 was found to elute
somewhat earlier than free T_4. The lower frame demonstrates
the relative protein concentration in each of the tubes. Fractions 1 to 3 correspond to the three protein peaks in order
from left to right.*

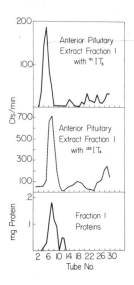

Fig. 2. *Rechromatography of fraction 1 anterior pituitary extract on Sephadex G-200 columns. The upper frame represents the radioactivity associated with $^{131}I\text{-}T_3$, the middle frame that activity associated with $^{125}I\text{-}T_4$, and the lower frame the relative protein concentration in each of the tubes.*

Sephadex G-200 column chromatography of the anterior pituitary extract incubated with radioiodinated T_3 showed slight variation from that of the T_4 behaviour. Consistently, peak 1 could be found centred around tube No. 6 (Fig. 1), analogous to that of T_4. However, no complete separation of peaks 2 or 3 could be obtained. The free T_3 fraction was found to centre around tube No. 22, peaking slightly earlier than the T_4 activity. Rechromatography of fraction 1, $^{131}I\text{-}T_3$ can be seen in Fig. 2. It corresponded well to that of fraction 1, $^{125}I\text{-}T_4$. Rechromatography of the fraction corresponding to peak 2, although it revealed some activity assoc-

iated with a corresponding protein peak, showed a marked dissociation of the bound activity into the free hormone peak
(Fig. 3). Rechromatography of the fraction corresponding to
peak 3 of the T_3 showed no distinct activity associated with
a corresponding protein.

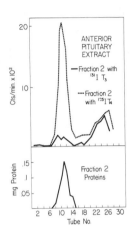

Fig. 3. *Rechromatography of fraction 2 anterior pituitary
extract using Sephadex G-200 columns. The upper frame represents the results for the radioactivity associated with ^{131}I-
T_3 and ^{125}I-T_4. The lower frame represents the corresponding
relative protein concentration.*

Simultaneous incubation of the anterior pituitary extract
with ^{131}I-T_3 and ^{125}I-T_4 showed essentially the same relation
as described for individual incubation. No change in the relative distribution of the individual peaks was noted whether
T_3 or T_4 were examined separately or simultaneously using
dual isotope technique. Therefore, in order to avoid duplic-
ation, only the results of the simultaneous incubation are
presented.

Column chromatography of bovine serum which was process-

ed in the same manner as the anterior pituitary extract revealed a peak count activity and a protein peak for T_3 and T_4,
centred around tube No. 9 (Fig. 5). This peak was indistinguishable from fraction 2 of the anterior pituitary extract.

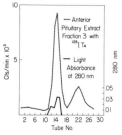

Fig. 4. *Rechromatography of fraction 3 anterior pituitary
extract using Sephadex G-200 columns. The radioactivity associated with* ^{125}I-T_4 *is shown with the corresponding relative
protein concentration measured by light absorption at 280 nm.*
^{131}I-T_3 *showed no distinct peak.*

An additional small protein peak could also be seen
centred around tube No. 6. This peak was not associated with
radioactivity on repeated examinations. At the region corresponding to fraction 3 of the anterior pituitary extract (Tubes
14-16), no associated proteins could be demonstrated, although
some activity could be seen, which appeared to trail the main
activity peak.

Sodium Dodecyl Sulfate (SDS) Acrylamide Gel Electrophoresis

Whole anterior pituitary extract and the three fractions
(1, 2, 3) which were obtained from the Sephadex G-200 column
were analysed by SDS acrylamide gel electrophoresis. Comparison was made with whole serum and serum aliquots eluted on
Sephadex G-200 columns which corresponded in elution to fractions 1-3 of the anterior pituitary extract. Electrophoresis
of the whole anterior pituitary extract revealed the presence

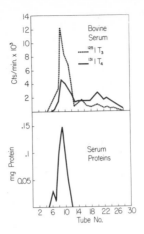

Fig. 5. *Sephadex G-200 column chromatography of bovine serum following incubation with* $^{131}I\text{-}T_3$ *and* $^{125}I\text{-}T_4$. *The radioactivity peaks in the upper frame are compared with the relative protein concentration in the lower frame.*

of multiple polypeptide fractions throughout the length of the gel. The relative mobility of BSA marker (M.W. 67,000) and pyronine-y dye (M.W. 302.8) are illustrated in Fig. 6. Comparison with bovine serum is demonstrated in the same figure. Major differences between the two are in the very slowly migrating fractions, particularly at the relative mobility of 0.13, and the rapidly migrating fractions, particularly at the relative mobility of 0.70.

The electrophoretic pattern of fraction 1 of the cytosol compared with fraction 1 serum can be seen in Fig. 7. Although at least thirteen peaks were observed in each of the studies, relative sizes of these peaks were significantly different.

Figure 8 represents the results obtained using fraction 2 of the cytosol and serum. The general pattern of these two studies is very similar, suggesting that the polypeptide chains are either of rather similarly structured proteins, or of identical origin.

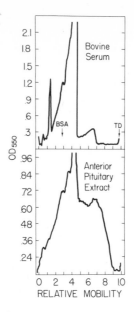

Fig. 6. *SDS acrylamide gel electrophoresis of bovine serum compared with that of the whole anterior pituitary extract. Migration distance of the tracing dye, pyronine-y (TD), and bovine serum albumin (BSA) are marked with arrows.*

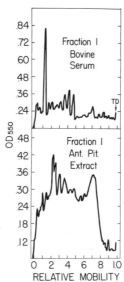

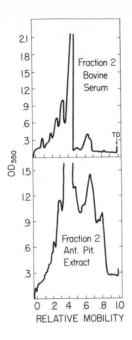

Fig. 8. *SDS acrylamide gel electrophoresis of fraction 2 of bovine serum with the corresponding fraction of anterior pituitary extract.*

The electrophoretic pattern of fraction 3 of the cytosol compared with fraction 3 of the serum can be seen in Fig. 9. Marked differences are observed in the migration pattern of the proteins in the two studies.

DISCUSSION

Chromatographic and electrophoretic studies of thyroid hormone binding to the anterior pituitary cytosol were performed. Using Sephadex G-200 column chromatography, three major protein fractions associated with thyroid hormone act-

Fig. 7. *SDS acrylamide gel electrophoresis of fraction of the anterior pituitary extract with the corresponding fraction of bovine serum.*

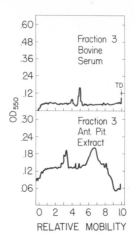

Fig. 9. *SDS acrylamide gel electrophoresis of fraction 3 of bovine serum with the corresponding fraction of anterior pituitary extract.*

ivity (assigned the numbers 1, 2 and 3) could be separated. Each of the obtained fractions could further be subdivided into multiple protein components using SDS acrylamide gel electrophoresis. A marked difference in the binding pattern of T_3 and T_4 to the cytosol is demonstrated using Sephadex G-200 chromatography. Whereas T_4 binds to all three fractions of the cytosol showing three distinct activity peaks (Fig. 1), the T_3 cytosol chromatography demonstrated only a distinct activity peak for fraction 1 (Fig. 1). The differences are accentuated when rechromatography of each of the fractions is performed. Strong binding for T_4 is demonstrated to all three fractions. However, high dissociation of the binding of T_3 for fractions 2 and 3 under the same conditions is apparent (Figs, 2,3,4). This indicates a marked difference in the affinity of the various fractions of the cytosol for T_3 and T_4. Simultaneous incubation of T_3 and T_4 did not change the basic

pattern from that observed with individual incubation. This
might suggest that the two hormones do not compete appreciably
on the cytosol and that they bind to different proteins. However, the marked batch to batch variation in the individual
sizes of the obtained peaks will necessitate a different approach to examine this question.

Comparison of the column chromatography of bovine serum
and that of the anterior pituitary extract revealed significant differences between the two. This was mainly true for
fractions 1 and 3. Whereas fraction 1 of the serum demonstrated a protein peak, the latter is not associated with a radioactivity peak as was fraction 1 of the anterior pituitary
extract. No activity peak in fraction 1 of the bovine serum
could be obtained when excess serum proteins were added to
the incubation mixture. Fraction 3 of the serum, on the other
hand, failed to reveal any protein peak, although some activity was seen trailing the main activity peak. The above indicates that the binding of thyroid hormones in fractions 1 and
3 was not merely due to serum protein contamination. In contrast, fraction 2 of the anterior pituitary cytosol cannot be
distinguished from that of the serum.

Similarly, when the findings of the SDS acrylamide gel
electrophoresis of the anterior pituitary cytosol and the
serum were compared, significant qualitative differences were
present for fractions 1 and 3. However, fraction 2 was remarkably similar for both preparations.

Whether fraction 2 of the anterior pituitary cytosol
binding of thyroid hormones is merely due to serum protein
contamination or not remains to be established.

Since it was first recognised that thyroid hormones accumulate preferentially in the anterior pituitary (7), several investigators have reported evidence for the binding of thyroid hormones to extracts of the anterior pituitary (9,16, 17). However, the site of action has not been established. At the present time, it is assumed that thyroid hormones stimulate formation of DNA dependent mRNA which in turn directs the synthesis of an inhibitor protein suppressing TSH production and release (18,19). Evidence favouring the existence of specific nuclear binding sites for T_3 within the anterior pituitary and other organs has been presented in animal experiments (20,21,22). It has been suggested that such binding sites which might be of limited capacity and close to saturation at endogenous concentration of thyroid hormones, affect the on-off release of TSH by saturation and desaturation. (11).

The role of cytoplasmic binding proteins in transport or regulation of thyroid hormones within the cell is not known. Since, however, for certain steroids it was shown (23,24) that cytoplasmic receptors facilitate the transport of the hormone to the nucleus, one might suspect that an analogous situation might be present for the thyroid hormones system. Evidence for the latter is yet outstanding.

Recent studies of T_3 and T_4 binding by the cytosol of porcine anterior pituitary indicate that at least two different binding sites for thyroid hormones are present. One of these has high specificity and low affinity for T_4, and the other has high affinity but low specificity for both T_3 and T_4 (17). We have been unable to duplicate such experiments using our pituitary preparation. Therefore, we chose to separate the proteins as reported in this paper prior to subjecting them for further analysis. Our finding that at least three different protein fractions bind T_4 is in agreement with the theoretical considerations of these authors.

Further investigation of the cytosol proteins and their possible role in the feedback inhibition of TSH secretion is presently in progress.

Acknowledgements
  The author wishes to thank Drs. M.T. Hayes and C.Y. Jung for their help and advice during the course of this work, and Miss S. Mancuso for her excellent technical assistance. Expert secretarial assistance was rendered by Miss M. Latchford.

R E F E R E N C E S

1. S. Reichlin *In* "The Thyroid" (S.C. Werner and S.H. Ingbar, eds), p. 95 (1971).

2. R.G. Hoskins, *J. Clin. Endocr.* <u>9</u>, 1429 (1949).

3. R. Guillemin, *Recent Progr. Hormone Res.* <u>20</u>, 89 (1964).

4. W. Vale, R. Burgus and R. Guillemin, *Proc. Soc. Exptl. Biol. Med.* <u>125</u>, 210 (1967).

5. J.J. DiStefano III and E.B. Stear, *Bull. Math. Biophys.* <u>30</u>, 1 (1968).

6. D. Sinha and J. Meites, *Neuroendocrinology,* <u>1</u>, 4 (1965).

7. D. Ford, H. Corey and J. Gross, *Endocrinology,* <u>61</u>, 426 (1957).

8. D.H. Ford, S. Kantounis and R. Lawrence, *Endocrinology,* <u>64</u>, 977 (1959).

9. R. Grinberg, *Endocrinology,* <u>75</u>, 281 (1964).

10. A.J. Eisenfeld, *Endocrinology,* <u>86</u>, 1313 (1970).

11. A.R. Schadlow, M.I. Surks, H.L. Schwartz and J.H. Oppenheimer, *Science,* <u>176</u>, 1252 (1972).

12. R.W. Henninger, F.C. Larson and E.C. Albright, *Endocrinology,* <u>78</u>, 61 (1966).

13. O.H. Lowry, N.J. Rosenbrough, A.L. Farr and R.J. Randall, *J. Biol. Chem.* <u>193</u>, 265 (1951).

14. G. Fairbanks, T.L. Steck and D.F.H. Wallach, *Biochemistry,*
     10, 2606 (1971).

15. T.S. Work and E. Work (eds) "Laboratory Techniques in
     Biochemistry and Molecular Biology", L. Fischer "An
     Introduction to Gel Chromatography", p. 166 (1971).

16. R. Grinberg, *Nature,* (Lond.) 205, 701 (1965).

17. S.B. Sufi, R.S. Toccafondi, P.G. Malan and R.P. Ekins,
     J. Endocr. 58, 41 (1973).

18. C.Y. Bowers, K.L. Lee and A.V. Schally, *Endocrinology,*
     82, 303 (1968).

19. C.Y. Bowers, K.L. Lee and A.V. Schally, *Endocrinology,*
     82, 75 (1968).

20. J.H. Oppenheimer, H.L. Schwartz, D. Koerner and M.I.
     Surks, *J. Clin. Invest.* 53, 768 (1974).

21. J.H. Oppenheimer, H.L. Schwartz, W. Dillman and M.I.
     Surks, *Biochem. Biophys. Res. Comm.* 55, 544 (1973).

22. J.H. Oppenheimer, *Mt. Sinai J. Med.* 40, 491 (1973).

23. B.W. O'Malley, *New Eng. J. Med.* Feb. 18, 370 (1971).

24. E.V. Jensen, T. Suzuki, T. Kawashima *et al. Proc. Nat.
     Acad, Sci.* 59, 632 (1968.

7. Interactions of Thyroxine with a Pituitary Cytosol Fraction

S.B. SUFI, P.G. MALAN AND R.P. EKINS

Department of Nuclear Medicine,

The Middlesex Hospital Medical School,

Nassau Street, London W1N 7RL, England.

INTRODUCTION

In an attempt to understand the molecular mechanism by which the thyroid hormones exert their metabolic effects, an analogy with the method of transport of the steroid hormones to their nuclear sites of action has been suggested (1). A number of reports have appeared in recent years which describe the binding of thyroxine and triiodothyronine to cytoplasmic and nuclear binding sites which display high affinity and, in some cases, high specificity (2-7). We have previously reported the binding characteristics of both the iodothyronine hormones with respect to an anterior pituitary cytoplasmic fraction (cytosol) (7). However, before attempting to isolate the binding components involved, we considered it to be necessary first to establish whether significant molecular modifications of T_4 occurred in the course of the binding reaction.

Two possible alterations might be supposed to occur to the iodothyronine structure: a general degradation of the molecule either by deamination or oxidative deamination of

the side chain, or by non-specific deiodination (8,9); alternatively, specific monodeiodination of T_4 to T_3 is possible.
The latter would be a particularly interesting phenomenon,
in view of accumulating evidence that T_3 is the metabolically
active thyroid hormone (1). As part of a study to determine
a possible role for the cytosol binding protein in the anterior
pituitary, where thyroid hormones exert feedback control on
thyrotrophin release, and also in an attempt to detect changes
which may occur to bound T_4, we have performed the studies
described in this paper.

METHODS AND RESULTS

Preparation of Anterior Pituitary Cytosol

Porcine pituitaries were collected from the slaughter
house directly into ice cold Krebs-Ringer phosphate buffer,
pH 7.4 (KRP buffer). In the laboratory, the tissue was resuspended in KRP buffer and was washed five times by stirring
for 10 min each time, to reduce contamination by serum proteins.
The anterior and posterior lobes were then dissected, and the
anterior lobes were again washed before homogenisation using
a Polytron for 10 sec. The homogenate was filtered through a
metal mesh, centrifuged at 1,000xg for 30 min to remove debris,
then at 100,000xg for 60 min to remove particulate cell components. The supernatant cytosol was finally aliquoted into
small containers and was stored at -20°C until required.
Protein concentration was determined by the method of Lowry
et al. (10).

Separation of Cytosol-bound from Free Thyroid Hormones

In order to study the binding characteristics of the
thyroid hormones to the cytosol components, it was first necessary to evaluate a procedure by which free hormone could be

separated from that which is bound. Various techniques were
examined to obtain maximum separation between bound and free
radioiodine labelled thyroid hormones, with a minimum of misclassification error (commonly called a "blank") in measuring
the two components. Short columns of Sephadex G-25 eluted at
$4^{\circ}C$ gave effective separation and yielded low misclassification
errors, but the technique was slow and was limited to a relatively small number of samples. Particulate adsorbents for
the free hormones which were examined included powdered silica,
a variety of grades of charcoal and talc, each of which was
tested in the presence or absence of a coating agent such as
gelatin, dextran or methylcellulose, to minimise adsorption
of cytosol proteins to the solid particles.

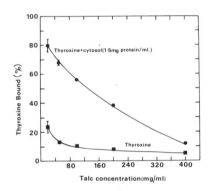

Fig. 1.*Talc separation of cytosol-bound and free ^{125}I-thyrox-*
ine. Tubes containing ^{125}I-thyroxine (515 fmol/ml) were incu-
bated in 500 μl buffer either in the presence or absence of
cytosol (750 μg protein). After equilibration of cytosol with
thyroxine, 100 μl of a suspension containing different amounts
of talc was added to all the tubes. They were immediately mixed
and then centrifuged, and the supernatant was separated from
the talc by aspiration. Radioactivity in the supernatant,
expressed as a percentage of the total, is plotted as thyroxine
bound on the ordinate.

Figure 1 shows the results of the experimental procedure which was used to check the effectiveness of uncoated talc in separating cytosol-bound from free thyroxine. Labelled thyroxine was equilibrated with the cytosol protein in a series of tubes, and a further series of tubes containing identical reagents, but no cytosol, was also prepared. Increasing amounts of talc were added to the tubes as a suspension in a constant volume of KRP buffer. Most of the labelled thyroxine was adsorbed to the talc in the absence of cytosol, but between 5 and 10% remained free in the supernatant, even at the higher concentrations of talc tested. Conversely, considerable adsorption of cytosol-bound label to talc occurred at high talc concentrations; consequently the amount selected for subsequent experiments was 20 µg of talc/µg cytosol protein/500 µl of incubation mixture. This yielded acceptable misclassification errors of bound-as-free and of free-as-bound. Premixing of talc with 0.1% gelatin effectively decreased cytosol adsorption but with a concomitant decrease in adsorption of free hormone, therefore this procedure was not used. Similar experiments were performed to validate the separation procedure for T_3 in the system; for both iodothyronine hormones the talc system was superior to all the others examined.

Kinetics of Thyroid Hormone Binding to Anterior Pituitary Cytosol.

(a) *Scatchard Analysis* : Since there was no other convenient way of characterising fresh cytosol preparations, we relied on determinations of the equilibrium constants for T_4 and T_3 obtained from Scatchard Plots of binding data at different concentrations of the ligand. A typical plot of bound to free ratio of $^{125}I-T_4$ versus the concentration of T_4 bound is shown

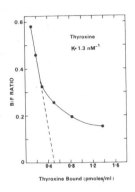

Fig. 2. *Scatchard plot of thyroxine binding to cytosol. Different concentrations of ^{125}I-thyroxine, in the range 0.3 to 20 pmol/ml, were incubated at 4°C for 60 min with cytosol (500 μg protein/ml). The talc procedure was used to separate the bound and free fractions.*

in Fig. 2. The slope of the tangent to this curve at zero hormone concentration yields an estimate of the equilibrium constant of high affinity binding sites for the hormone: the intercept of the tangent at this point with the concentration axis is indicative of their concentration (11). The mean equilibrium constant (±S.D.) for the T_4 interaction was 2.7 ± 1.7 nM^{-1}, and for T_3 it was 0.42 ± 0.18 nM^{-1}, determined for each of different cytosol preparations at 4°C.

(b) *Association Reaction :* In order to determine the incubation times required to establish equilibrium in subsequent binding studies, the association of ^{125}I-thyroxine with cytosol was determined at 4°C and also at 20°C, as shown in Fig. 3. Concentrations of reagents used were of the same order or lower than those employed subsequently. Binding of hormone to the cytosol was extremely rapid using the reagent concentrations shown in the legend to Fig. 3, and the association rate was

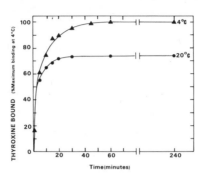

Fig. 3. *Association of* [125]*I-thyroxine with cytosol at 4°C and at 20°C. Tubes containing cytosol (500 µg /ml) were incubated with* [125]*I-thyroxine (260 fmol /ml) for various time intervals. At the end of the incubation period cytosol-bound and free thyroxine were separated by adding a suspension containing 5 mg talc /100 µl to each 500 µl of incubation mixture.*

too rapid to determine accurately, even when the concentrations were decreased by one-half. Within about 5 min at both temperatures, half-maximal binding was achieved, while maximum binding and equilibration of the reactants occurred by about 30 min at 20°C and by 60 min at 4°C, and remained constant for up to 4 hr of incubation. Binding of T_4 at 20°C attained a value only about 70% of that observed at 4°C: this effect was not thought to be due to the talc separation procedure employed, since virtually identical results for separation of bound and free thyroid hormones were obtained at either temperature using Sephadex gel filtration. Association rate curves for T_3 binding at 4°C were very similar to those of T_4, using the same concentrations of reagents, except that a lower percentage of ^{125}I-triiodothyronine was bound.

Effect of Temperature on Thyroxine Bound to Cytosol

The influence of temperature on the amount of T_4 bound

to cytosol was investigated further. Equilibration of ^{125}I-
T$_4$ with anterior pituitary cytosol for 3 hr at 22°C reduced
binding to 50% of that observed at 4°C, as is shown by the
first two bars in Fig. 4. To determine whether the decreased
binding observed at 22°C was due to changes in either the
association or dissociation rate constants, cytosol and labelled thyroxine were equilibrated at 22°C for 90 min and then
were allowed to re-equilibrate at 4°C for a further 90 min.

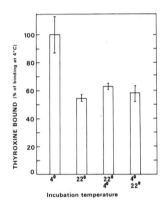

Fig. 4. *Effect of temperature on thyroxine binding to cytosol. Cytosol (400 µg /ml) and ^{125}I-thyroxine (500 fmol /ml)
were incubated either at 22ºC or at 4ºC for 3 hr. At the end
of this time the fraction of thyroxine bound is shown in the
first two experiments in the figure. In the second part of
the figure incubation was performed for 90 min at each temperature. Error bars indicate ± S.E.M. (n = 5).*

This result is shown by the third bar in Fig. 4, and a slight
but not statistically significant increase in binding was
observed when compared with that found after incubation at
22°C for 180 min. A further control experiment is shown in Fig.
4 in which two 90 min incubations were performed, the first
at 4°C and the second at 22°C; only about 60% of the maximum

binding achieved at 4°C was observed. Similar results were obtained when incubation was performed at 37°C instead of 22°C, and these results suggested a temperature effect either on ^{125}I-T$_4$ degradation or on the cytosol binding site.

Effect of Temperature on the Cytosol Component

In these experiments, cytosol was incubated at either 4°C or at 37°C, but in the absence of labelled thyroxine. The cytosol was first subjected to similar temperature changes to those described in Fig. 4, and subsequently the cytosol was incubated at 4°C with ^{125}I-T$_4$ for one hour. The results are shown in Fig. 5, and no effect of prior incubation of cytosol for up to 3 hr at 37°C was observed on the binding of labelled thyroxine, subsequently after re-equilibration at 4°C. It is therefore possible that changes observed in T$_4$ binding at higher temperatures might be due either to degradation of labelled T$_4$ or that a temperature dependent conformational change occurs only when T$_4$ is bound. The latter implies an essentially irreversible effect of T$_4$ binding at higher temperatures, that causes an allosteric effect which prevents hormone binding to a second site on the molecule: alternatively, dissocation of subunits of the cytosol protein, which themselves do not bind T$_4$, may occur.

Conversion of ^{125}I-Thyroxine to ^{125}I-Triiodothyronine

(a) *Chromatographic System:* A histogram of a typical one-dimensional chromatogram of ^{125}I-T$_4$, following incubation with cytosol for 24 hr at 37°, is illustrated in Fig. 6. Good resolution of T$_4$ and T$_3$ peaks was obtained, and separation from other labelled iodothyronines was considered to be reasonable for a one-dimensional separation system. Radioactive peaks were identified with reference to authentic carrier compounds

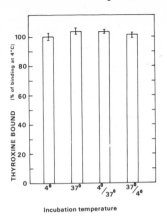

Fig. 5. *Effect of temperature on cytosol. Cytosol (400 μg/ml) was incubated for 3 hr at either 4°C or 37°C, or it was incubated for 90 min at each of these temperatures. Tubes were then quickly cooled to 4°C and allowed to equilibrate with ^{125}I-thyroxine (500 fmol/ml) for a further 1 hr. The fraction of ^{125}I-thyroxine bound was determined as described in the legend to Fig. 3. Error bars indicate ± S.E.M. (n = 5).*

(obtained from Sigma Chemical Co.) which were visualised on the chromatogram by ultraviolet absorption and by spraying with diazotised sulphanilic acid. Mono- and di-iodotyrosine remain near the origin, while iodide migrates to a position between the origin and thyroxine. A check on the results obtained by one-dimensional chromatography was made using a two-dimensional system (12), and sufficiently reliable quantitation of T_4 and T_3 present was obtained to justify using chromatography in only a single dimension in subsequent experiments, providing that the positions of radioactive peaks were carefully matched with the respective carrier compounds.

(b) *Purity of* ^{125}I-*Thyroxine*: All batches of ^{125}I-T_4 (The Radiochemical Centre, Amersham, England) used in these studies were checked for purity by chromatography in *tert*.amyl alcohol-hexane-2M ammonia before use. Table 1 summarises the amounts

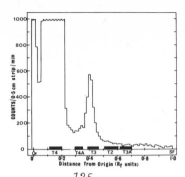

Fig.6. *Chromatography of* ^{125}I*-thyroxine incubated with cytosol. Cytosol (35 mg /ml) and* ^{125}I*-thyroxine (170 pmol/ml)
were incubated for 24 hr at 37°C. Two volumes of alkaline (NaOH
ethanol containing iodothyronine carrier compounds (1 mg /ml)
were added, and 75 μl of the supernatant was streaked on to
Whatman 31ET paper. The chromatogram was developed in a descending system using* <u>tert.amyl alcohol-hexane-2M ammonia</u> *(5:1:
6)*[12] *for 6-8 hr at* <u>25°C</u>*. Carrier iodothyronines, located by
ultraviolet absorption, are shown as black bars on the abs-
cissa. Radioactive measurements were performed after cutting
the paper into 5mm-wide strips.
Or = origin, T₄ = thyroxine, T₄A = tetraiodothyroacetic acid,
T₃ = 3',3,5-triiodothyronine, T₂ = 3,5-diiodothyronine, T₃A =
3',3,5-triiodothyroacetic acid, S F = solvent front.*

of the radioactive components present as a percentage of the
total radioactivity on the chromatogram. All preparations were
at least 93% ^{125}I-T_4, and the major contaminants observed were
iodide and T_3, with less than 1% tetraiodothyroacetic acid
(T_4A).

(c) *Apparent conversion of* ^{125}I*-thyroxine to* ^{125}I*-Triiodo-
thyronine.*

In these studies, labelled T_4 was incubated in the dark
with anterior pituitary cytosol for 24 hr at 37°C. Three control
experiments were performed : either (a) cytosol, or (b) labelled
T_4 was incubated alone; ^{125}I-T_4 or cytosol, respectively, was
then added immediately before chromatography, and (c) ^{125}I-

Table 1.   *Chromatography of* ^{125}I-T_4

In tAM OH–HEX ANE–2M–NH$_4$OH

SPOT	% OF TOTAL	±S.D.
Origin + I⁻	3.0	0.5
T_4	94.8	1.4
T_4A	0.8	0.2
T_3	1.3	0.1
T_2	0.18	0.03
T_3A	0.15	0.04
Total :	100.2	

All batches of ^{125}I-thyroxine were checked
chromatographically for radiochemical purity
before use, as described in the legend to Fig. 6.

T_4 was incubated in the presence of heat–denatured cytosol.
Each of these controls yielded statistically indistinguishable
results, and the mean of the controls was used to compare with
the test incubation results. Since ^{125}I-T_4 is randomly labelled
on either the 3' or 5' position, measurement of the mono–deiodination product at either of these positions would represent
only half of the T_3 generated. Multiplication by a factor of
two is thus required to convert the change in radioactivity
measured to reflect the molar proportion of T_3 produced.

   The apparent conversion of ^{125}I-T_4 to ^{125}I-T_3 for fourteen separate experiments is summarised in Table 2. This shows
the mean of duplicate chromatograms for each experiment. The
percentage conversion is quite variable and ranges from 0.2%

Sufi et al.

Table 2.   "Apparent" Conversion of $^{125}I\text{-}T_4$ to $^{125}I\text{-}T_3$
By Anterior Pituitary Cytosol (24 h, $37^{\circ}C$)

Expt. No	% $^{125}I\text{-}T_3$ On Chrogm		Apparent % Conversion
	Control	Test	
1	0.9	1.4	1.0
2	1.7	1.8	0.3
3	1.0	5.8	9.6
4	1.8	1.9	0.2
5	2.2	2.7	1.0
6	1.3	1.7	0.8
7	1.4	2.2	1.6
8	1.3	2.1	1.6
9	1.2	1.9	1.4
10	1.4	3.7	4.6
11	1.4	1.8	0.8
12	1.6	1.9	0.6
13	2.0	2.2	0.4
14	1.5	2.1	1.2

Cytosol (500 µg/ml) was incubated with ^{125}I-thyroxine
for 24 hr at $37^{\circ}C$ in the dark. The percentage of ^{125}I-
triiodothyronine formed was estimated chromatographically as described in the legend to Fig. 6. Control
experiments performed, and the method for obtaining
apparent percent conversion are described in the text.
Using all the available data, mono-deiodination of
thyroxine to triiodothyronine was highly significant
($P < 0.5\%$)

to 10%, with a mean of 1.4%, and the control chromatograms
showed between 1 and 2% of radioactivity in the T_3 position.
These differences could be due in part to variability between

the different cytosol preparations; however, when a one-sided
t-test was performed on the data, which included the duplicate
chromatogram results, highly significant mono-deiodination of
T_4 by the cytosol was obtained (P < 0.5%).

Since non-specific deiodination of thyroxine is known to
occur in cytosol preparations (9), it is possible that the
increase in T_3 observed may merely reflect increased non-
specific deiodination of T_4. When an analysis of variance
was performed on the data shown in Fig. 7, relating the change
in percent T_4 observed in test compared with control chromatograms with the apparent percentage conversion to T_3, no
significant correlation could be found between these two
variables.

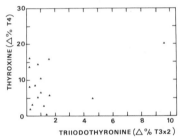

Fig. 7. *Plot showing the lack of correlation between thyroxine degradation and triiodothyronine formation, following
incubation of* [125]*I-thyroxine with cytosol as described in
the footnote to Table 2. The changes observed on test, as
compared with control chromatograms, for thyroxine and triiodothyronine radioactivity are plotted as the y-axis and x-
axis, respectively.*

Addition of a 100-fold excess of T_4 to the cytosol during
the incubation at 37°C with [125]$I-T_4$ did not reduce the mono-
deiodination of labelled hormone. Similarly, the addition of
propylthiouracil or methylmercaptoimidazole to the incubation

mixture in some preliminary experiments had only a slight
effect on decreasing the amounts of T_4 converted to T_3.

DISCUSSION

While thyroid hormones are known to modulate the effects
of thyrotrophin releasing hormone on the pituitary by a feedback mechanism, it is not yet known whether control is exerted
equally by T_4 and T_3, or whether T_4 must first be converted to
T_3. In a recent review, Oppenheimer and Surks (1) outline the
present evident which suggests that only T_3 may be hormonally
active, with T_4 acting largely as a pro-hormone. The site of
action of the thyroid hormones may be at the nucleus in most
tissues (1,13), but their site of action in anterior pituitary
thyrotroph cells has not yet been defined and this site may
well be extranuclear.

We have previously demonstrated that cytosol from porcine
anterior pituitaries contains protein components which bind
both T_4 and T_3; however, these binding sites have a higher
affinity for T_4 ($K = 2.7$ nM^{-1}) than for T_3 ($K = 0.42$ nM^{-1}).
The equilibrium constants reported here for anterior pituitary
cytosol are one or two orders of magnitude lower than those
reported for iodothyronine binding to nuclei of cultured GH_1
cells (4), but this does not rule out the possibility that the
cytosol binding component fulfils a transport or metabolic
role.

These results contrast with the *in vivo* binding of T_3
and T_4 to the rat anterior pituitary reported by Schadlow *et
al.* (3): rapid saturation of ^{125}I-T_4 binding sites was observed
while T_3 uptake was much slower and achieved a higher binding
capacity, but only the latter iodothyronine was displaced by

excess unlabelled hormone. Samuels and Tsai (4) have reported
that cytosol prepared from cultured GH_1 cells contains only
non-specific, low affinity binding sites for T_3. These results
and our own are not necessarily incompatible with those of
Oppenheimer's group, however, since intracellular compartment-
alisation of each of the thyroid hormones, which is most
probable in the intact gland, would be destroyed when the
tissue is homogenised and the cytosol is studied in the absence
of other subcellular particles.

Association and dissociation rates of the two iodothyronines
with the anterior pituitary cytosol were found to be quite
rapid (7). However, T_4 binding to cytosol at $4^{\circ}C$ was greater
than at $22^{\circ}C$ or $37^{\circ}C$ as was shown in Figs 3 and 4. Specificity of thyroxine binding to the cytosol presumably requires
similar molecular configurations to those which are required
for binding of T_4 to serum thyroxine binding globulin (TBG)
or prealbumin (TBPA). The characteristics of T_4 interaction
with cytosol and the serum proteins are quite similar, although
the cytosol binding component has been shown to be distinguish-
able from them by chromatography (7). Thyroxine binding to
serum TBG and TBPA has been intensively studied, and the
specificity of this interaction requires the presence of the
hydrophobic tetraiodobiphenyl ether structure, and the hydro-
philic phenolic hydroxyl and alanyl side-chain groupings (14).
If the iodothyronine/protein interaction is primarily one
between hydrophobic sites, one would expect higher binding of
hormone at $22^{\circ}C$ or $37^{\circ}C$ than at $4^{\circ}C$, on purely thermodynamic
grounds. Since the reverse was observed it is possible that
electrostatic interactions are of primary importance. Increased
dissociation of thyroxine from TBG in the presence of inc-

reasing chloride or phosphate concentrations (15), which would
tend to suppress electrostatic interactions, suggest that the
latter forces may in fact be involved.

However, the experiments describing the effects of temperature on the binding of thyroxine (Figs. 4 and 5) suggest
that a more fundamental alteration may be taking place, either
to labelled thyroxine or to the cytosol-thyroxine complex.
The first possibility that the decrease in thyroxine bound at
$22^{\circ}C$ or $37^{\circ}C$ could have resulted from destruction or deiodination of the iodothyronine molecule was examined. In fourteen
experiments with different cytosol preparations, quite variable
but statistically significant mono-deiodination of T_4 to T_3
was observed (Table 2). Production of T_3 from T_4 could not
have arisen fortuitously by "non-specific" deiodination, since
there was no correlation between the amount of T_4 degraded
and the amount of T_3 formed. The mean conversion of T_4 to T_3
was only 1.4% and the overall decrease in labelled T_4 in the
presence of cytosol in these experiments varied from nearly
zero up to about 15% (Fig. 7). However, this change is insufficient to account for the 50% decrease in binding of T_4
observed at $22^{\circ}C$ compared with the amount bound at $4^{\circ}C$ (see
Fig. 4).

Very similar figures for conversion of T_4 to T_3 have been
reported by Refetoff *et al.* (12) who studied the metabolism
of the iodothyronines in cultured human fibroblasts. One
reason for the low mono-deiodination observed by both Refetoff
and ourselves may have been that the preparations were not
dialysed to remove a natural iodothyronine deiodinase inhibitor
which has been reported to be present in a variety of tissues
(16). Alternatively, the low levels of deiodination might

reflect contamination of the cytosol preparation with microsomal components which are known to contain deiodinase activity (16). Another possibility occurs that an acceptor molecule
may not be present to remove triiodothyronine as it is formed,
and so product inhibition of deiodinase activity prevents
further deiodination of T$_4$.

In conclusion, deiodination or degradation of labelled
T$_4$ is probably not sufficient to account for the decrease in
hormone bound to cytosol at 22°C compared with 4°C. The
significant, but quantitatively minor mono-deiodination of T$_4$
to T$_3$ observed could be due to the presence of deiodinase
inhibitors (16), the absence of an acceptor molecule for the
T$_3$ produced, or even to contamination of the cytosol preparation
by small amounts of microsomal components of the cells. The
inability of labelled hormone to rebind to cytosol, when the
cytosol-thyroxine complex which was formed at 22°C is re-
incubated at 4°C, suggests that a temperature dependent alteration has occurred to the cytosol-thyroxine complex. Even though
the cytosol-thyroxine association rate is rapid at 4°C or 20°C,
the results shown in Fig. 4 suggest that the re-association
of labelled hormone to cytosol, already carrying hormone bound
at 22°C, is extremely slow and is greater than 90 min. Attempts
to explain these results suggest that a temperature-dependent
allosteric effect occurs to the cytosol protein when it binds
T$_4$. At 22°C, but not at 4°C, a second binding site for T$_4$,
either on the same molecule or on a dissociated subunit, is
altered in such a way that it will no longer bind T$_4$. These
observations are consistent with an effect of temperature on
the free energy of the thyroxine-cytosol interaction, and
this phenomenon is at present under further investigation.

Acknowledgements. We should like to thank Drs. B.L. Brown and R.S. Toccafondi (Florence) for their helpful advice throughout this study, and Mrs. S.M. Ellis, Miss S. von Borcke and Miss N. Wechsler for their assistance with certain parts of this work.

R E F E R E N C E S

1. J.H. Oppenheimer and M.I. Surks, *In* "Handbook of Physiology : Endocrinology", (R.O. Greep and E.B. Astwood, eds), Vol. 3, pp. 197-214 (1974).

2. J.H. Oppenheimer, D. Koerner, H.L. Schwartz and M.I. Surks, *J. Clin. Endocr. Metab.* 35, 330-333 (1972).

3. A.R. Schadlow, M.I. Surks, H.L. Schwartz and J.H. Oppenheimer, *Science, N.Y.*, 176, 1252-1254 (1972).

4. H.H. Samuels and J.S. Tsai, *Proc. Nat. Acad. Sci., U.S.A.* 70, 3488-3492 (1973).

5. J.R. Tata, L. Ernster and E.M. Suranyi, *Biochim. Biophys. Acta,* 60, 461-479 and 480-491 (1962).

6. R. Grinberg, *Endocrinology,* 75, 281-283 (1964).

7. S.B. Sufi, R.S. Toccafondi, P.G. Malan and R.P. Ekins, *J. Endocr.* 58, 41-52 (1973).

8. L. van Middlesworth, *In* "Handbook of Physiology : Endocrinology" (R.O. Greep and E.B. Astwood, eds), Vol. 3, pp. 215-231 (1974).

9. J.R. Tata, *Biochim. Biophys. Acta.* 28, 95-99 (1958).

10. O.H. Lowry, N.J. Roseborough, A.L. Farr and R.J. Randall, *J. Biol. Chem.* 193, 265-275 (1951).

11. H.O. Feldman, *Anal. Biochem.* 48, 317-338 (1972).

12. S. Refetoff, R. Matalon and M. Bigazzi, *Endocrinology,* 91, 934-947 (1972).

13. J.R. Tata, L. Ernster, O. Lindberg, E. Arrhenius, S. Pederson and R. Hedman, *Biochem. J.* 86, 408-428 (1963).

14. K.A. Woeber and S.H. Ingbar, *In* "Handbook of Physiology : Endocrinology" (R.O. Greep and E.B. Astwood, eds), Vol. 3, pp. 187-196 (1974).

15. S.W. Spaulding and R.I. Gregerman, *J. Clin. Endocr.*

Metab. <u>34</u>, 974-982 (1972).

16. S. Nakagawa and W.R. Ruegamer, *Biochemistry*, <u>6</u>, 1249-1261 (1967).

F

8. The Effect of Inhibiting Triiodothyronine Production from Thyroxine by Propylthiouracil on the Physiological Activity of Thyroxine in Thyroidectomised Rats*

ROZ D. FRUMESS AND P. REED LARSEN

Division of Endocrinology and Metabolism,
Department of Medicine,
University of Pittsburgh School of Medicine,
Pittsburgh, Pennsylvania, U.S.A.

INTRODUCTION

In addition to its goitrogenic actions within the thyroid gland, 6-n-propylthiouracil (PTU) has repeatedly been shown to reduce the physiological effectiveness of exogenously administered L-thyroxine (T_4) in the rat. Concomitant administration of PTU leads to decreased effects of T_4 on liver, heart and kidney mitochondrial α-glycerolphosphate dehydrogenase (αGPD) activity (1-3), and impairs T_4-induced suppression of TSH release from the pituitary (4-6). This effect of PTU has been associated with its inhibition of the peripheral deiodination of T_4 (7-12).

Recently, Oppenheimer, Schwartz and Surks demonstrated that extrathyroidal conversion of tracer T_4 to 3,5,3'-triiodo-L-thyronine (T_3) occurs in the rat (13), and that this conversion is inhibited by PTU (14). Since recent studies

* *Supported by Grant 14283 from NIAMDD. P.R. Larsen is a Career Development Awardee of the U.S. Public Health Service, Grant 70401.*

estimate that two thirds of the T_3 utilised per day in iodine
sufficient rats arises from T_4 (15), inhibition of this
important pathway for T_3 production by PTU would provide an
attractive explanation for its observed antagonism to the
biological actions of T_4. This would be compatible with the
original speculation of Gross and Pitt-Rivers that, in order
to be metabolically active, T_4 must first be deiodinated to
T_3 (16). If this view is correct, one would expect administration of PTU to thyroidectomised rats maintained on physiological replacement doses of T_4 to result in lower T_3 levels
as well as decreased hormonal activity when compared to rats
given T_4 alone.

M E T H O D S

Surgically thyroidectomised (with parathyroid
reimplantation) or sham-operated Sprague Dawley male rats
(Zivic Miller) were maintained on Purina rat chow and tap
water ad lib, at a constant temperature of 75 ± 1°F. They were
left untreated for 4-8 weeks to allow the thyroidectomised
animals to become hypothyroid. Three sets of experiments were
then performed to study the effect of PTU on the biological
action of T_4. In each of these experiments half of the thyroidectomised animals were given daily intraperitoneal injections of PTU in 2.0 ml of physiological saline alkalinised with
NaOH (pH 8.5) at a dose of 1 mg/100g body weight/day. The
remaining animals received control injections of the vehicle.
These injections were started 1 day prior to and continued
throughout the course of the hormone injections. Injections
were used to avoid variations in PTU intake which might occur
with administration of the drug in the diet.

Experiment A : At the time of thyroidectomy, rats in this
study weighed 150–200 g. After 8 weeks, by which time growth
had been on a plateau for 2 weeks, the thyroidectomised rats
were divided into six groups of 9–10 animals of equal mean
weight (256 g). The experimental groups were given subcutaneous T$_4$ (0.8 or 1.6 µg/100g/day) with or without PTU.
The dose of 0.8 µg T$_4$/100g/day was chosen because it approximated the calculated daily T$_4$ production rate based on our
previous studies (15). To control for nonspecific toxic
effects of PTU as well as for any direct effect of PTU on TSH
levels, one group of thyroidectomised rats received PTU alone.
The other two control groups consisted of untreated thyroidectomised and sham-operated rats. Injections were continued
for five days and each rat was identified and weighed every
other day. Animals were killed by cardiac puncture after
chloroform anesthesia and the necks were examined for any
thyroid remnants. Serum T$_4$ was measured in duplicate at two
dilutions by methods previously described (17). The method
was modified to use 10 and 5 µl aliquots of rat serum in place
of human serum. Serum T$_3$ was measured by methods and modifications described previously using duplicate aliquots of 100
and 50 µl (15). Sera containing small quantities of T$_3$ (<20 ng
/100 ml) were reassayed using 200 and 100 µl samples. Rat
serum TSH was measured in duplicate at two dilutions by the
procedure described in the protocol supplied with the rat TSH
immunoassay materials kindly donated by the National Institute
of Arthritis and Digestive Diseases. Equal numbers of control
and experimental samples were included in all assays to
minimise interassay variation. Mean normal values ± SD for

Zivic Miller male Sprague Dawley rats weighing 200 g or more
are : 3.7 ± 0.89 µg T_4/100 ml; 38 ± 17 ng T_3/100 ml; 191 ± 249
µU TSH/ml. The dialysable fractions of T_3 and T_4 (DFT_3 and DFT_4)
were determined in duplicate by the method of Oppenheimer
et al. with minor modifications (19). Absolute free T_3 and T_4
concentrations are the product of the dialysable fractions
and individual total T_3 and T_4 concentrations.

Experiment B : To study the effect of PTU on liver mitochondrial αGPD, rats of mean weight 400-500 g at the time of
surgery were treated as above, except that only 1 dose of T_4
(0.8 µg/100g/day) was used and rats were treated for 10 and
15 days. Liver mitochondrial αGPD activity was determined by
the method of Lee and Lardy(20). Since only 5 mitochondrial
samples, performed in duplicate, could be assayed at one time,
one representative from each of the differently treated groups
was run in each assay to minimise interassay variation. The
same control sample was also determined with each assay and
no significant variation in this sample was noted. Rats were
killed and assays performed as described above.

Experiment C : Rats of starting weight 150-200 g were used
in this experiment. Starting four weeks after thyroidectomy
these rats received two equal subcutaneous doses of T_3 each
day at 08.00 and 17.00 h. (total dose of 0.1 µg T_3/100g/day)
with and without PTU. This dose was estimated to be about
two-thirds of the daily T_3 production rate (15). A third
group was untreated. After twelve days of treatment, assays
of liver αGPD, T_3, T_4 and TSH were carried out as above.

All statistical analyses were performed using Student's
"t" test for unpaired samples (21).

RESULTS AND DISCUSSION

Figure 1 compares serum T4, T_3 and TSH concentrations
and growth rate (±SEM) in thyroidectomised rats maintained
on 0.8 µg T_4/100g/day ± 1 mg PTU/100g/day for 5 days (experiment A). Serum T_4 was higher and serum T_3 lower in ten rats
receiving PTU + T_4 than in ten rats receiving T_4 alone. In
spite of the higher T_4 in PTU treated rats, TSH levels were
significantly higher in this group. In addition, growth rate
was slower in the group receiving PTU + T_4.

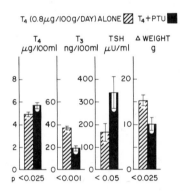

Fig. 1. *Serum T_4, T_3 and TSH concentrations and weight changes
in thyroidectomised, hypothyroid rats after 5 days treatment
with T_4, with or without, propylthiouracil. Results are shown
as mean ± standard error.*

Figure 2 compares these parameters in nine rats treated
with 1.6 µg T_4/100g/day with 10 rats who received 1.6 µg T_4/
100g/day + PTU. Again, TSH was higher in the group receiving
PTU, in spite of the higher T_4 and corresponding with the
lower T_3 found in this group. Weight gain was not different
in these two groups, but since both were similar to that
observed in rats receiving 0.8 µg T_4/100g/day it is possible

that maximum growth rate had already been attained at that
dosage.

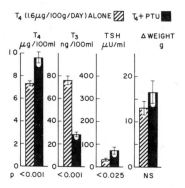

Fig. 2. *Serum T_4, T_3 and TSH concentrations and weight changes
in thyroidectomised hypothyroid rats after 5 days treatment
with T_4 with, or without, propylthiouracil. Results are shown
as mean ± standard error.*

The lower T_3 concentrations associated with PTU administration demonstrate directly that PTU inhibits the peripheral conversion of T_4 to T_3 in the rat, confirming the
tracer studies of Oppenheimer *et al.*(14). Using previously
published kinetic data for normal and PTU-treated rats (14)
it is possible to quantify this inhibition by calculating the
rate of conversion of T_4 to T_3 in thyroidectomised rats
maintained only on T_4 with the equation

$$\text{CONVERSION RATE} = 100 \times \frac{T_3 \text{ turnover (mol/day)}}{T_4 \text{ turnover (mol/day)}}$$

The conversion rate in rats treated with 0.8 µg T_4/100g
per day for five days was 18.3 ± 0.6 (SEM)%, and this was
reduced to 8.0 ± 0.7% in the presence of PTU corresponding
to 56.3% inhibition of conversion. PTU inhibited conversion

by 71.1% in rats treated with 1.6 µg T_4/100g per day, reducing
the rate of conversion from 24.9 ± 1.2% to 7.2 ± 0.5%.
Although the conversion rates calculated from the present data
are slightly higher than that determined with isotopic techniques (16.9%), the per cent inhibition of conversion due to
PTU is in good agreement with the value of 60% previously
reported (14).

Data from older rats treated with 0.8 µg T_4/100g per day
for 10 and 15 days in experiment B were pooled. Except for
the T_3 levels in the PTU + T_4 group, which were lower at 15
than at 10 days, there were no significant differences in the
results within the groups at the two time periods. Again, PTU
treatment was associated with higher serum T_4 (9.3 ± 0.7 vs
6.6 ± 0.7 µg/100 ml, p<0.025), lower serum T_3 (16 ± 3 vs 30 ±
2 ng/100 ml, p<0.005) and higher serum TSH (220 ± 33 vs 88 ±
24 µU/ml, p<0.01).

In these three experiments, higher TSH levels are
associated with low T_3 and high serum T_4 in rats maintained
on PTU + T_4. This finding is contrary to what one might anti-
cipate if T_4 *per se* is the active hormone with regard to
TSH suppression. The results are consistent with the work of
Schadlow *et al.* who demonstrated specific high affinity,
limited capacity binding sites for T_3 but not for T_4 in the
nuclei of pituitary cells (22).

Although these data indicate that serum TSH varies
inversely with serum T_3 as opposed to serum T_4, the results
do not completely rule out a direct though apparently minor
role of T_4 in TSH suppression. If one compares the 1.6 µg T_4
+ PTU group (9.6 ± 0.5 µg T_4/100ml; 28.2 ng T_3/100 ml; 70 ±

15 µU TSH/ml) with rats receiving 0.8 µg T_4 alone in experiment A (4.9 ± 0.2 µg T_4/100 ml; 37 ± 1 ng T_3/100 ml; 165 ± 41 µU TSH/ml), it is apparent that higher TSH levels (p<0.05) in the latter are associated with a lower serum T_4 (p<0.001) and a higher mean serum T_3 (p<0.005). This implies that T_4 can, in large enough quantities, suppress TSH release directly. It may be a biological demonstration of the low affinity (only one-tenth as great as that of T_3) with which T_4 has been shown to bind to receptors in the pituitary (22).

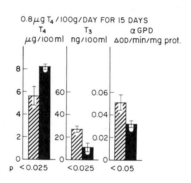

Fig. 3. *Serum T_4 and T_3 concentrations and hepatic mitochondrial α-glycerolphosphate dehydrogenase activity in thyroid-ectomised, hypothyroid rats receiving T_4 with or without propylthiouracil for 15 days. Results are shown as mean ± standard error.*

Since liver mitochondrial αGPD activity is considered to be a sensitive index of the thyroid state in rats (2,20), this parameter was assayed in rats treated for 15 days in experiment B. As shown in Fig. 3, the four rats treated with 0.8 µg T_4/100g per day + PTU exhibited lower αGPD activity in spite of a higher serum T_4 concentration when compared to four rats who received T_4 alone. The lower enzyme activity correlated with the lower T_3 concentration found in the PTU treated group. Therefore, inhibition of T$_3$ production from T$_4$ is also associated with decreased αGPD activity in hypothyroid rats, in addition to decreased TSH suppression and growth as demonstrated above. Rats treated with 0.8 μg T$_4$/100g per day alone showed no significant differences in αGPD activity or in serum T$_4$, T$_3$ or TSH concentrations when compared to the sham-operated rats, demonstrating that this course of treatment appeared to return these rats to the euthyroid state.

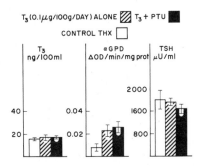

Fig. 4. *Serum T$_3$ and TSH concentrations and hepatic mitochondrial α-glycerolphosphate dehydrogenase activity in thyroidectomised, hypothyroid rats after 12 days treatment with T$_3$ with, or without, propylthiouracil. Results in untreated rats are shown for comparison and all are given as mean ± standard error*

Although PTU inhibits the deiodination of T$_3$ (8,9,12,14) it has not been shown to antagonise the metabolic effects of T$_3$ (1,23). Figure 4 demonstrates that there was no significant difference in αGPD activity in rats receiving 0.1 μg T$_3$/ 100g per day with or without PTU, although these values were significantly (p<0.05) higher than the activity in untreated thyroidectomised rats. The presence or absence of PTU also

did not influence T_3 or TSH concentrations in T_3-treated rats
and these were not different from those observed in untreated
thyroidectomised animals.

In order to insure against the possibility that PTU has
effects other than on peripheral T_3 production and that these
might have been responsible for our observations, control groups
of thyroidectomised rats treated only with PTU without T_4
were compared to untreated thyroidectomised rats in experiments A and B. No systematic effects of PTU on control animals
not given T_4 were noted suggesting that PTU had no non –
specific effects on the assays. In addition, since PTU has
been shown to inhibit conversion by approximately 60%, the
fact that thyroidectomised rats maintained on twice the
replacement dose of T_4 (1.6 µg T_4/100g/day) with PTU had T_3
levels within the normal range in addition to normal TSH
values and growth rate implies that PTU treatment had no
nonspecific influence on these parameters. PTU has previously
been shown to have no direct inhibitory action on the synthesis
of αGPD in rat liver (1). The findings of Oppenheimer *et al.*
(14) that chronic PTU administration decreased the distribution volume of T_3 by one-half with only slight alteration
in the total degradation rate of labeled T_3, would result in
inappropriately high serum T_3 concentrations, not low as
reported here. Griessen and Lemarchand-Bereaud recently
demonstrated that PTU increased the half-life of [131] I-TSH
by 50% after 17 days treatment in intact rats (16). Since
these authors reported that PTU also increased the volume
of distribution of TSH with no resulting change in plasma
clearance, serum TSH levels should still be an accurate
reflection of TSH production rates.

It has been suggested that PTU might antagonise the activity of T_4 by increasing the binding of T_4 to serum proteins, thereby decreasing the free T_4 concentration. Serum DFT_3 and DFT_4 were determined in the animals in experiment A to evaluate any possible influence of PTU on the binding of hormone to rat serum proteins. There was no significant difference between the 6 sham-operated rats ($0.073 \pm 0.004\%$ DFT_4, $0.42 \pm .05\%$ DFT_3), 10 rats receiving 0.8 µg T_4 alone ($0.065 \pm 0.004\%$ DFT_4, $0.40 \pm 0.01\%$ DFT_3), 10 rats receiving 0.8 µg T_4 + PTU ($0.67 \pm 0.004\%$ DFT_4, $0.44 \pm 0.02\%$ DFT_3) and 10 rats receiving 1.6 µg T_4 + PTU ($0.073 \pm 0.008\%$ DFT_4), $0.40 \pm 0.01\%$ DFT_3). Thus, there is no evidence that PTU treatment alters the affinity of T_3 or T_4 for rat serum proteins.

Despite these considerations, since the ultimate mechanism of action of thyroid hormone is not known, the possibility that PTU inhibits T_4 action at this serum protein site as well as inhibiting T_4 to T_3 conversion must remain as a possible, though remote, explanation.

The demonstration that inhibition of T_3 production from T_4 by PTU is associated with decreased thyromimetic effects of T_4 suggests that T_4 must first be converted to T_3 for expression of its maximum biological activity. Although this is important from a theoretical viewpoint, it must be noted that treatment with T_4 and PTU still caused a return of these animals to a near euthyroid status at least in terms of serum TSH levels. There are two possible explanations for this observation. Since T_4 to T_3 conversion is only inhibited 60%, the T_3 generated from conversion still taking place in the presence of PTU may be responsible for the remaining hormonal activity. Alternatively, T_4 may have some intrinsic activity at least as regards inhibition of pituitary TSH release.

R E F E R E N C E S

1. W.W. Hoffman, D.A. Richert and W.W. Westerfield.
    Endocrinology, 78, 1189 (1966).

2. W.R. Ruegamer, W.W. Westerfield and D.A. Richert.
    Endocrinology 75, 908 (1964).

3. W.R. Ruegamer, J.S. Warren, M. Barstow and W. Beck.
    Endocrinology 81, 277 (1967).

4. G.M. Jagiello and J.M. McKenzie, *Endocrinology*, 67,
    451 (1960).

5. F. Escobar del Rey, G. Morreale de Escobar, M.D. Garcia
    Garcia and J. Mouriz Garcia, *Endocrinology*, 71, 859
    (1962).

6. M. Griessen and T. Lemarchand-Bereaud, *Endocrinology*,
    92, 166 (1973).

7. L.E. Braverman and S.H. Ingbar, *Endocrinology*, 71, 701,
    (1962).

8. G. Morreale de Escobar and F. Escobar del Rey,
    Endocrinology, 71, 906, (1962).

9. P.P. Van Arsdel, Jr. and R.H. Williams, *Am. J. Physiol.*
    186, 440, (1956).

10. S.L. Jones and L. Van Middlesworth, *Endocrinology*, 67,
    855 (1960).

11. F. Escobar del Rey and G. Morreale de Escobar,
    Endocrinology, 69, 456 (1961).

12. L. Van Middlesworth and S.L. Jones. *Endocrinology*, 69,
    1085 (1961).

13. H.L. Schwartz, M.I. Surks and J.H. Oppenheimer,
    J. Clin. Invest. 50, 1124 (1971).

14. J.H. Oppenheimer, H.L. Schwartz and M.I. Surks,
    J. Clin. Invest. 51, 2493 (1972).

15. G.M. Abrams and P.R. Larsen, *J. Clin. Invest.* 52,
    2522 (1973).

16. J. Gross and R. Pitt-Rivers, *Recent Prog. Horm. Res.* <u>10</u>, 109, (1954).

17. P.R. Larsen, J. Dockalova, D. Sipula and F.M. Wu. *J. Clin. Endocrinol.* <u>37</u>, 177 (1973).

18. P.R. Larsen, *J. Clin. Invest.* <u>51</u>,1939 (1972).

19. J.H. Oppenheimer, R. Squef, M.I. Surks and H. Haver. *J. Clin. Invest.* <u>42</u>, 1769 (1963).

20. Y-P Lee and H.A. Lardy. *J. Biol. Chem.* <u>240</u>, 1427 (1965).

21. G.W. Snedecor and W.G. Cochran. *Statistical Methods (ed. 6).* Iowa State University Press, Ames, Iowa, U.S.A. (1967).

22. A.R. Schadlow, M.I. Surks, H.L. Schwartz and J.H. Oppenheimer, *Science,* <u>176</u>, 1252 (1972).

23. J. Mouriz, G. Morreale de Escobar and F. Escobar del Rey. *Endocrinology,* <u>79</u>, 248 (1966).

9. Sporadic and Familial Partial Peripheral Resistance to Thyroid Hormones

B.-A. LAMBERG, R. SANDSTROM, S. ROSENGARD, P. SAARINEN
AND D.C. EVERED

Endocrine Research Unit, University of Helsinki,
Minerva Foundation, the 3rd Department of Medicine,
University of Helsinki, the Central Hospital of Middle
Ostrobothina and the Department of Medicine,
Royal Victoria Infirmary, University of Newcastle-upon-Tyne.

INTRODUCTION

Hereditary defects of thyroid hormone synthesis causing goitre and hypothyroidism, and of the thyroid hormone transport proteins are well known (1,2,3). Recently attention has been paid to the failure of action of thyroid hormones in peripheral tissues. Refetoff *et al.* (4,5) described a new type of familial goitre in which the primary failure is apparently an inborn peripheral resistance to the action of thyroid hormones. This syndrome is characterised by deaf-mutism, delayed bone maturation with stippled epiphyses, raised levels of thyroid hormones in the blood, and goitre. Since then a somewhat similar family was reported by Agerbaek (6) and two singular cases by Bode *et al.* (7) and Lamberg (8) in which the defect seems not to have been as pronounced as in the cases of Refetoff *et al.* (5).

In 1971 and 1972 two patients were observed at the Thyroid Outpatients Department, University Central Hospital, Helsinki,

who presented with an initially inexplicable elevation of the
total and free thyroxine levels in the blood although being
euthyroid. Further studies made it evident that these two
subjects had a partial peripheral resistance to thyroid hormones. One of them had congenital goitre without hereditary
trends and a report of this case has already appeared elsewhere (8). The other patient had no goitre but the defect was
familial. The present report gives a summary of relevant data
of the first case together with some additional information,
and a presentation of the second case with a family study.

M E T H O D S

The serum protein-bound iodine (PBI) was determined with
the Auto-Analyser Technicon N-56 method (normal range 4.0 -
8.5 µg/100ml), the total thyroxine (T_4) by the competitive
protein binding technique (9) (3.9 - 10.7 µg/100ml), free
thyroxine (FT_4) according to Liewendahl *et al.* (10) (2.3 -
6.7 ng/100ml), total triiodothyronine (T_3) according to Hesch
and Evered (11) (79 - 172 ng/100ml), uptake of radioactive
triiodothyronine by Sephadex (T_3U) according to Hansen (12)
(80 - 120% of normal), urinary excretion of hydroxyproline
(dU-HOP) according to Kivirikko *et al.* (13) (8 - 22 mg/m^2/day),
the binding capacity of the thyroxine binding globulin (TBG_{cap};
15 - 27 µg/100ml) and pre-albumin ($TBPA_{cap}$; 110 - 390 µg/100ml)
with the agarose-gel technique (14), serum thyrotrophin (TSH)
by radioimmunoassay (15) (1.6 - 6.9 µU/ml) and the long-acting
thyroid stimulator (LATS) with the McKenzie bioassay (16).

In addition, the following special tests were used.

Thyrotrophin releasing hormone (TRH) stimulation test
(17) : 200 µg of synthetic TRH (Hoffman-LaRoche, Basle) was
injected intravenously. Samples of serum were drawn at zero

time and after 20 and 60 min and the TSH concentrations were measured from these samples. When serum T_3 was measured in addition to TSH additional serum samples were drawn after 120 and 180 min. In this laboratory (Endocrine Research Unit) an increment of 3-30 µU/ml TSH is regarded as a normal response (17).

The potassium perchlorate discharge test was carried out by measuring the thyroidal uptake every hour for 4 hours, after which 200 mg of potassium perchlorate was administered orally and the uptake measured three times during the next 2 hours.

The T_3 suppression test was carried out by oral administration of 100 µg T_3 daily in five divided doses for 7 days. Thyroidal uptake as well as PBI and TSH were measured before and after the test.

Thyroxine degradation was measured according to the principles described by Ingbar and Freinkel (18) and Sterling and Chodos (19). 50 µCi of radioactive thyroxine (Radiochemical Centre, Amersham) was administered intravenously, serum samples were drawn daily for 10 days, and their radioactivity measured. The thyroidal uptake of liberated radioiodine was not blocked. PBI, T_4 and the butanol-extractable PBI (BEI) were measured before the test, and during the test PBI was determined in four samples of serum.

The thyroxine distribution volume, the half-life and daily fractional turnover-rate were calculated in conventional manner, and from these values the extrathyroidal hormone pool and the daily turnover of T_4 was estimated. Normal mean values are :

The extrathyroidal thyroxine pool calculated from PBI values : 508 - 548 µg iodine (18,19,20,21), 488-549 µg iodine/

1.73 m^2 (19,22,23), and from T$_4$ values : 635 µg T$_4$ (24).

The daily turnover of thyroxine calculated from PBI values : 52 - 89 µg iodine/day (18,19,20,21), 49 - 51 µg iodine 1.73 m^2/day (19,22,23), 0.75 µg iodine/kg/day (19), and from T$_4$ values 82 - 95 µg T$_4$/day (24,25,26).

C A S E   R E P O R T S

Case 1

Patient studies. The patient, a female clerk aged 25, had goitre at birth. Her development was normal. At age 12 sub-total thyroidectomy was performed for nodular goitre and at age 17 she was re-operated. On both occasions she was clinically euthyroid although she had constantly elevated PBI values. She was then treated with thyroid preparations until autumn 1971, the PBI values remaining elevated and the patient eu-thyroid. In spring 1972 after she had been off any thyroid treatment for more than 3 months more specific thyroid studies were commenced at the Thyroid Outpatients Department and the 3rd Department of Medicine, University Central Hospital, Helsinki.

The patient was clinically euthyroid, the clinical diag-nostic index (27) (CDI) was 0 and + 6 points, dU-HOP 13 mg/m^2/day, the serum cholesterol 258 mg/100ml, the BMR -9% and the red blood cell glucose-6-phosphate dehydrogenase, the content of reduced glutathione (GSH) and the GSH stability were all normal indicating an euthyroid state (28,29). There were no signs of renal disease and the liver enzymes were normal. X-rays of the bones revealed no abnormality. Tbe thyroid was judged to be about 30 g by palpation, the 24 h thyroid uptake of radioactive iodine was 50%, in the T$_3$-suppression test the uptake decreased from 51 to 17% and the serum TSH from 2.5 to

Table 1.   *Specific thyroid studies in case 1.*

PBI (a)	15.7	T_4 distribution volume, litres		7.15
BEI (a)	12.7	T_4 half-life in blood, days		6.20
T_4 (a)	18.0	T_4 fractional daily turnover-rate		0.11
FT_4 (b)	12.8	T_4 extrathyroidal pool, µg(1)		1290 (910)
T_3, (b)	315	turnover, µg/day		198 (100)
T_3U, %	132	turnover, µg/1.73 m^2/day		218 (110)
TBG_{cap}, (a)	26.8	turnover, µg/kg/day		4.0 (2.0)
$TBPA_{cap}$, (a)	187	T_4 and T_3 antibodies (2)		neg.
LATS	neg.			

(a) µg/100ml   (b) ng/100ml

(1) Values calculated from BEI values are in parentheses.

(2) Kindly determined by Prof. B.N. Premachandra, St. Louis.

Lamberg et al.

Table 2.   *Response to TR H in case 1.*

	basal	20 min	60 min	120 min
Spring 1972				
TSH, µU/ml	4.5	20.0	25.0	–
Summer 1972				
TSH, µU/ml	6.0	22.8	16.7	7.8
T_3, ng/100ml	315	315	350	430

Table 3. *Thyroid parameters during T_4 treatment in case 1.*

Dose T_4, µg/day (1)	None	165	275	440
		3 wk	3 wk	3 wk
PBI, µg/100 ml	18.2	20.2	22.7	21.2
T_4, µg/100ml	–	24.3	30.2	29.3
FT_4, ng/100ml	–	12.3	20.5	17.7
T_3, ng/100ml	–	230	310	267
T_3U, %	93	95	117	127
24 h uptake, %	–	–	38	14
TSH, µU/ml	–	5.1	4.1	3.2
Increment after TRH, TSH, µU/ml	–	8.8	9.9	3.5

(1) During this treatment the patient was taking oral contra-
    ceptives.

1.4 μU/ml, thyroglobulin antibodies were once positive at
1/25 titre, fine needle biopsy of the thyroid showed normal
findings.

A detailed account is given in a previous publication (8)
but the studies on thyroid hormones and the response to TRH
are summarised in Tables 1 and 2. At the end of these studies
the patient was given increasing amounts of thyroxine. Unknown
to the authors she had started to use contraceptive pills
(Neo-Delpregnin^r, Novo, Copenhagen) when the trial started.
Due to this her TBG_{cap} increased to 32.4 μg/100ml, the $TBPA_{cap}$
remaining unchanged. During the thyroxine trial she remained
euthyroid, the CDI was -5 and -7 points, dU-HOP 11.6 - 12.2
$mg/m^2/day$, and serum cholesterol 258-290 mg/100ml. Relevant
data are summarised in Table 3.

Family studies. The family pedigree is shown in Fig. 1. In
addition to the proband, 35 members of the family were screened
by PBI determinations and in a few instances by measuring T_4.
All were initially approached by a questionnaire with specific
questions as regards thyroid disturbances and 22 were later
clinically examined. The patient's mother had goitre at pu-
berty and one uncle had been treated for goitre. No other
instances of thyroid problems were found. The thyroid hormone
level was normal in all cases.

Case 2.

Patient studies. The patient was a male student aged 21 who
suffered from Prurigo Besnier since early childhood, but at
no time had goitre been observed and his development had
been quite normal. Consanguinity between parents was not reported. There were some thyroid problems in the family (see
below).

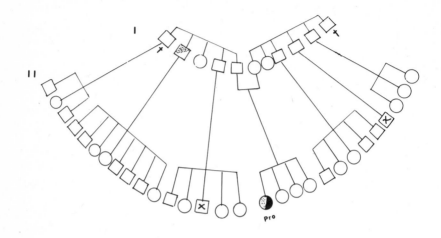

Fig. 1. *Pedigree of the family of case 1. Stippled area indicates presence of goitre, black area elevated levels of thyroid hormones. x = not examined. Pro = proband.*

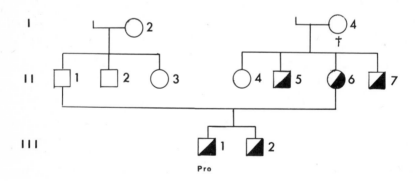

Fig. 2. *Pedigree of the family of case 2. Stippled area indicates presence of goitre or other thyroid disease, black area elevated levels of thyroid hormones. Pro = proband.*

During military service at age 21 he was hospitalised
for prurigo. He complained of nervousness, fatigue, increased
demand for sleep and breathlessness of $\frac{1}{2}$ - 1 year's duration.
PBI was determined a few times being always elevated (9.2 -
11.3 µg/100ml) and the T_3 uptake by Sephadex varied from 114
to 123%. He was therefore sent for further examinations to
the Thyroid Outpatients Department, University Central Hospital
in May, 1971, where he has since then been studied at intervals.

He was clinically entirely euthyroid and the CDI (27)
varied from 0 to 11 points. The thyroid appeared normal on
palpation, thyroid scintigram showed slightly more accumulation
in the right lobe but otherwise diffuse distribution of the
radioactive iodine. X-rays showed nothing abnormal in the trachea
or in the chest, the electrocardiogram was normal and the
pulse rate 52 beats/min. BP was 120/20. Routine haematological
studies and urine analysis showed normal findings. There were
no signs of renal disease and the liver enzymes were normal.
The red blood cell glucose-6-phosphate dehydrogenase, GSH and
GSH stability were all normal and compatible with an euthyroid
state (28,29). The alkaline phosphatase was slightly elevated
being 56 IU/ml which was thought to be due to bone growth
since the urinary excretion of hydroxyproline at the time of
the first study was also slightly elevated (Table 4). Serum
proteins were normal with normal electrophoretic findings.
Fine needle biopsy of the thyroid showed normal cytology with
a slight increase in lymphocytes but no signs of chronic thyroiditis.

During the period from May 1971 to September 1973 the
patient was restudied several times. He remained euthyroid and
the CDI varied from 0 to + 6 points. Results from these studies

Table 4.   *Some thyroid data in case 2.*

	1971 summer	1971 autumn	1972	1973
PBI, µg/100ml	9.4	10.7	11.7	10.5
BEI, µg/100ml	-	-	10.6	-
T_4, µg/100ml	16.5	12.5	11.7	13.3
FT_4, ng/100ml	8.6	8.9	7.4	9.2
T_3, ng/100ml	-	-	150	182
T_3U, %	115	113	119	116
TBG_{cap}, µg/100ml	-	19.7	21.4	-
$TBPA_{cap}$, µg/100ml	-	-	239	-
Thyroglobulin antibodies	neg.	1/10	neg.	neg.
Antimicrosomal antibodies	neg.	neg.	neg.	neg.
T_4 and T_3 antibodies (1)			neg.	neg.
dU-HOP mg/m^2/day	25	-	18	-
Serum cholesterol mg/100ml	250	-	193	205
24 h uptake of ^{131}I	41	-	-	37
after T_3-suppression	12	-	-	-
LATS	neg.	-	-	-

(1) Kindly determined by Prof. B.N. Premachandra, St. Louis.

Table 5.   *Response to TRH in case 2.*

	basal	20 min	60 min	120 min	180 min
Oct. 1971					
TSH, μU/ml	6.0	50.2	20.6		
Sept. 1972					
TSH, μU/ml	5.7	23.5	16.4		
May 1973					
TSH, μU/ml	4.5	31.5	23.5	9.2	8.2
T_3, ng/100ml	182	188	250	300	316

Table 6.   *Thyroxine turnover study in case 2.*

T_4, μg/100ml	11.7	
BEI, μg/100ml	10.6	
T_4 distribution volume, litres	10.0	
T_4 half-life in blood, days	6.2	
T_4 fractional daily turnover-rate	0.128	
T_4 extrathyroidal pool, μg (1)	1170	(1060)
turnover, μg/day	150	(136)
turnover, μg/1.73 m^2/day	134	(121)
turnover, μg/kg/day	1.94	(1.75)
Patient's weight, kg	77.5	
height, cm	176	

(1) Values calculated from BEI values are in parentheses.

are compiled in Tables 4-6. Finally the patient was treated with increasing amounts of thyroxine. During the first 3 weeks he was given 220 µg per day, for the next 3 weeks 330 µg per day, and for the following 2 months 440 µg per day. At intervals clinical evaluations and thyroid studies were carried out as seen in Table 7. He remained euthyroid the whole time as judged from the clinical appearance, the CDI, the dU-HOP and the serum cholesterol level.

Table 7. *Thyroid parameters during T_4 treatment in case 2.*

Dose T_4, µg/day	None	220	330	440
		3 wk	3 wk	2 mo
PBI, µg/100ml	10.5	9.9	11.7	16.5
T_4, µg/100ml	13.3	14.2	13.9	18.6
FT_4, ng/100ml	9.2	12.6	11.5	17.9
T_3, ng/100ml	182	217	–	244
T_3U, %	116	152	147	198
24 h uptake, %	37	30	21	2.4
TSH, µU/ml	4.5	5.9	3.4	< 1.0
Increment after TRH, TSH, µU/ml	27.0	20.3	7.1	0.6
Serum cholesterol, mg/100ml	205	170	162	182
dU-HOP, mg/m^2/day	–	19	12	13
CDI	+6	–11	–2	–11

Family studies. The family pedigree is shown in Fig. 2. Subjects II, 2 and II, 3 were approached by a questionnaire only, but all the others were also clinically examined. A specific form for hyperthyroidism was used (30) and the CDI evaluated. In addition, specific thyroid studies were carried out as seen

in Table 8. Liver enzymes in the blood and dU-HOP were determined in all subjects submitted to the clinical examination.
Each subject will be presented with short comments.

Subject, I, 2, female, 74, had congestive heart failure
and arterial hypertension; spontaneous hypothyroidism had been
diagnosed 8 years previously. She was taking 100 µg thyroxine
per day. The increased thyroglobulin antibody titre and the
TSH level and the TRH-response pattern indicated hypothyroidism
due to chronic thyroiditis.

Subject, I, 4, female, deceased, was reported to have
had goitre.

Subjects II, 1, male 53, II, 2, male 50 and II, 3, female
47, euthyroid, had no goitre.

Subject II, 4, female, 58. A visible goitre was noted 15
years previously, but she had received no thyroid treatment.
The thyroid on palpation was about 40 g, and she was clinically
euthyroid (CDI -5 points, serum cholesterol 197 mg/100ml,
dU-HOP 17 mg/m^2/day).

Subject II, 5, male 56. Goitre observed at age 20, sub-
total thyroidectomy at age 43 for toxic goitre. At the time
of examination euthyroid and the thyroid of normal size. (CDI
-13 points, serum cholesterol 288 mg/100ml, dU-HOP 12 mg/m^2/day).

Subject II, 6, female, 51, had a goitre since childhood.
In 1970 some signs and symptoms of mild hyperthyroidism were
noted (PBI 12.0 and 12.7 µg/100ml). She was considered slightly
hyperthyroid and was initially treated with carbimazole after
which she received 7 mCi radioactive iodine in the spring 1971.
In spite of constantly elevated PBI values she has been considered euthyroid after that. At the time of examination, the
thyroid was of normal size and she was euthyroid (CDI -7 points,

Lamberg et al.

Table 8. *Thyroid Studies in*

Subject	PBI (a)	T_4 (a)	FT_4 (b)	T_3 (b)	T_3U %	TBG_{cap} (a)
I, 2	5.7			80		
II, 1	6.2					
II, 4	5.0	6.6		110	98	25.0
II, 5	8.7	7.9 10.8[e] 14.0[f]	6.0	212 257[e]	119	19.0
II, 6	11.5	11.7 12.5[e] 19.5[f]	6.9	245 257[e]	103	21.5
II, 7	11.2	17.1 13.8[e] 22.0[f]	11.8	240[e]	110	22.5
III, 1 (pro)	10.5	13.3	9.2	182	116	19.7
III, 2	10.9	10.5 11.2[e] 16.8[f]	7.0	167 307[e]	94	20.0

(a) µg/100ml;   (b) ng/100ml;   (c) Maximal increment

(d) The values given refer to haemagglutination
measurements. The results by complement fix-
ation tests were all negative. These determinations were kindly carried out by Prof.
K. Aho using his method (39).

the Family of Case 2.

TBPA cap (a)	TRH stimulation: TSH			μU/ml (c)	Thyroid antibodies (d)
	basal	20min	60min		
	29.0	110	72.0	79.0	1/40000
100	2.3	8.1	4.7	4.7	
130	5.0	20.0	25.0	20.0	
130	7.8	35.0	25.0	27.2	1/2500
108	4.1	20.0	20.0	15.9	
239	4.5	31.5	23.5	27.0	
120	5.8	21.0	16.0	15.2	1/10

(e) These determinations were made in 1974, other values are from 1973. (f) denotes T_4 values obtained simultaneously by radioimmunoassay.

Note. T_4 and T_3 antibodies were kindly determined by Prof. B.N. Premachandra. From the same samples thyroglobulin antibodies were also determined, being negative in all cases, as were the results for T_4 and T_3 antibodies.

serum cholesterol 288 mg/100ml, dU-HOP 44 mg/m^2/day).

Subject II, 7, male 46, had no goitre and was euthyroid (CDI -6 points, serum cholesterol not determined, dU-HOP 26 mg/m^2/day).

Subject III, 2, male, 18, had a normal thyroid and was clinically euthyroid, (CDI -6 points, serum cholesterol 165 mg/100ml, dU-HOP 15 mg/m^2/day).

In all subjects the liver enzymes were normal.

Comments. Although the proband's paternal grandmother had chronic thyroiditis with spontaneous hypothyroidism, the inheritable thyroid condition seems to be confined to his mother's family. There is both goitre and elevated thyroid hormone levels with euthyroidism to be found. The proband's brother and one uncle (II, 7) have elevated serum thyroid hormone concentrations but they are euthyroid and they have no goitre. His mother and one uncle had been considered hyperthyroid before this study but this is retrospectively impossible to confirm and the possibility remains that they only had nontoxic goitre and elevated PBI values. The liver enzymes were normal in all cases which rules out marked liver diseases. Interestingly subjects II, 6 and II, 7 had increased urinary excretion of hydroxyproline the reason of which is not apparent. The inheritance of the elevation of thyroid hormones is apparently dominant.

DISCUSSION

The characteristic features common to both probands were euthyroidism with raised concentrations of total and free T$_4$ and total T$_3$ levels in the blood with normal hormone binding capacity of the thyroxine binding proteins and normal thyroid-pituitary relationships. The extrathyroidal thyroxine pool was raised considerably above normal and the daily turnover increased to 150-200 μg which is about twice the normal mean value (18-26). This increase was even more striking when related to body surface area or body weight (19,22,23). In spite of this both patients were euthyroid as evidenced by the clinical examination on several occasions, normal CDI, serum cholesterol, red cell enzymes (28,29) and, when related to age, also the urinary excretion of hydroxyproline (31). Furthermore, the response to TRH was essentially normal. The probands differed in the following respects : the presence of goitre in case 1 and its absence in case 2, and the familial inheritance in case 2.

The tissues in these subjects must be in some way unresponsive to thyroid hormones as evidenced by the constant elevation of the T_4 and T_3 levels in the blood. The anterior pituitary must be one of the unresponsive tissues since the TSH concentration and the response to TRH were essentially normal. Apparently the partial resistance to thyroid hormones at the pituitary level must have brought about increased formation of thyroid hormones which fits with the increased turnover of T_4. It may be presumed that after an initial increase of TSH secretion a new homeostatic situation developed by which a euthyroid state was maintained and the blood TSH decreased to a normal level. Some variation in the TSH level and in the response to TRH occurred in both cases which may be indicative of constant adjustment of the thyroid-pituitary relationship. In case 1 the first TRH-stimulation test showed a slightly delayed increase in the TSH level and in case 2 the increase in the first test was definitely abnormally high. One consequence of such a compensatory mechanism would be in

G

the long run the development of goitre but this will evidently
depend on the severity of the underlying metabolic defect.
This is probably the cause of the presence of goitre in case
1 and its absence in case 2. It can be assumed that the interaction of TSH with thyroid tissue was normal since there was
a normal increase in the T_3 concentration after stimulation
with TRH in both cases.

The resistance to thyroid hormones was also apparent from
the observations made during treatment with T_4. In case 1 the
24 h thyroidal uptake of radioactive iodine decreased from
about 50% to 14% with a dose of 440 µg T_4 per day and in case
2 from about 40% to 21% with 330 µg per day. In normal conditions a daily dose of 280 µg T_4 will effectively suppress both
the thyroidal radioiodine uptake and the serum TSH level (32,
33). Case 1 was probably slightly more resistant to thyroid
hormones than was case 2. Indications of this are, for instance,
the difference in the levels of T_4, FT_4 and T_3 in these cases
and the presence of goitre in case 1. In both cases, however,
the uptake was effectively suppressed in the standard T_3-sup-
pression test when 100 µg of T_3 was given for 7 days. This
would mean that, after all, the resistance in these cases was
not very marked and certainly of lesser degree than in the
cases studied by Refetoff *et al.* (4,5) and by Agerbaek (6).
On the other hand, a daily dose of 330-440 µg T_4 per day should
correspond to about 80-110 µg T_3 per day when taking into
consideration that only about 60% of orally administered T_4
is absorbed (32) in contrast to T_3 and that some 30-40% of T_4
will be converted to T_3 after absorption (34).

The level of free thyroxine may be elevated in chronic
liver diseases, in some other serious illnesses as well as in

high altitude, with or without concomitant changes in the
thyroxine binding proteins (22,23,25,35-37). Similar changes
have been also reported in inherited increase of TBG (38). In
the cases studied no indications of such alterations were
present. The same applies to the members of the family of
case 2.

Case 1 is apparently a single sporadic case of partial
peripheral resistance to thyroid hormones with congenital
goitre similar to the patient reported by Bode *et al.* (7). In
spite of careful search no other cases were found in her
family and the possibility of a sporadic mutation has to be
considered. In the family of case 2, however, the partial
resistance was evidently inherited in an autosomal dominant
way in contrast to the family described by Refetoff *et al.* (5)
in which the inheritance was autosomal recessive. Goitre was
observed only in the oldest members of the proband's mother's
family and it is therefore possible that the defect is so mild
in this family that a long time is required before it will be
manifested as a goitre if no other goitrogenic factors inter-
vene. It can be assumed that the development of goitre in connection with peripheral resistance to the action of thyroid
hormones is due to the action of TSH the secretion of which
is presumably not normalised before a new homeostatic situation
has developed, as discussed above. It is of interest that the
response of TSH to the injection of TRH in this family was on
the whole fairly brisk, the increment in the TSH level being
in most cases well above the normal mean. This may be some
indication of the constant adjustment of the thyroid-pituitary
axis discussed. Whether subjects II, 5 and II, 6 really had
hyperthyroidism or only high PBI values with non-toxic goitre

is difficult to assess retrospectively. It is of interest to note a slight increase in the urinary excretion of hydroxy-proline in subjects II, 6 and II, 7 in the absence of hyper-thyroidism. This could possibly be an expression of a variable resistance as discussed by Refetoff *et al.* (5) and by Agerbaek (6) some tissues being possibly more resistant than others.

There was no indication of a defect in the conversion of T_4 to T_3 although such a possibility was strongly considered in case 2 initially when the first T_3 concentration value was in the normal range. The T_4/T_3 ratio which is normally (34) about 70 was 57 in case 1 and 73-78 in case 2.

The mechanism by which the resistance to thyroid hormones is brought about is not yet solved although some experiments have been carried out on the tissue level (3,5,7). Problems related to hormone receptors or intermediate biochemical reactions may be involved (5). Further studies on these patient are therefore required. A search for circulating T_3 and T_4 antibodies was kindly carried out in our cases by Prof. B.N. Premachandra but no such were detected. Autoimmune phenomena seem therefore not to be involved.

Acknowledgements.

The authors want to thank Prof. B.N. Premachandra, M. D. St. Louis, U.S.A. for performing the search for T3 and T4 anti-bodies, Prof. K. Aho, M. D. for determination of the thyroid antibodies, Dr. R. Pelkonen, M. D. for performing and Dr. M. Lehtinen for evaluating the thyroid biopsies, Mrs. H. Toivonen, M.Sc. for determination of the thyroxine degradation rates and Mrs. M.-L. Kuhanen for the TSH assays.

Human TSH and TSH antiserum were donated by the Pituitary Agency of the National Institutes of Health, Bethesda, Mary-land, the human TSH reference standard A came from the National Institute of Medical Research, London and synthetic TRH was supplied by Hoffman-LaRoche, Basle.

This study was aided by grants from the National Research

Council for Medical Sciences of the Finnish Academy, the Sigrid Juselius Foundation, the Medicinska Understods-foreningen Liv och Halsa and the Nordic Insulin Foundation.

REFERENCES

1. J.B. Stanbury, *Rec. Progr. Hormone. Res.* 19, 547 (1968).

2. I.B. Weinstein and F.D. Kitchin *In* "The Thyroid" (S.C. Werner and S.H. Ingbar, eds), pp. 383-405 (1971).

3. S. Refetoff and L.J. DeGroot *In* "Handbook of Physiology", section 7 "Endocrinology, vol. 3 "Thyroid" (M.A. Greer and D.H. Solomon, eds), pp. 161-178 (1974).

4. S. Refetoff, L.T. DeWind and L.J. DeGroot, *J. Clin. Endocr. Metab.* 27, 279-294 (1967).

5. S. Refetoff, L.J. DeGroot, B. Benard and L.T. DeWind, *Metabolism* 21, 723-756 (1972).

6. H. Agerbaek, *Israel J. Med. Sci.* 8,12 (1972). Abstr. of paper presented at the 5th Annual Meeting of Europ. Thyroid Ass., Jerusalem, Sept. 1973.

7. H.H. Bode, M. Danon, B.D. Weintraub, F. Maloof and J.D. Crawford, *J. Clin. Invest.* 52, 776-782 (1973).

8. B.-A. Lamberg, *Lancet,* I, 854-857 (1973).

9. K. Liewendahl, R. Ruutu and B.-A. Lamberg, *Acta.Med. Scand.* 194, 341-348 (1973).

10. K. Liewendahl, J. Totterman and B.-A. Lamberg, *Acta Endocr.* 67, 793-800 (1971).

11. R.D. Hesch and D.C. Evered, *Brit. Med. J.* I, 645-648 (1973).

12. H.H. Hansen, *Scand. J. Clin. Lab. Invest.* 18, 240-244 (1966).

13. K. Kivirikko, O. Laitinen and D.J. Prockop, *Analyt. Biochem.* 19, 249-255 (1967).

14. O.P. Heinonen, B.-A. Lamberg and J. Virtamo, *Acta Endocr.* 64, 171-180 (1970).

15. A. Gordin and P. Saarinen, *Acta Endocr.* 71, 24-36 (1972).

16. B.-A. Lamberg, A. Gordin, M. Viherkoski and G. Kvist, *Acta Endocr.* 62, 199-209 (1969).

17. A. Gordin, P. Saarinen, R. Pelkonen and B.-A. Lamberg, *Acta Endocr.* 75, 274-285 (1974).

18. S.H. Ingbar and N. Freinkel, *J. Clin. Invest.* 34, 808-819 (1955).

19. K. Sterling and R.B. Chodos, *J. Clin. Invest.* 35, 806-813 (1956).

20. R.I. Gregerman, G.W. Gaffney and N.W. Shock, *J. Clin. Invest.* 41, 2065-2074 (1962).

21. M. Inada, K. Koshiyama, K. Torizuka, H. Akagi and T. Miyake, *J. Clin. Endocr. Metab.* 24, 775-784 (1964).

22. M. Inada and K. Sterling, *J. Clin. Invest.* 46, 1275-1282 (1967).

23. D. Bellabarba, M. Inada, N. Varsano-Aharon and K. Sterling, *J. Clin. Endocr. Metab.* 28, 1023-1030 (1968).

24. C. Pittman, J.B. Chambers and V.H. Read, *J. Clin. Invest.* 50, 1187-1196 (1971).

25. J. McConnon, V.V. Row and R. Volpe, *J. Clin. Endocr. Metab.* 34, 144-151 (1972).

26. W. Jubiz, A.H. Bigler, L.F. Kumagai and C.D. West, *J. Clin. Endocr. Metab.* 34, 1009-1015 (1972).

27. J. Crooks, I.P.C. Murray and E.J. Wayne, *Quart. J. Med.* 28, 211-234 (1959).

28. M. Viherkoski and B.-A. Lamberg, *Scand. J. Clin. Lab. Invest.* 25, 137-143 (1970).

29. P. Vuopio, M. Viherkoski, E. Nikkila and B.-A. Lamberg, Ann. Clin. Res. 2, 184-186 (1970).

30. B.-A. Lamberg, O.P. Heinonen, M. Viherkoski, A. Aro, K. Liewendahl, K. Kvist, O. Laitinen and P. Knekt, *Acta Endocr.* Suppl. 146 (1970).

31. J. Uitto, O. Laitinen, B.-A. Lamberg and K. Kivirikko, *Clin. Chim. Acta* 22, 583-591 (1968).

32. T.H. Oddie, D.A. Fisher and D.J. Epperson, *J. Clin. Endocr. Metab.* 25, 1196-1206 (1965).

33. G.E. Cotton, C.A. Gorman and W.E. Mayberry, *New Engl. J. Med.* 285, 529-533 (1971).

34. P.R. Larsen, *Metabolism,* 21, 1073-1092 (1972).

35. J.H. Oppenheimer, *New Engl. J. Med.* 278, 1153-1162 (1968).

36. G. Bernstein and J.H. Oppenheimer, *J. Clin. Endocr. Metab.* 26, 195-201 (1966).

37. M.I. Surks, *J. Appl. Physiol.* 21, 1185-1190 (1966).

38. J.A. Thomson, E.M. Meredith, S.G. Baird, W.R. McAinsh and J.H. Hutchison, *Quart. J. Med.* 41, 49-61 (1972).

39. K. Aho, P. Virkola and O.P. Heinonen, *Acta Endocr.* 68, 196-202 (1971).

10. Four Compartment Model of Thyroxine Metabolism

C.H.G. IRVINE

University College of Agriculture, Lincoln College,
Canterbury, New Zealand.

INTRODUCTION

Peripheral thyroxine (T_4) metabolism has been investigated in many species by following the disappearance of labelled T_4 from plasma (1-5). However the information obtained is usually limited to the noncompartmental analysis of the area under the curve, permitting determination of T_4 secretion rate and transit time of a T_4 particle (6). Alternatively the data can be analysed by a one compartment method which determines fractional turnover from the final slope of the plasma curve, and the volume of distribution from the extrapolation of the slope to zero time (1-4); however these measurements can give quite spurious answers (see later). While a system of 3-pool analysis has been suggested (5) there are serious insufficiencies in the model proposed, and no validation of it by collateral studies of tissue or extravascular uptakes, specific activities (SA) etc. Furthermore, the whole application of compartmental analysis unsupported by such data has been challenged by the finding that the SA of extravascular albumin measured directly bore no relationship to the prediction based on compartmental analysis of the accepted model, or of any other model (7). In this paper a model for analysing peripheral

T_4 metabolism is proposed which gives results which are consistent with the measurements of extravascular T_4 made in the dead (8) and living (9) animal.

M A T E R I A L S   A N D   M E T H O D S

Sheep subjects were 6 male Romneys, 1-3 years old weighing 55-70 kg. Experiments were done indoors at 11-18°C in small pens. General management was as described previously (9,10). It was necessary to prevent recycling of the ^{125}I-iodide derived from ^{125}I-T_4 breakdown. The maximum amount of iodide which could be tolerated without physiological disturbance, 5 mg/day, still allowed 3.7% of the ^{125}I released from ^{125}I-T_4 to be taken up by the thyroid (10). Additional thyroid block was obtained by twice daily s.c. injection of thyroxine sodium pentahydrate 1 μg/kg. At this dose the mean plasma T_4 was raised by an average of 8% over the first 4 hr following injection, and not at all over the remaining 8 hr. Although the thyroid was secreting sufficient T_4, and presumably T_3, to maintain normal plasma levels its ^{125}I uptake was slightly below 1% of the ^{125}I released from ^{125}I-T_4 catabolism. This regime gave no evidence of toxicity or interference with peripheral T_4 metabolism (author's unpublished data).

Sheep were given i.v. 10 μCi ^{125}I-T_4 (Radiochemical Centre, Amersham, England), purified by dialysis (8). Where information on iodide kinetics was required ^{131}I iodide was given concurrently.

Six ml blood samples were collected into heparinized tubes at 2,5,10,20,40 min, 1,2,4,6,8,12,18,24,36,48,60,72,84, and 96 hr and radioactivity from 3 ml plasma was measured in a 2 channel Packard autogamma spectrometer before and after precipitation of serum proteins with trichloracetic acid.

After deduction of ^{125}I as iodoprotein (see later) TCA pre-cipitable ^{125}I was regarded as T_4. Samples were counted to give an accuracy of ± 1%. The results were expressed as the fraction of the dose/litre plasma. Since the plasma volume was measured by this method (see later) the fraction of the dose in the plasma compartment was calculated. At representative time intervals, a 12 ml sample was collected and the plasma not required for trichloracetic acid precipitation was extracted with acid butanol-chloroform-ammonia and chromatographed in tertiary pentanol-ammonia (8).

To define T_4 kinetics accurately it was necessary to determine the fraction of the dose in the extravascular ex-changeable T_4 space at a point in time before and after equi-libration, usually at 18 and 48 hr. This was determined by subtracting from the dose given the sum of the following quantities :

(1) $^{125}I-T_4$ in plasma

(2) ^{125}I in collected urine and faeces plus any non-exchange-able ^{125}I that has not yet left the excretory organs, e.g. urinary and alimentary systems.

(3) ^{125}I given as $^{125}I-T_4$ and subsequently degraded to other labelled compounds which are retained in th body at the time of measurement, e.g. $^{125}I-T_3$, ^{125}I-iodoprotein, ^{125}I-iodide, $^{125}I-T_4$ conjugates.

These losses of $^{125}I-T_4$ from the exchanging compartments were determined as follows.

Urine and faeces were collected twice daily with additional collections as described later. ^{125}I was measured as described previously, before and after iodide separation (10). ^{125}I no

longer present as exchangeable T_4, either because of degradation or passage into non-exchanging areas of the gut or urinary
system, was calculated at 18 and 48 hrs from the following
information :

(1) Earlier experiments in sheep with urinary catheters showed
that the urinary SA after ^{125}I given as T_4, its conjugates or
iodide, peaked 1 hr after its plasma peak (10, and author's
unpublished data). Therefore a 1 hr delay was believed to
occur between the entry of these products into blood and their
actual recovery from the bladder. Faecal T_4 is derived from
T_4 which enters the gut in the small intestine, or is excreted
as conjugate in bile (10). When ^{125}I as T_4, its conjugate or
iodide was infused into the duodenum, faecal SA peaked 18 hr
later (10). The same delay occurred between i.v. administration
and the SA peak in faeces in biliary fistulated sheep. Therefore
faecal ^{125}I was regarded as having left the exchanging compartments 18 hr earlier. In the present experiment each passage
of urine was collected during the periods 12-30 hr and 44-46
hr, and faecal bags were changed 6 hourly over the periods
30-54 hr and 60-84 hr. ^{125}I thus collected was graphed so that
even without induced evacuation or catherization it was possible
to correct for ^{125}I stored in the bladder or rectum at 18 and
48 hr. Thus faecal and urinary ^{125}I was related to the time
it left the exchanging compartments.

(2) It was necessary to determine if any products of $^{125}I-T_4$
metabolism were still within body tissues since such ^{125}I is
not in the exchanging $^{125}I-T_4$ system. No T_4 conjugates have
been found in plasma or tissues of sheep after extensive
investigation (8-10, and further unpublished data from this
laboratory). In contrast significant amounts of ^{125}I-iodide

have been found in extracellular fluid after i.v. ^{125}I-T$_4$.
Plasma ^{125}I-iodide was measured by dialysing 1 ml for 1 hr at
room temperature against 1 ml phosphate buffer containing 200
mg IRA 400 resin. The volume of the iodide space and the
fractional transfer rate from this space into urine, k_{UI}, were
measured by standard methods (11) after i.v. ^{131}I-iodide, 4
μCi, given with ^{125}I-T$_4$. ^{125}I iodide retained in the iodide
space at any time, $q^{125}{}_I{}^-$, was measured as the product of
the plasma ^{125}I-iodide and the iodide space. However when the
plasma ^{125}I-iodide was less than 10% of total plasma ^{125}I
this method was not regarded as sufficiently accurate. In
this case, $q^{125}{}_I{}^-$ was obtained also by analytical or graphical
differentiation of the cumulative urinary ^{125}I-iodide excretion curve, q_{UI}, after which the differential $dq_{UI}(t)/dt$
was divided by the fractional transfer rate from the iodide
space into urine, i.e.

$$q^{125}{}_I{}^-(t) = \frac{dq\mathrm{UI}(t)}{dt} \cdot \frac{1}{K\mathrm{UI}}. \quad (11)$$

Two other degradation products of ^{125}I-T$_4$ which may accumulate
in the body are ^{125}I-T$_3$ and ^{125}I-iodoprotein (12). While some
conversion of T$_4$ to T$_3$ does occur in the sheep (13), the
plasma and tissue levels of ^{125}I-T$_3$ were less than 0.5% of
^{125}I-T$_4$ when measured by chromatography of representative
48 hr samples and were disregarded (8, and author's unpublished data). Significant levels of ^{125}I-iodoprotein were
found after 48 hr and appropriate corrections were made (8).

Calculation of $^{125}I\ T_4$ kinetics

Some information may be obtained without any assumptions
being made about compartments and models. The area under the
^{125}I-T$_4$ plot of time against % dose per μg was used to measure

the T_4 secretion rate (6).

The semilogarthmic plot of the plasma curve was then resolved by "curve peeling" (14). The resulting sum of exponentials, $\Sigma C_n e^{-\lambda t}$, was then fed into an iterative curve fitting programme and run until the residual sum of squares decreased by less than 1% between successive iterations. From this sum of exponentials the space of instantaneous mixing, presumably plasma, was determined as $V_p = 1/\Sigma C_n$. The rate constant of exit of $^{125}I\text{-}T_4$ from plasma was obtained as $\Sigma C_n \lambda_n / \Sigma C_n$. Initially I used the best fir for 3 terms because computations for a 3-pool system were available, (5,11). However when the experimental data were compared with the points obtained by fitting 3 or 4 terms the residual sum of squares was 2.89% and 0.91% respectively of the total sum of squares. The much better fit for 4 terms is illustrated graphically in Fig. 2. and shows that 4 terms are required.

Further useful information could be obtained only by fitting the data to a model. Although valid criticism has been levelled at physiological modelling (15), a model was justified in the present case because :

(1)   The extensive data obtained reduced experimental imprecision to a minimum.

(2)   The plasma $^{125}I\text{-}T_4$ curve could be fitted almost perfectly to a sum of real exponential terms.

(3)   Extensive post-mortem data from sheep showed that body tissues could be grouped into four types depending on the rate of equilibration of $^{125}I\text{-}T_4$ after i.v. injection, and the SA of T_4 after equilibration. These are (8) :

(a) Plasma which equilibrates in 1-2 min

(b) Liver, kidney, lung, heart, which equilibrate in 0.5

-1 hr

(c) Gut, its exchangeable contents and its related glands which equilibrate in approximately 4 hr

(d) Muscle, brain and skin which equilibrate in 32–64 hr.

Between sheep the equilibration time for any one tissue type was very similar but in any one sheep the times for different tissues were quite dissimilar (8,9). Therefore a 4 compartment model was used in which compartment 1 = plasma, 2 = liver, kidney, 3 = gut, 4 = muscle, brain, skin, with possible bidirectional exchange between compartment 1 and each of the others, possible final loss of stable and tracer T_4 from all compartments except 1, initial entry into compartment 1 only, and no direct movement between 2, 3 and 4 (Fig. 1). The justification for this model is discussed later.

Since techniques for obtaining a unique solution of a 4-compartment system could not be found in the available literature, the following method was developed.[*] Total turnover rates (k_{ii}) for each pool i were determined from the differential equations describing the tracer behaviour of the system outlined where there is no direct transfer between compartments 2,3 and 4 (see Fig. 1).

$$\frac{dq_1}{dt} = -k_{11}q_1 + k_{12}q_2 + k_{13}q_3 + k_{14}q_4$$

$$\frac{dq_2}{dt} = k_{21}q_1 - k_{22}q_2$$

$$\frac{dq_3}{dt} = k_{31}q_1 - k_{33}q_3$$

[*] *Full details can be obtained from the author.*

$$\frac{dq_4}{dt} = k_{41}q_1 - k_{44}q_4$$

where q_i is the quantity of tracer in compartment i and k_{ij} is the fraction of q_j transferred to compartment i per unit time. k_{oj} is the fractional rate of irreversible loss from q_j. These equations were solved by Laplace transforms (5).

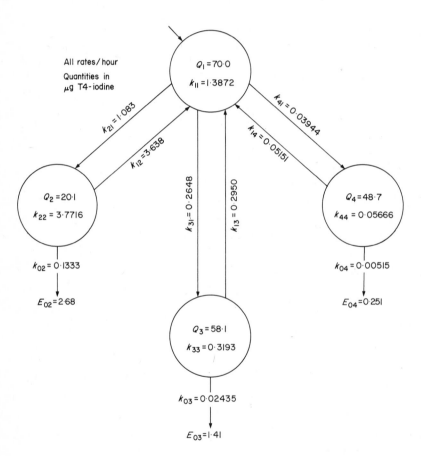

Fig. 1. *Parameters of thyroxine kinetics determined from a typical experiment.*

A 4 x 4 matrix which is an expansion of the 3 x 3 matrix of
Sharney *et al.* (16) was used to express q_1, the amount of ^{125}I
T_4 in pool 1 at any time, in terms of the coefficients and exponents of the plasma curve. Turnover rates of each pool and
the total amount of T_4 degraded, or secreted, per hour could
then be determined. However, to obtain transfer rates between
pools and the amounts degraded in each pool, further information
was required. Therefore the sum of the ^{125}I-T_4 in all compartments, $(q_1 + q_2 + q_3 + q_4)$, at 18 and 48 hr was determined
from the dose given minus the amount which had left the exchangeable T_4 space. After subtracting q_1, it was possible to
use the matrices of q_2, of q_3 and of q_4 to derive transfer rates
between compartments and also solve the model uniquely for all
compartment sizes, specific activities and degradation rates
in each compartment. Total degradation is equal to production
or secretion rate in the steady state. Thus all the physio-
logically useful parameters of the system were obtained. While
this method is based on the approach of Sharney *et al.* (5,16)
for the 3-pool system, it avoids an assumption made by Sharney
et al. (5), i.e. that faecal collection measures T_4 degraded
in pool 2 (liver), and that urinary collection measures irreversible loss from pool 3 (lymph and other body water). This
assumption is invalid and quite incorrect but without it a
unique solution to even the 3 compartment system is not possible
using the method of Sharney *et al.* (16). Although the liver is
regarded as a major organ in T_4 degradation in man, the results
of Sharney *et al.* (5) show that 1.43 µg is degraded daily in
the liver and from 46.2 to 96.9 µg, depending on the model used,
in lymph and other body water. The present method of using
$(q_2 + q_3 + q_4)$ at 2 time intervals was developed to avoid

this error, and was also necessary to solve uniquely the more complex 4-pool system.

T_4 loading experiments

After the experiment described, 1 mg T_4 was given by subcutaneous injection followed by 0.25 mg 12-hourly, to two of the sheep. Plasma free and total T_4 concentration was measured daily by the Sephadex binding method (17) and competitive protein binding respectively (18). After 2 days 20 µCi ^{125}I-T$_4$ was given i.v. and ^{125}I-T$_4$ kinetics were measured as before.

Human experiments

Experiments similar to the sheep experiments were done in 1966 and reported earlier(3). However, as indicated, kinetic analysis could not be done because the data would not fit the 3 exponential term system of Lewallen *et al.* (11) for reasons which were not then clear. However the original data do fit a 4 term exponential perfectly. Experimental details were as follows (3) :

Three normal male volunteers, two 21-year-olds and one 42-year-old, were given 15 µCi ^{131}I-T$_4$ and blood, faecal and urinary samples were taken for 7 days and processed as for sheep. Iodide 4 mg daily was given to reduce the SA of recycled ^{131}I. Iodide space and fractional transfer rate into urine were obtained from the extensive data in the literature (11,19,20). Iodoprotein was not measured originally but recent findings suggest that it would be approximately 0.03% dose/litre after 1½ half lives compared with a plasma ^{131}I-T$_4$ concentration of 2.5% dose/litre, so it would have no significant effect on the results.

R E S U L T S

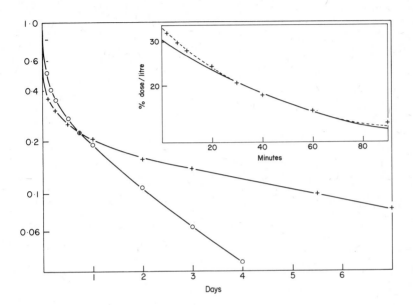

Fig. 2. *Experimental values expressed as fraction of dose in plasma. Not all data points are shown. Crosses = man; circles = sheep.*

Inset are human data. (+) experimental values. Continuous line is best 3-pool fit; dotted line is best 4-pool fit.

SHEEP

$q_1(t) = 0.2437e^{-4.8991t} + 0.3271e^{-5354t} + 0.1573e^{-.08006t}$
$+ 0.2719e^{-.02019t}$ 4-pool system − residual s.sq. = 0.91% of total s. sq.

$q_{11}(t) = 0.4353e^{-2.357t} + 0.2365e^{-.1015t} + 0.3282e^{-.02043t}$
3-pool system − residual s. sq. = 2.89% of total s.sq.

MAN

$q_1(t) = 0.2277e^{-3.3387t} + 0.4065e^{-1.2260t} + 0.1684e^{-.0748t}$
$+ 0.1974e^{-.00526t}$ 4-pool system − residual s.sq. = 0.056% of total s. sq.

$q_1(t) = 0.6095e^{-1.4123t} + 0.1736e^{-.0641t} + 02169e^{-.00531t}$
3-pool system − residual s.sq. = 0.98% of total s.sq.

For a typical sheep the plasma ^{125}I-T$_4$ curve was best fitted by the sum of exponentials $0.10783e^{-4.8991t} + 0.14472e^{-.53542t} + 0.06960e^{-.08006t} + 0.12032e^{-.020193t}$ (Fig. 2). The C's were normalized to give $c_1 = 0.2437$, $c_2 = 0.32707$, $c_3 = 0.15730$, $c_4 = 0.27193$. Plasma volume was $1/\Sigma C_n = 2.26$ litres and since plasma T_4 iodine was 3.1 µg/100ml, plasma ^{125}I-T$_4$ was .2263 and .1065 of the dose at 18 and 48 hours respectively. ^{125}I-T$_4$ loss was

via urine .072 and .160, via gut .104 and .290, into thyroid .0030 and .0081, remaining in body as ^{125}I-iodide .179 and .199. ^{125}I-T$_4$ remaining in the exchanging T_4 space, $(q_2 + q_3 + q_4)$ was therefore .4158 and .2534.

From these date the turnover rates, transfer rates, pool sizes, SA, losses from compartments and the T_4 secretion rate, as shown in Fig. 1, have been calculated.

The results obtained for 6 sheep, given as means and standard deviations, where k_{ii} = fractional turnover rate/hr for compartment i, and k_{ij} = fractional transfer rate/hr into compartment i from compartment j, were as follows :

$k_{11} = 1.404 \pm .028$, $k_{22} = 3.862 \pm .61$, $k_{33} = 0.303 \pm .066$, $k_{44} = 0.0528 \pm .008$. Fractional transfer rates between compartments were : $k_{12} = 3.705 \pm .81$, $k_{21} = 1.230 \pm .099$, $k_{13} = 0.277 \pm .051$, $k_{31} = 0.1363 \pm .028$, $k_{14} = 0.04755 \pm .0089$, $k_{41} = 0.03685 \pm .0061$. Fractional irreversible loss from each compartment : $k_{02} = 0.1567 \pm .038$, $k_{03} = 0.0258 \pm .0093$, $k_{04} = 0.00525 \pm .0021$. Mean compartment sizes were (in µg T_4 iodine) : $Q_1 = 79.8$, $Q_2 = 25.1$, $Q_3 = 35.9$, $Q_4 = 55.7$. Mean irreversible loss from each compartment was : $E_{02} = 3.933$ µg T_4 iodine/hour, $E_{03} = 0.9262$, $E_{04} = 0.292$. Total loss was 5.152 µg T_4 iodine/hour which is equal to the T_4 secretion rate under the steady state. At equilibrium the SA of pool 2, compared with plasma = 1, was 1.00, pool 3 = 1.11, pool 4 = 1.48.

In the two sheep given loading doses of stable T_4 the normal plasma total and free T_4 of 3.6 µg/100ml and 2.9 ng/100 ml (Sheep 27) and 4.6 µg/100ml and 3.1 ng/100 ml (Sheep 9) were raised to 12.0 µg and 13.8 ng (Sheep 27) and 11.8 µg and 11.9 ng (Sheep 9). Both sheep showed similar changes in T_4 kinetics. For sheep 27 the post-T_4 values were (pre-T_4 values in brackets) : k_{11} 3.01705 (1.3872), k_{22} 7.99595 (3.7716) k_{33} 0.5111 (0.3193), k_{44} 0.06468 (0.05666), k_{12} 7.80891 (3.638), k_{21} 2.43675 (1.083), k_{13} 0.48269 (0.2950), k_{31} 0.53110 (0.2648), k_{14} 0.06125 (0.05151), k_{41} 0.04930 (0.03944). Fractional rates of irreversible loss were : k_{02} 0.18704 (0.1333), k_{03} 0.02841 (0.02435), k_{04} 0.00343 (0.00515). Compartment sizes were (µg T_4 iodine) : Q_1 233.0 (70.0), Q_2 71.0 (20.1), Q_3 242.1 (58.1), Q_4 177.6 (48.7). Amounts of irreversible loss were : E_{02} 13.28 µg T_4 iodine/hour (2.68), E_{03} 6.88 (1.41), E_{04} 0.609 (0.251).

The results were very similar for each human subject so the data were averaged. The plasma curve fitted the expression $q_1(t) = 0.2277\ e^{-3.3387t} + 0.4065\ e^{-1.2260t} + 0.1684\ e^{-.0748t} + 0.1974\ e^{-.00526t}$. Turnover and transfer rates/hr were : k_{11} = 1.2724, k_{22} = 2.7663, k_{33} = 0.56466, k_{44} = 0.04143, k_{21} = 0.3960, k_{12} = 2.7582, k_{31} = 0.7928, k_{13} = 0.5505, k_{41} = 0.0836, k_{14} = 0.03955, k_{02} = 0.0081, k_{03} = 0.0142, k_{04} = 0.00188. Irreversible loss was : E_{02} = 0.186 µg T_4-I/hr, E_{03} = 3.18 µg T_4-I/hr, E_{04} = 0.605 µg T_4-I/hr. Compartment sizes were : Q_1 = 160.1 µg T_4-I, Q_2 = 22.9 µg T_4-I, Q_3 = 224 µg T_4-I, Q_4 = 322 µg T_4-I. Total loss or secretion rate was 3.97 µg T_4-I/h.

DISCUSSION

A very good fit of the plasma $^{125}I\text{-}T_4$ curve was obtained
with the sum of 4 real exponential terms. This suggests that
the T_4-containing areas of the body fall into 4 compartments
within which the SA of tracer is the same at any time, although
it differs significantly between compartments. There is no
implication of an anatomical or physiological connection between tissues within a compartment, e.g. brain and muscle. It
is clear that within a tissue, e.g. muscle, some $^{125}I\text{-}T_4$ will
be in interstitial fluid (ISF) or in the subcellular tubular
system which is an extension of it, some will be in the cell
cytoplasm, in microsomes, nuclei and mitochondria (21). Any
delay in distribution throughout a tissue might result in
significant difference in the SA of T_4 within that tissue.
This could conceivably result in the SA of the ISF of a slowly
equilibrating tissue, e.g. muscle, being similar to the intracellular SA of a more rapidly equilibrating tissue, e.g. gut.
This could invalidate both the postulated allocation of such
whole tissue to a single compartment, and also the assumption
that the only transfer between compartments occurs via plasma.
Therefore the uniformity of SA within a tissue was investigated
by comparison of the SA of whole tissue with that of its ISF.
Because of its contiguity to the bloodstream the SA of ISF
should show the maximum difference from the mean tissue SA.
Comparisons were made for several tissues at several intervals
after i.v. $^{125}I\text{-}T_4$ using ISF SA data reported from this laboratory (9) and whole tissue SA data obtained post mortem
on the same sheep and on others from the same flock (8). These
SA curves for liver, gut and muscle are compared in Fig. 3.
Figure 3 also shows the SA for each compartment using the

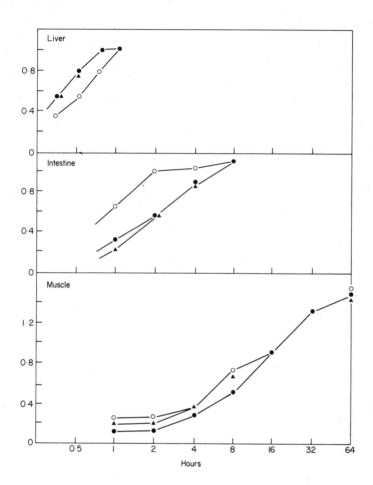

Fig. 3. *Equilibration of* ^{125}*I-T$_4$ in various areas as determined in the living sheep; from autopsy at various times after*
^{125}*I-T$_4$; and from calculations using the 4-pool system. Dots
= calculated SA of q$_1$; circles = SA of whole tissue; triangles
= SA of regional lymph.*
*All results are expressed on the basis that the SA of plasma
= 1, at each time.*

exponents, coefficients, k and Q values calculated as described above. Reasonably good agreement was found at all times between the SA of whole liver, hepatic lymph and pool 2. The SA of gut lymph and pool 3 also agreed reasonably well but at the earliest intervals gut wall had a significantly higher SA. This could conceivably be due to the large amount of exchanging $^{125}I-T_4$ within the gut lumen (see later) which takes longer to equilibrate and thus lowers the earlier SA values for compartment 3 below those found for gut wall. Nevertheless at no time does the SA of any of these areas within compartment 3 approach that of a slower or faster compartment. Therefore the heterogeneity of the SA within this compartment would not invalidate the compartmental concept described. Excellent agreement was found at all times between the SA of muscle tissues, of lymph derived largely from muscle, and of compartment 4.

The compartment sizes calculated by this method are comparable with those obtained by post mortem studies on similar sheep (8). For example, liver, kidney and lung contained 0.34 as much T_4 as the plasma pool while the calculated Q_2 was 0.32 of Q_1. The muscle, skin and brain contained 0.45 of plasma while Q_4 was 0.79 of Q_1; however the body tissues measured at post mortem accounted for only 23.4 kg of the 40 kg body weight An appreciable part of the difference would be made up of fat which had an SA of 1.48 of plasma at equilibrium and therefore would equilibrate at the same slow rate as compartment 4. Tendons, ligaments, other fibrous tissue and cartilage would also contribute to the difference between T_4 in muscle, skin and brain as found on post mortem, and the value for Q_4 obtained by calculation. The gut wall contained only 0.17 as much T_4 as plasma whereas Q_3 was 0.45 of plasma. The gut of herbivores contains a moderately large amount of T_4 which appears to exchange across the epithelium (8). This would account for much of the difference between T_4 in the gut wall and Q_3. It is possible that direct transfer between peripheral compartments 2 and 3 could occur if ^{125}I-T_4 excreted in bile was resorbed into the ISF or cells of the gut via an entero- hepatic circulation. This would invalidate the assumption that $k_{32} = 0$. I have found that no resorption of biliary T_4 or its degradation products occurs in the sheep (10) and although an enterohepatic circulation was originally postulated for the rat (22) more recently Cottle (23) and Galton and Nisula (24) have shown that no resorption of biliary T_4 occurs in this species. At present there is no evidence for an enterohepatic circulation of T_4 in any species. This was confirmed for sheep and man where k_{32} calculated as described elsewhere was not significantly different from zero.

The SA at eqilibrium for almost all body tissues has been given elsewhere (8). When these data obtained by direct measure- ment were compared with SA values calculated by compartmental analysis, the SA of pool 2, expressed on the basis that SA of plasma = 1, was 1.00 compared with 1.00 found for liver, kidney and lung. For pool 3 it was 1.11 compared with 1.07 for gut wall; the slower equilibration of gut contents which comprise over 50% of pool 3 could account for this difference. The SA of pool 4 was 1.48 while the SA of muscle tissue inclusive of ISF was 1.51, of skin 1.35, of brain 1.78, and of fat 1.48. The high SA of these areas, which contain 30% of the body's T_4 pool, illustrates the error introduced by determining the volume of distribution (VD) of T_4 by extrapolation to zero time of the final slope of the plasma disappearance curve, a method which is valid only if the SA throughout the VD is identical. In the example used above the total T_4 pool was 196.9 µg and since the plasma concentration was 3.1 µg/100ml, VD was 6.35 litres. By the extrapolation method VD is obtained as $1/C_4 = 1/0.12032 = 8.31$ litres. Any parameters derived from VD determined by the extrapolation method, e.g. T_4 secretion rate, are also in error.

The plasma disappearance curve after labelled T_4 i.v. has been studied in many species including man (1,3,5) and sheep (4). None of the workers have reported more than 3 exponential terms and consequently believe that not more tħn 2 compartments exchange directly with plasma. This is surprising in view of the fact that it has been universally found that there is a large liver pool which reaches or is very close to equilibrium by 60 min (ref. 25, Fig. 1 for man, review by Tata (26) for other species). This circumstance would give a steep initial fall in the plasma $^{125}I\text{-}T_4$ which would require the exponent of the first term to exceed 3; however exponents above 1.5 have not been reported. Some workers (27) have found that the initial volume of distribution of T_4 is significantly larger than albumin, although in both cases it should be equal to the plasma volume. This could be explained if an insufficient number of early samples were taken so that distribution into a rapidly equilibrating compartment was overlooked in the analysis. This is confirmed in reports in which frequent early samples were taken (25,28) which gave a plasma curve up to 6 hr which was identical with my Fig. 2. The fractional decrease of $^{125}I\text{-}T_4$ in the plasma of 23 normal humans determined during the period 5-20 min as 0.015 ± .006/min (29) was

identical to my results. In a further report from the same
laboratory (28) the zero time intercept of the final slope
(obtained by taking plasma volume as 4% body weight and
dividing by the volume of distribution) was 0.214 compared
with 0.199 in my data; their final slope was 0.106/day compared
with 0.125 for my younger subjects.

Although these data of Musa *et al.* (28) were not fitted
to a sum of exponentials the very close similarity to my data
except in the final slope indicate that 4 slopes, including
an initial very fast component, would be necessary. Initially
I thought that this initial fast component might be due to
slow mixing in slowing moving areas of plasma such as spleen,
venous reservoirs, etc. However the plasma curve after ^{125}I-
albumin in sheep (9) and man (11) does not show this steep
component; therefore slow mixing in plasma of a protein-bound
substance was excluded. This steep initial slope is likely to
be due to equilibration of ^{125}I-T$_4$ in the liver, kidney, etc.
and must be included in any kinetic analysis. It might be noted
that the number of compartments is determined somewhat arbitrarily by deciding how many compartments should be used to fit
the residual values after the first 2 curve peels. Once this
decision is made even the most sophisticated computerised
curve-fitting procedures cannot alter the number of terms.
The present data, as well as all the others I have examined
from several species, could be much better fitted by 2 additional components after the first 2 peels, as indicated by
the reduction in the (residual/total) sum of squares of deviations from 0.0289 for a 3-pool system to 0.0091 for a 4-pool
system in the sheep and from 0.0098 to 0.00056 in man. However
because one component often gives reasonable approximation for

the limited number of samples usually taken during the first
20 min, and possibly because of the additional complexity of
4-pool models an exchangeable system of 3 or even 2 pools has
been used.

In man the results differ from those of the sheep in that
the most rapidly equilibrating pool is pool 3 in which the
transfer rate from plasma, k_{31}, is 0.79. This is similar to
the mean plasma to liver transfer rate of 0.71 in 2 subjects
studied by Nicoloff and Dowling (30), to the 0.74 calculated
from the externally monitored one way hepatic clearance of
31 ml/min and a plasma volume of 4% body weight (28,29), but
less than the 0.93 obtained similarly by Cavalieri and Searle
(25). It appears that in man the liver is the major component
of compartment 3 which contains 1.4 times as much T_4 as plasma,
consistent with the results of Cavalieri and Searle (25),
Oppenheimer *et al.* (27) and Musa *et al.* (28), but much larger
than the liver T_4 estimate of Nicoloff and Dowling (30). The
major component of compartment 2 in man may be gut since it
has a more rapid entry rate from plasma than in the sheep but
a much smaller pool size. Both differences are consistent
with known physiological and anatomical differences in these
species. The parameters of compartment 4 in man closely re-
semble those of the sheep so it probably has the same components.

While the above discussion may vindicate the present
method as a facile technique for investigating T_4 kinetics
using perfect data, it is relevant to consider the extent to
which reasonable experimental error may affect the results.
Plasma organic ^{125}I was counted to ± 1% and labelled iodoprotein and T_3, which made up less than 5% of the organic

^{125}I could be measured with sufficient accuracy to give the
plasma ^{125}I-T$_4$ measurements an accuracy comparable to that of
total organic ^{125}I. Because the 19 samples measured always
fell on a smooth curve, random errors were easily detected
and checked. The T$_4$ secretion rate may therefore be measured
with a high degree of accuracy. When a 4-term exponential was
fitted to the plasma data the error sum of squares was less
than 1% so it seems reasonable to expect these parameters also
to be measurable with a high degree of accuracy. The calculation
of the compartmental turnover rates, k_{11}, k_{22}, k_{33}, and k_{44}
is of such a format that any error in the input parameters,
the c's and λ's, leads to a comparable or only slightly increased error in the turnover rates. However calculation of
the intercompartmental transfer rates requires additional
information about urinary and faecal and thyroidal ^{125}I and
^{125}I retained in the body as iodide. Faecal ^{125}I collected
may be measured with an accuracy comparable to plasma. Estimation of ^{125}I in gut which has been irreversibly lost from
the exchanging T$_4$ space but has not yet been collected is
subject to considerable error in herbivora in which this is
a large fraction. Experience from sheep post mortems has shown
that in 50% of sheep the retained gut ^{125}I would differ by
more than 12% from the amount predicted using the technique
described above. At 18 h this would give an error of 0.009
in the estimate of $(q_2 + q_3 + q_4)$ and at 48 h the figure would
be 0.004 (author's unpublished data). Urinary ^{125}I excreted
and retained can be estimated with high accuracy. Although
measurement of thyroidal ^{125}I is not so accurate, the amount
in the thyroid, less than 1% of the dose, is so small that
the error in $(q_2 + q_3 + q_4)$ would be insignificant. ^{125}I-iodide

in the iodide space was measured by two quite different methods
which gave good agreement. However, because the amount in
the iodide space is large, these measurements should be made
very carefully. A large extrathyroidal iodide pool is unique
to the sheep which has a very low rate of iodide clearance by
the kidney (H.D. Purves, pers. comm. 1963, confirmed by author's
unpublished data which show a renal iodide clearance of 0.0113
/h in the sheep compared with 0.087 (19), 0.074 (11), and
0.083 (20) in man). Furthermore in the sheep the extrathyroidal
iodide space is approximately 100% of body volume (author's
unpublished data) most of which is in the gut (8), compared
with 38.6% (19), 34% (11) and 35% (20) in man. A 5% error
in measuring the ^{125}I in the iodide space would be of no
significance in other species but would be the major source
of error in measuring $(q_2 + q_3 + q_4)$ in the sheep. Such an
error, together with a 10% error in the same direction in
measuring ^{125}I retained in the gut would give a 4.3% error in
$(q_2 + q_3 + q_4)$ at 18 h and 5.9% at 48 h in typical sheep data.
Errors in opposite directions would be almost totally compen-
sating. Assuming the errors were non-compensatory, errors in
the derived parameters would be :k_{12}, k_{21}, Q_2, k_{02} and E_{02}
less than 1%; k_{13}, k_{31}, Q_3 approximately 3%; k_{03} and E_{03}
approximately 30%; k_{14}, k_{41}, Q_4 approximately 10%; k_{04}, E_{04}
approximately 50%. Because of difficulties in accurate est-
imation of retained ^{125}I in the gut and iodide space, calculation of irreversible loss from pools 3 and 4 is subject to
considerable error in the sheep; in other herbivora they would
be considerably reduced, and in carnivora they should be minimal. Results obtained for other parameters should be of acceptable accuracy in all species. Although the T_4 secretion rate

is obtained by ΣE_{Oi}, errors in individual E_{Oi} values have no
effect on their sum, which is the same irrespective of the
values of $(q_2 + q_3 + q_4)$ used.

The very good agreement between compartmental sizes,
SA in compartments and rates of equilibration when measured
by compartmental 4-pool analysis and by post mortem and ISF
measurements support the use of compartmental analysis as a
means of investigating peripheral T_4 metabolism in subjects
with minimal experimental interference.

It should be emphasised that although the results obtained
were quite consistent between the sheep used, these were
selected from a uniform line and there was minimal variability
in the experimental conditions. It is quite possible that
other species and even other breeds of sheep could have
different parameters. In fact this technique could be useful
in the study of differences in T_4 kinetics between species
and under different physiological, environmental and pathological conditions. The use of this technique to show changes
in T_4 kinetics during acute exposure to an elevated total
and free T_4 concentration illustrates its potential in this
respect. While this was more in the nature of a pilot experiment, and idiosyncrasies in the species used reduced the
precision of the results, several marked changes in parameters
deserve comment. The fractional turnover rates of compartments
1 and 2 were more than doubled, for compartment 3 it was increased 60% while for compartment 4 it increased by only 14%.
Since these rates can be measured very precisely, this indicates a real difference in the way the liver, gut and muscle
handle a T_4 load. The irreversible loss from each compartment,
E_{Oi} was increased to 5.0 times control for compartment 2, 4.8

for compartment 3, and 2.5 for compartment 4. In muscle de-iodination is the only pathway of metabolism, in gut direct excretion into the lumen is also possible and in the liver conjugation mechanisms which have a high capacity are found also.

This method should be useful in examining the changes in T_4 distribution and metabolism in various areas in response to the effects of changes in free and total T_4, of substances which affect plasma and cellular binding, and of altered metabolism in organs which degrade T_4 such as exercising muscle and cirrhotic liver.

Acknowledgement.
  I wish to thank Mr. B. M.Lawson for his extensive, versatile and expert technical assistance in many aspects of this work.

REFERENCES

1. K. Sterling, J.C. Lashof and E.B. Man, *J. Clin. Invest.* **33**, 1031, (1954).

2. C.H.G. Irvine, *J. Endocrinol.* **39**, 313, (1967).

3. C.H.G. Irvine, *J. Clin. Endocrinol.* **28**, 942 (1968).

4. K. Vohnout, S.L. Hansard and E.L. Morton, *Amer.J. Vet. Res.* **29**, 657 (1968).

5. L. Sharney, R.L. Segal, A.E. Dumont, A. Girolami and S. Silver, *J. Mt. Sinai Hosp.* **33**, 396 (1965).

6. A. Rescigno and E. Gurpide, *J. Clin. Endocrinol. Metab.* **36**, 263 (1973).

7. J. Katz, A.L. Sellars, G. Bonorris and S. Golden, Plasma Protein Metabolism (Rothschild, M.A. and T. Waldmann, eds.) Academic Press, New York. p. 129 (1970).

8. C.H.G. Irvine, *Endocrinology*, **94**, 1060 (1974).

9. C.H.G. Irvine, *J. Clin. Invest.*

10. C.H.G. Irvine, *Endocrinology*, **85**, 662 (1969).

11. C.G. Lewallen, M. Berman and J.E. Rall, *J. Clin. Invest.*

<u>38</u>, 66 (1959).

12. M.I. Surks and J.H. Oppenheimer, *J. Clin. Invest.* <u>48</u>, 685 (1969).

13. D.A. Fisher, I.J. Chopra and J.H. Dussault, *Endocrinology*, <u>91</u>, 1141 (1972).

14. G.L. Brownell, M. Berman and J.S. Robertson, *Int. J. Appl. Rad. Isotopes*, <u>19</u>, 249 (1968).

15. E. Gurpide and J. Mann, *J. Clin. Endocrinol.* <u>30</u>, 707 (1970).

16. L. Sharney, L.R. Wassreman, N.R. Gevirtz, L. Schwartz, R. Levitan, A.M. Garcia, D. Leavitt and D. Tendler, *J. Mt. Sinai Hosp.* <u>33</u>, 236 (1965).

17. C.H.G. Irvine, *J. Clin. Endocrinol.* <u>38</u>, 655 (1974).

18. C.H.G. Irvine, *J. Clin. Endocrinol.* <u>38</u>, 468 (1974).

19. L.J. DeGroot, *J. Clin. Endocrinol.* <u>26</u>, 149 (1966).

20. M. Berman, E. Hoff, M. Barandes, D.V. Becker, M. Sonenberg, R. Benua and D.A. Koutras, *J. Clin. Endocrinol.* <u>28</u>, 1 (1968).

21. R.W. Heninger, F.C. Larson and E.C. Albright, *Endocrinology*, <u>78</u>, 61 (1966).

22. A. Taurog, *in* Brookhaven Symp. Biol., Brookhaven National Laboratory, New York, 1955, No. 7, p. 11.

23. W.H. Cottle, *Amer. J. Physiol.* <u>207</u>, 1063 (1964).

24. V.A. Galton and B.C. Nisula, *J. Endocrinol.* <u>54</u>, 187 (1972).

25. R.R. Cavalieri and G.L. Searle, *J. Clin. Invest.* <u>45</u>, 939 (1966).

26. J.R. Tata, Distribution and metabolism of thyroid hormones. *In* The Thyroid Gland (R. Pitt-Rivers and W.R. Trotter, eds). Butterworths, London, 1964, p. 163.

27. J.H. Oppenheimer, G. Bernstein and J. Hasen, *J. Clin. Invest.* <u>46</u>, 762 (1967).

28. B.U. Musa, R.S. Kumar and J.T. Dowling, *J. Clin. Endocrinol.* <u>29</u>, 667 (1969).

29. J.T. Dowling, W.G. Appleton and B.U. Musa, *J. Clin. Endocrinol.* <u>28</u>, 1503 (1968).

H

30. J.T. Nicoloff and J.T. Dowling, *J. Clin. Invest.* <u>47</u>, 26 (1968).

11. Physiological Significance of Nuclear Receptor Sites

J.H. OPPENHEIMER, H.L. SCHWARTZ, M.I. SURKS,[+]
D.H. KOERNER AND W. DILLMAN

Endocrine Research Laboratory, Division of Endocrinology,
Department of Medicine,
Montefiore Hospital and Medical Center,
and the Albert Einstein College of Medicine,
Bronx, New York, U.S.A.

INTRODUCTION

Following the initial report of limited capacity nuclear binding sites for L-triiodothyronine (T_3) in rat liver and kidney (1) a substantial body of information has been accumulated regarding the nature and significance of these sites. T_3 bound to nuclear sites exchanges rapidly with cytoplasmic T_3 pools (2). The sites have a low capacity (approximately 0.6 ng T_3/mg DNA) but an exceedingly high affinity (4.6 x 10^{11} L/M) for T_3. They have been characterised as nonhistone nucleoproteins with a probable molecular weight of 60–65,000 (3). Samuels and Tsai (4) have shown similar nuclear sites in tissue cultures of GH_1 cells derived from rat pituitary

Supported by NIH Grant No. 15421-14 and Department of the Army Contract No. DA 49-193-MD-2967.

+ *Recipient, Research Career Development Award K04-AM 19502-01A1.*

tumours and from human lymphocytes. Cytoplasmic binding sites
are not required to translocate T_3 to the nucleus since nuclear binding can be readily demonstrated in isolated nuclei
incubated in an aqueous medium (5,6). More recently, solub-
lised nucleoproteins have also been shown to react with T_3
to form T_3 protein complexes similar to those observed under
in vivo conditions as well as in incubation experiments in
isolated nuclei (7,8,9).

The demonstration of limited-capacity high-affinity
nuclear binding sites in itself, however, does not prove that
the sites in question are important in initiating hormonal
action. Accordingly, we have carried out a number of studies
to test the hypothesis that nuclear binding sites are true
receptors, i.e. the starting points in the sequence of biochemical reactions terminating in the expression of hormonal
activity at the cellular level.

STUDIES OF ANALOGUES

A correlation has been established between hormonal
action of individual analogues as demonstrated by conventional bioassay procedures and the ability of such analogues to
bind to the nuclear sites. Nuclear binding has been assessed
by two techniques: A. Increasing doses of nonradioactive T_3
and thyroid hormone analogues together with ^{125}I-T_3 have
been injected intravenously into intact rats and the displacement of ^{125}I-T_3 from hepatic nuclear sites measured,
(10); B. Isolated nuclei have been incubated with tracer
quantities of ^{125}I-T_3 together with varying concentrations
of unlabeled T_3 and thyroid hormone analogues.

The results of both approaches indicate that MIT and DIT

do not displace radioactively labeled T_3 from nuclei, that
compounds with two iodine substituents in the 3' and 5' positions such as L-thyroxine (T_4) and tetrac (the acetic acid
analogue of T_4) are considerably less effective in displacing
T_3 than compounds with a single bulk substitution in the
phenolic ring such as T_3, triac (the acetic acid analogue of
T_3), and isopropyl T_2. Whereas isopropyl T_2 is known to be a
potent thyromimetic substance, triac is substantially less
effective than T_3 in most bioassay systems. This discrepancy,
however, is easily resolved. Thus, triac appears to be more
rapidly metabolised than T_3. In experiments in which equi-
molar doses of triac and T_3 were injected into animals (8)
it was shown that whereas the nuclear displacement by triac
and T_3 were comparable at 30 mins, the effects of triac were
more rapidly dissipated, presumably because of an increased
rate of fractional metabolism of triac. Recent tracer experiments with labeled T_3 and triac in our laboratory have in
fact shown that the fractional removal rate of triac from
plasma and nuclei is twice that of T_3(11). Thus duration of
occupancy of nuclear sites by the test analogues as well as
the affinity of the nuclear sites for the analogue are important determinants of the biologic potency of the substance.
D-T_3 exhibited 7/10th of the displacement potency of L-T_3
in liver nuclei, but only 3/10th that of L-T_3 in heart nuclei.
This tissue difference may account for the selective decrease
in serum cholesterol in experimental animals and in patients
treated with D-T_3 (12). Reverse T_3, 3,3',5'-triiodothyronine,
does not displace radioactive T_3 from nuclei ; neither does
reverse T_3 exhibit thyromimetic effects. In fact, reverse

T_3 antagonises the calorigenesis of thyroxine (13). Our findings thus suggest that this antagonism does not result from a competition between reverse T_3 and thyroid hormones at the nuclear level.

Table 1. *Comparison of Relative Binding of T_3 Analogues*

		Nucleus	
Analogues	Cytosol K_A/K_{T_3}	*In Vivo* RDP	*In Vitro* K_A/K_{T_3}
L-T_3	1.00	1.0	1.0
L-T_4	.33	.10	.10
Reverse T_3	.07	0	.001
Triac	.16	1.0	1.6
Isopropyl-T_2	.02	1.0	1.0

Cytosol K_A/K_{T_3} = Ratio of association constants of of analogues to that of T_3 (14).

RDP = Relative Displacement Potency determined by *in vivo* experiments (10).

In Vitro K_A/K_{T_3} = Ratio of nuclear association constants of analogues to T_3 determined *in vitro* (6).

The avidity of analogues for nuclear sites differs markedly from that exhibited by cytosol binding proteins (14). Relative to T_3, both triac and isopropyl-T_2 are comparatively weakly bound to cytosol binding proteins (Table 1). This differs markedly from the relative binding of these analogues by nuclear sites. Cytosol binding differs in other ways from nuclear binding. Whereas nuclear binding sites appear to constitute a high affinity, low capacity system, cytosol binding is characterised by high capacity and low affinity (14). As indicated above, cytoplasmic binding proteins do not appear to be involved in the translocation of T_3 to the nucleus.

The striking correlation between biologic function and nuclear binding has been confirmed in recent collaborative studies with Dr. Eugene Jorgenson in which some 40 T_3 analogues were examined for biologic and displacement activity (15). Thus, the distal orientation of the phenolic ring is important both for nuclear binding and biologic activity. Non-halogenated compounds which showed weak thyromimetic activity also demonstrate weak displacement activity.

NUCLEAR BINDING OF T_3 BY OTHER TISSUES

A second line of evidence pointing to the biological significance of nuclear sites is based on an analysis of nuclear binding in various rat tissues (16). The nuclear binding capacities of liver, kidney, heart, adenohypophysis, brain, spleen and testis were determined by *in vivo* displacement techniques which have previously been described (2). The results are indicated in Table 2. Although specific binding sites were demonstrated in all tissues studied, a wide variation in their concentration was encountered in individual tissues. The number of binding sites was particularly low in spleen and testis, two tissues which are generally presumed to be unresponsive to thyroid hormone by conventional biochemical criteria (increased

Table 2. *Nuclear T₃ Binding Characteristics of Rat Tissues (From Reference 16).*

Tissue	DNA[A] Recovery (%)	Total DNA/g tissue (mg)	Nuclear T₃[B] (% total T₃)	Binding ng/mg DNA	Capacity normalised to liver (= 1)	Binding ng/g tissue	Capacity normalised to liver (= 1)	$\frac{K_i}{K_h}$ [C]
Liver	59	2.90	12.9	.61	1.00	1.77	1.00	1.0
Brain	31	1.55	13.5	.27	0.44	0.42	0.24	0.7
Heart	26	2.01	15.4	.40	0.65	0.80	0.45	1.0
Spleen	56	17.27	13.0	.018	0.03	0.31	0.18	1.2
Testis	23	9.56	3.0	.0023	0.004	0.022	0.01	---
Kidney	42	4.93	9.0	.53	0.87	2.61	1.47	0.6
Ant.Pit.	84	8.33	52.6	.79	1.30	6.58	3.72	1.0

[A] Number of animals studied and range: liver, (8)(52–62); brain, (3)(24–32); heart, (5)(17–28); spleen, (3)(48–63); testis, (3)(22–28); kidney, (2)(38–45); anterior pituitary, (5)(76–90).

[B] Corrected for DNA Losses

[C] Ratio of nuclear association constant of given tissue (i) to association constant of liver (h). Data for testis are not sufficiently precise to allow calculations.

oxygen consumption and enhanced levels of the mitochondrial enzyme α-glycerolphosphate dehydrogenase in tissues from hormone-treated animals). Brain also appears to be unresponsive to hormone by these biochemical criteria, but it is apparent from Table 2 that the number of binding sites per g of tissue as well as per mg of DNA lie in an intermediate position between those tissues known to be responsive such as pituitary, liver, kidney and heart on the one hand and spleen and testis on the other. It is therefore difficult to be certain whether the failure to demonstrate increased oxygen consumption of the brain after T_3 injection is due exclusively to a reduction of the level of binding sites per g of tissue or whether other factors are also operative. The comparatively low concentration of nuclear sites in spleen accords well with the recent report by Samuels and Tsai of a relatively low density of specific nuclear sites in human lymphocytes (17).

The same set of studies allowed us to calculate the percentage of the total number of nuclear sites which are occupied under endogenous physiological levels of circulating T_3. Thirty-five to 50% of the sites are occupied under the normal physiological state. The similarity in the percentage of occupancy of nuclear sites in the various tissues implies that the nuclear association constant in these tissues is the same (Table 2). Thus, whereas the number of binding sites per mg DNA or per nucleus differs widely among the various tissues, the sites themselves appear identical.

Lastly, it was possible for us to calculate from these data the percentage of the total cellular T_3 which is associated with the specific nuclear site (Table 2). Of considerable interest to us was the finding that whereas less than

16% of the total cellular T_3 was bound to the specific nuclear
sites in other tissues, fully 52% of total cellular T_3 was
bound to specific nuclear sites in the anterior pituitary.
The high percentage of binding sites in the anterior pituitary was due both to the high concentration of nuclear sites
per mg DNA as well as to the high content of DNA in the pituitary. The large fraction of cellular T_3 in the anterior pituitary explains why we were able to demonstrate specific binding of T_3 in the pituitary without preliminary subcellular
fractionation, whereas this was impossible in the other tissues studied (18).

NUCLEAR BINDING SITES IN HYPER-
THYROIDISM AND HYPOTHYROIDISM.

Recent experiments from our laboratory have indicated
that hyperthyroidism *per se* is not associated with any changes
in nuclear binding capacity. This was demonstrated by determining the capacity using *in vivo* displacement techniques in
animals rendered hyperthyroid three days after the injection
of 1-3 mg of T_3 I.V. The hyperthyroid state of the animal
was confirmed by the level of mitochondrial a-glycerolphos-
phate dehydrogenase which was approximately three times the
normal euthyroid level. In three separate experiments the
average binding capacity of control animals was 0.48 ng/mg
DNA whereas the average binding capacity in the hyperthyroid
group was 0.44 ng/mg. The difference was not statistically
significant. Similarly, animals rendered hypothyroid, either
following combined thyroidectomy and radioiodine treatment,
or after a one-month course of PTU, showed no change in the
nuclear binding capacity. If one assumes that nuclear binding

sites constitute the exclusive intiating sites of hormonal action, it follows that the number of binding sites in a given tissue should constitute a constraint for maximal response by the tissue to the administration of thyroid hormone. This expectation was met by the results of recent experiments carried out in our laboratory. Thus, we have shown that the increase in α-glycerolphosphate dehydrogenase activity was independent of the dose of T_3 injected as long as the nuclear sites were occupied for the experimental period.

Our findings thus strongly suggest the concept that an interaction of T_3 with nuclear sites constitutes the initiating event leading to the transcription of the genome, the synthesis of new RNA, and finally, to the synthesis of new protein in the sequential order first described by Tata and associates (19). More recently Baxter *et al.* (21) have reported that T_3 binds specifically to that subfraction of chromatin which appears active in transcription. Of fundamental importance in elucidating the mechanism of action of thyroid hormones at a cellular level will be the identification of the protein or proteins which are synthesised in response to the enhanced transcription.

R E F E R E N C E S

1. J.H. Oppenheimer, D. Koerner, H.L. Schwartz and M.I. Surks, *J. Clin. Endocr. Metab.* 35, 330-333 (1972).

2. J.H. Oppenheimer, D. Koerner, M.I. Surks and H.L. Schwartz, *J. Clin. Invest.* 53, 768-777 (1974).

3. M.I. Surks, D. Koerner, W. Dillman and J.H. Oppenheimer, *J. Biol. Chem.* 248, 7066-7072 (1973).

4. H.H. Samuels and J.S. Tsai, *Proc. Nat. Acad..Sci. U.S.A.*, 70, 3488-3492 (1973).

5. H.H. Samuels and J.S. Tsai, *J. Clin. Invest.* <u>53</u>, 656-659, (1974).

6. D. Koerner, M.I. Surks and J.H.Oppenheimer, *J. Clin. Endocr. Metab.* <u>38</u>, 706-709 (1974).

7. H.H. Samuels, J.S. Tsai and J. Casanova, *Science*, <u>184</u>, 1188-1191, (1974).

8. P. Thomopoulos, B. Dastuge and N. Deter, *Biochem. BioPhys. Res. Comm.* <u>58</u>, 499-506,(1974).

9. J. Torresani and L.J. DeGroot, Abstract 81, 56th Annual Meeting, Endocrine Society Program, 1974, p. A-96.

10. J.H. Oppenheimer, H.L. Schwartz and M.I. Surks, *Biochem. Biophys. Res. Comm.* <u>55</u>, 544-550 (1973).

11. B. Goslings, H.L. Schwartz, W. Dillman, M.I. Surks and J.H. Oppenheimer, Abstract 79, 56th Annual Meeting, Endocrine Society Program, 1974.

12. C.M. Greenberg, B. Blank, F.R. Pfeiffer and J.P. Pauls, *Am. J. Physiol.* <u>205</u>, 821-826 (1973).

13. C.S. Pittman and S.B. Barker, *Endocrinology*, <u>64</u>, 466-468 (1959).

14. W. Dillman, M.I. Surks and J.H. Oppenheimer, *Endocrinology*, <u>96</u>, 492-498 (1974).

15. D. Koerner, H.L. Schwartz, M.I. Surks, J.H. Oppenheimer and E.C. Jorgenson, Program, American Thyroid Association, Abstract (1974).

16. J.H. Oppenheimer, H.L. Schwartz and M.I. Surks, *Endocrinology*, <u>95</u>, 897-903 (1974),

17. J.S. Tsai and H.H. Samuels, *J.Clin. Endocr. Metab.* <u>38</u>, 919-922 (1974).

18. A.R. Schadlow, M.I. Surks, H.L. Schwartz and J.H. Oppenheimer, *Science*, <u>176</u>, 1252-1254, (1972).

19. J.R. Tata, L. Ernster, O. Lindberg, E. Arrhenius, S. Pedersen and R. Hedman, *Biochem. J.* <u>86</u>, 408-428 (1963).

20. J.R. Tata *In* Handbook of Physiology, 7, "Endocrinology", vol. B, Thyroid (M.A. Greer and D.H. Solomon, eds) Chapter 26, pp.469-477, American Physiol. Soc., Washington, D.C. (1974).

21. J.D. Baxter, M.A. Charles, G. Rytfel, B.J. McCarthy
     and K.M. Macleod. Program 66th Annual Meeting, American
     Society for Clinical Investigation, Abstract 14, p. 4a
     (1974).

12. The Effect of Thyroid Hormone on Adenyl Cyclase—A Potential Site for Thyroid Hormone Action

RICHARD B. GUTTLER, CAROL L. OTIS, JAMES W. SHAW,

DWIGHT W. WARREN AND JOHN T. NICOLOFF.

University of Southern California School of Medicine, Department of Medicine, Los Angeles, California.

INTRODUCTION

The observation in 1918 by Goetsch that adrenalin caused tachycardia, increase in blood pressure, and tremulousness in hyperthyroidism in a dose which he claimed had no effect on normal subjects was the primary impetus for 60 years of research aimed at understanding the thyroid-adrenal axis (1). This simple finding which was touted as a diagnostic test for hyperthyroidism unfortunately resulted in severe and occasionally fatal complications, such as thyroid storm and uncontrolled tachyarrhythmias. However, in spite of this, his observation has been confirmed and is considered an important concept in endocrinology. The mechanisms to explain his findings, however, are still unknown. The evolution of theories regarding this effect go from altered sympathetic nerve activity in the early 1900's to the present theory of enhanced cyclic AMP response to catecholamines. Limited *in vitro* and *in vivo* studies

Supported in part by USPH Grant AM-11727, General Clinical Research Center Grant RR-43, and a Special NIH Grant AM-53097 (Dr. Richard B. Guttler).

have suggested that this may be the mechanism to explain Goetsch's original observations. The present studies were designed to evaluate the response of adenylate cyclase cyclic AMP generating system to various hormonal stimuli on the face of alterations in the thyroid hormone concentration. This was accomplished by using a sensitive protein binding assay for urine and plasma cyclic AMP (2) in assessing the response to epinephrine and other cAMP mediated hormones.

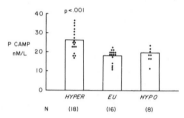

Fig. 1. *Fasting, resting, supine plasma cyclic AMP values in hyper, hypo, and euthyroid subjects.*

Figure 1 shows the resting plasma cAMP concentration in nanomoles/litre in 18 hyperthyroid, 16 euthyroid and 8 hypothyroid subjects. It can be seen that the hyperthyroid group had a minimal but significant ($p < .001$) elevation in their supine resting plasma cAMP concentration when compared to euthyroid subjects. However, there was no significant difference in the concentrations observed in the hypothyroid patients compared to the euthyroid subjects.

Epinephrine-thyroid hormone interrelationships.

We next evaluated the thyroid hormone effects on cyclic AMP generation to epinephrine administration by measuring the plasma cAMP response as shown in Figure 2. This study was performed on 5 hyperthyroid, 4 hypothyroid and 5 euthyroid subjects given epinephrine at a dose of 0.05 µg/kg/min. over

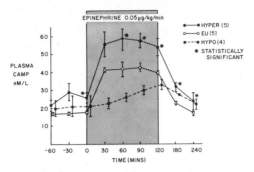

Fig. 2. *Response of plasma cyclic AMP concentrations to epinephrine infusion in hyper, hypo, and euthyroid subjects.*

a 2-hour period by infusion pump. The dose of epinephrine chosen was shown by Murray and Kelly (3) to produce an enhanced response, as measured by pulse pressure multiplied by the pulse, in the hyperthyroid subjects with minimal side effects. It can be clearly seen that there is both an increased peak rise in plasma cAMP concentration and a sustained augmentation of plasma cAMP in the hyperthyroid group compared to the euthyroid group. Plasma cAMP concentration in both groups returned to the basal state with similar disappearance slopes upon completion of the infusion. However, the hypothyroid group demonstrated a minimal rise in plasma cAMP which occurred toward the completion of the infusion and an apparent delayed disappearance from the plasma at the completion of the infusion. Plasma epinephrine concentrations, measured by the fluorimetric method of Renzini (4), were equivalent following the epinephrine infusion in all groups studied.

Similar, but more significant results were obtained when evaluating the urinary cyclic AMP excretion during epinephrine infusion as is shown in Fig. 3. The basal and epinephrine

Guttler et al.

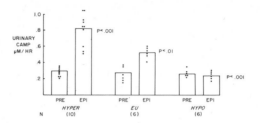

Fig. 3. *Comparison of urinary cyclic AMP excretion rates before (PRE) and after epinephrine infusion (EPI) in hyper, hypo, and euthyroid subjects.*

stimulated urinary cyclic AMP excretion in μMoles/hour is shown for 10 hyperthyroid, 6 euthyroid, and 6 hypothyroid subjects. There was no difference in the basal hourly cAMP excretion noted in the three groups. However, there is a marked augmentation in cAMP excretion in the hyperthyroid group when compared to euthyroid which is significant at a p level of <.001, and it can be noted that the hypothyroid group had complete failure to respond to epinephrine infusion. The urinary cAMP excretion response to epinephrine is significant in that the urinary values are an integrated measure of nucleotide production and excretion and may, therefore, reflect altered production rates in hyper- and hypothyroidism.

Figure 4 compares the thyroid hormone concentration as measured by adjusted thyroxine iodine to the peak plasma cAMP response to an epinephrine infusion in a group of 10 patients with varying thyroid functional states. It can be seen that there is a positive correlation between the serum thyroxine iodine and the peak plasma cAMP response to epinephrine. This correlation was significant at a p level of < .001 and with an r value of 0.917.

Figure 5 illustrates a study designed to determine if

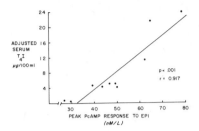

Fig. 4. *Correlation of adjusted serum thyroxine concentration (free thyroxine index) to the maximal plasma cyclic AMP response to 1.0 mg of intravenously administered glucagon.*

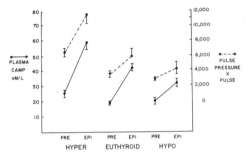

Fig. 5. *Comparison of basal (PRE) and epinephrine (EPI) response on plasma cyclic AMP (solid line) and pulse pressure x pulse index (dotted line). Note positive correlation between plasma cyclic AMP levels and cardiovascular response to epinephrine.*

plasma cAMP alterations paralleled the end organ cardiovascular response to epinephrine. It can be noted that the plasma cAMP concentrations correlated closely with the cardiovascular index measured as the pulse pressure x pulse before and after epinephrine infusion in a series of hyperthyroid, euthyroid, and hypothyroid subjects. The correlation data relating to cAMP production and cardiovascular effects are consistent with the view that the altered cAMP generating system is responsible for Goetsch's original observation of augmented

cardiovascular response to a given dose of epinephrine in
clinically toxic hyperthyroid subjects. To determine if plasma
cAMP response to epinephrine can be reversed with beta blockade,
the comparison of the combined infusion of propranolol (10 mg
/hour) concurrently with epinephrine (0.05 µg/kg/min) to epinephrine alone in 6 hyperthyroid and 5 euthyroid subjects was
performed. These studies are illustrated in Fig. 6. The hyperthyroid group showed a significant blunting in cyclic AMP
during the combined infusion. This is in contrast to the total
abolition of cAMP response seen in the euthyroid subjects.

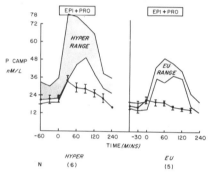

Fig. 6. *Comparison of plasma cyclic AMP response to epinephrine (EPI) with (solid line) and without (shaded area) propranolol (PRO) infusion at 10 mg/hour in hyperthyroid (HYPER)
and euthyroid (EU) subjects. Note that propranolol can completely block epinephrine induced cyclic AMP rise in euthyroid
but not hyperthyroid subjects.*

In preliminary studies, the infusion of 20 mg of propranolol per hour was able to completely blockade the effects
of epinephrine induced elevations in cAMP in hyperthyroid
subjects. Thus, a higher dose of propranolol would appear to
be necessary to block cAMP generation in thyrotoxic subjects.
The cause of this disparity in dosages required to block cAMP
production is presently under study.

In summary, these studies on catecholamine-thyroid inter-relationships suggest that there is a modulating influence of thyroid hormone on altering the ability of adenylate cyclase to respond to an appropriate hormonal stimulus. Also that the minimally increased basal plasma cAMP concentrations seen in hyperthyroid subjects may be an effect of heightened catecholamine sensitivity in hyperthyroidism and finally that beta blockade reversed the cAMP response to epinephrine.

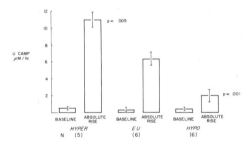

Fig. 7. *Effect of bovine parathyroid hormone in altering urinary cyclic AMP excretion in hyper, hypo, and euthyroid subjects.*

Parathyroid hormone-thyroid hormone interrelationships:

To determine if thyroid hormone excess or insufficiency has an influence on other cAMP mediated systems, 200 units of bovine parathormone of a similar lot number was injected intravenously in 5 hyperthyroid, 6 euthyroid, and 6 hypothyroid subjects as depicted in Fig. 7. It can be noted that there is a similar response as was seen with the epinephrine infusion, in that there is an augmentation of cAMP excretion in the hyperthyroid subjects and blunting in the hypothyroid subjects. These findings are consistent with the work of Alexander *et al.* (5) who have shown an exaggerated end-organ response to parathormone administration in thyrotoxicosis when serum calcium elevation was the parameter studied.

Guttler et al.

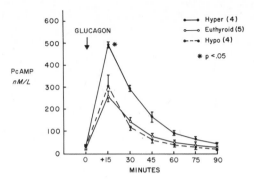

Fig. 8. *Comparison of plasma cyclic AMP response to an intra-venous pulse dose of glucagon in hyper, hypo and euthyroid subjects.*

Glucagon-thyroid hormone interrelationships :

Figure 8 depicts the plasma cAMP response to 1 mg of glucagon administered intravenously. It can be noted that the hyperthyroid group again had a significant augmented response in peak plasma cAMP, but in contrast to epinephrine and para-thormone, there was no blunting in the peak plasma cAMP response noted in the hypothyroid group.

Plasma cAMP disappearance rates in hyper- and hypothyroidism

To determine if there were differences in turnover rate of cAMP in plasma which might account for the abnormalities in cAMP generation seen in hyper- and hypothyroidism, the following analysis was performed. Depicted in Fig. 9 is the plasma disappearance of cAMP from the peak concentration obtained following 1 mg of glucagon in 4 hyperthyroid, 4 hypothyroid, and 5 euthyroid subjects. As can be noted, the disappearance rate of plasma cAMP from the peak value post-glucagon is essentially the same in the various thyroid states. The $t_{\frac{1}{2}}$ values for cAMP disappearance varied from 16.5 min

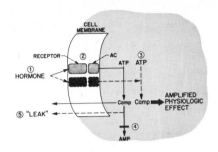

Fig. 9. *Theoretical sites where thyroid hormone may act to alter cyclic AMP production.*

in the hyperthyroid subjects to 18 min in the hypothyroid subjects. This similarity in t½ values would certainly support the contention that changes in plasma cAMP values probably serve as an excellent index for alterations in cAMP blood production rate regardless of thyroid status.

DISCUSSION

Figure 9 summarises the potential sites where thyroid hormone may alter the ability of the adenylate cyclase systems to generate cyclic AMP to hormonal stimuli with resultant heightened or dampened physiological response at the end organ. Thyroid hormone may increase the hormone receptor affinity or the amount of receptor protein as shown by ①. It may increase the membrane bound enzyme adenylate cyclase itself, its activity, or affect the transducer in the membrane in a manner similar to that recently described by Rodbell for GPT or guanidine triphosphate (6) shown by ②. Thyroid hormone may increase the delivery of ATP to the site of conversion to cyclic AMP as shown by ③ or affect the degradation of cAMP by altering the activity of specific phosphodiesterases as shown in ④. All of which would result in augmented physio-

logical rsponse. Also it may affect membrane permeability to
cyclic AMP with resultant leak out of the cell as shown in ⑤ .
Additionally, it might affect divalent cation messengers like
calcium or magnesium with resultant effect on cAMP generation.
The nucleotide leak theory probably is untenable due to the
fact that there are physiological effects which parallel the
rise in cyclic AMP, suggesting a primary intracellular elevation as shown by the cardiovascular response to epinephrine
and the calcium elevation to parathormone. Therefore, plasma
cAMP concentration is probably a reflection of increased
intracellular nucleotide generation or production rate. Phosphodiesterase inhibition by thyroid hormone excess has been
reported *in vitro* and recently studies by Stouffer *et al.* (7)
have suggested that a high affinity phosphodiesterase is
activated in hypothyroid states with resultant rapid cAMP degradation. Therefore, high concentrations of thyroid hormone
may result in inhibition of this phosphodiesterase. Studies
by Ismail-Beigi and Edelman (8) have shown that the ATP to ADP
ratios are low in the thyroid hormone treated liver tissue *in
vitro* in spite of probable increased ATP production and thus
augmented ATP delivery for cAMP production is a possibility
as a site of the major thyroid hormone effect. Recently, Rodbel
et al. (6) have noted that GTP may act upon a transducer in
the cell membrane with amplification of the cAMP produced to
glucagon stimulation in liver tissue. Therefore, thyroid
hormone may produce its effects by affecting GTP concentrations
or acting directly in a similar manner.

These thyroid hormone induced alterations noted in the
adenylate cyclase AMP generating systems may explain the
clinically significant alterations in catecholamine effective-

ness in thyroid disorders first described by Goetsch in 1918. Many other aberrations in endocrine function seen in thyroid disorders, for example, hypercalcaemia, metabolic bone disease, glucose intolerance in hyperthyroid subjects, and the norepinephrine resistance seen in myxoedema could be due to thyroid hormone mediated alterations in the cyclic AMP generating system.

R E F E R E N C E S

1. E. Goetsch, *N.Y. State J. Med.*, 18, 259, (1918).

2. A.G. Gilman, *Proc. Nat. Acad. Sci.*, 67, 305, (1970).

3. J.F. Murray and J.J. Kelly, *Ann. Int. Med.*, 51, 309, (1959).

4. V. Renzini, C.A. Brunori and C. Valori, *Clin. Chem. Acta.*, 30, 587 (1970).

5. M.T. Harrion, R.McG. Harden and W.D. Alexander, *J. Clin. Endocrinol. & Metab.*, 24, 214, (1964).

6. M. Rodbell, M.C. Lin and Y. Salomon, *J. Biol. Chem.*, 249, 59, (1974).

7. J.F. Stouffer, K.J. Armstrong, R. Van Inwegen, W.J. Thompson and G.A. Robison, Program of The Endocrine Society Meeting, June 12-14, 1974. Abstract #133.

8. F. Ismail-Beigi and I.S. Edelman, *Proc. Nat. Acad. Sci.*, (USA) 67, 1071, (1970).

13. Effects of Altered Thyroid Function upon Hepatic L-Triiodothyronine Aminotransferase Activity in Rats

DORIAN TERGIS, NORMAN FISHMAN,* M.D. AND RICHARD S. RIVLIN, M.D.

Department of Medicine, Francis Delafield and Presbyterian Hospitals, and Institute of Human Nutrition, College of Physicians and Surgeons of Columbia University, New York, New York, 10032, U.S.A.

INTRODUCTION

An enzyme has recently been detected in various rabbit tissues which transaminates the thyroid hormones, L-triiodothyronine (T_3) and L-thyroxine (T_4) (1,2). This enzyme is located in the soluble fraction of the cell, and preferentially utilises T_3 rather than T_4. With pyruvate as a substrate, the enzyme exhibits specificity for T_3.

This newly-described enzyme, L-triiodothyronine aminotransferase, is distinct from another thyroid hormone transaminase reported earlier by Nakano (3,4). The latter enzyme is mitochondrial in location, exhibits a relative specificity for T_4 rather than for T_3 and does not act upon nitrated tyr-

This work was supported by grants from the USPHS (AM 15265 and CA-12126) and from the Stella and Charles Guttman Foundation.

* *Present address : Department of Medicine, Washington University School of Medicine, St. Louis, Missouri, 63110, U. S.A.*

osines even with α-ketoglutarate as the amino group acceptor.

The physiological role of both of these transaminates
is largely unknown. The present report summarises recent investigations in this laboratory which attempt to define a role
for L-triiodothyronine aminotransferase in thyroid hormone
economy and to determine any effects of altered thyroid function upon enzyme activity.

MATERIALS AND METHODS

Animals.

All studies were performed using male white rats of the
Holtzman strain. T_4 and T_3 were administered by intraperitoneal injection at varying dose levels and for varying periods
of time. In each instance control rats of the same age and
sex received injections of isotonic saline of the same volume
and pH as that of the hormone solutions.

Hypothyroidism was achieved by the administration of a
single intraperitoneal injection of ^{131}I, 300 μCi/100g body
weight, to rats which had fed on a low iodine diet for four
weeks after the time of weaning (5). These animals were utilised at least two months after administration of radioactive
iodine.

Preparation of Tissue.

Rats were sacrificed by a blow to the head followed by
decapitation and exsanguination. Organs were promptly removed
and placed on ice until homogenisation on the same day as
sacrifice. Each organ was homogenised in a Teflon tissue
grinder for a period of two minutes with two volumes of a
Tris-HCl buffer solution at pH 7.8. The buffer solution also
contained KCl, magnesium acetate, sucrose and mercaptoethanol
(1,2). Homogenates were then passed through two layers of

cheesecloth to remove cellular debris. An aliquot was removed
and frozen overnight for assay the following day. Under these
conditions no appreciable loss of enzyme activity occurred.

Enzyme Assay

The procedures developed for the assay of L-triiodothyronine aminotransferase activity in rabbits (1,2) were found
to be suitable for assay of the enzyme in rat tissues with
only minor modifications. Advantage was taken of the ability
of the enzyme with α-ketoglutarate as the amino group acceptor
to act upon 3,5-dinitro-L-tyrosine as a substrate, thereby
producing the stable coloured compound, 3,5-dinitro-p-hydroxy-
phenylpyruvic acid, which could be determined by simple
spectrophotometric assay. The data obtained were expressed as
milliunits/mg protein, with each milliunit of enzyme activity
representing 1 nanomole of product formed per min under the
standard conditions of the assay.

Protein concentrations were measured in duplicate by the
method of Lowry *et al.* (6), employing a standard solution of
bovine serum albumin.

R E S U L T S

Tissue Distribution.

Initial experiments determined the tissue distribution
of L-triiodothyronine aminotransferase in adult male rats.
High enzyme activity was demonstrable only in liver and kidney.
Low but measurable activity was detected in brain, lung,
heart, testes and spleen. Virtually no activity was demonstrable in the skeletal muscle of the hind limb, the blood
serum, the thyroid gland or the anterior pituitary gland. In
preliminary measurements made of the brains of newborn animals,
very low enzyme activity was recorded, similar to that prev-

iously measured in brains of adult animals.

Age Effects

Observations were made of the hepatic activity of L-triiodothyronine aminotransferase in rats from birth to 130 days of age. Significant enzyme activity was detectable at the time of birth. There was a progressive increase in activity of this enzyme during the time period studied, and L-triiodothyronine aminotransferase activity in animals 130 days of age was approximately 50% greater than that noted in animals within several hours of birth.

T_4 *and* T_3 *Administration.*

The effects of treatment of normal adult animals with large doses of T_4 and T_3 upon the hepatic activity of L-triiodothyronine aminotransferase are shown in Table 1. In this experiment, normal adult animals 130 days of age were divided into two groups, half receiving daily injections of T_4, 100 μg/100g body weight, and the remainder receiving daily injections of isotonic saline of the same volume and pH as that of the hormone solutions. After eight days of treatment, the animals were sacrificed and hepatic enzyme activity was determined. T_4 in these pharmacological doses increased enzyme activity from 18.7 ± 1.2 to 29.7 ± 2.2 milliunits/mg protein. This difference was highly significant (p < 0.001) (7).

The daily administration of pharmacological doses of T_3 (25 μg/100 g) for the same 8-day period increased enzyme activity from 20.4 ± 0.8 to 27.6 ± 1.3 milliunits/mg protein. This difference was also significant (p < 0.01). The magnitude of the increase in L-triiodothyronine aminotransferase activity produced by T_4 and T_3 under these conditions was similar. Subsequent experiments have determined that increases in the

Table 1. *Effects of Administration of T$_4$ and T$_3$ to Normal Adult Male Rats upon the Hepatic Activity of L-Triiodothyronine Aminotransferase.*

Treatment Group	Number of Animals	Hormone* Dose Given	L-Triiodothyronine Aminotransferase Activity (milliunits/mg protein)
Saline	7	-	18.7 ± 1.2 **
T$_4$	7	100μg/100g	29.7 ± 2.2 (p<0.001)
Saline	9	-	20.4 ± 0.8
T$_3$	9	25μg/100g	27.6 ± 1.3 (p<0.01)

* *All animals received daily i.p. injections for 8 days.*

** *Values are expressed as Mean ± S.E.M.*
   (Data from Reference 7).

activity of L-triiodothyronine aminotransferase can be produced by much lower doses of either T$_4$ or T$_3$. Doses of T$_4$ of approximately 15 μg/100 g and of T$_3$ of 5 μg/100 g, when administered daily to normal adult animals for 8 days, increase enzyme activity significantly. A study of the time required for T$_4$ to achieve an increase in the hepatic activity of L-triiodothyronine aminotransferase has revealed that increases occur earlier than 8 days after starting treatment. Daily administration of T$_4$ for three days significantly increases enzyme activity.

In view of the fact that both liver and kidney have much greater activities of L-triiodothyronine aminotransferase than any of the other organs studied, as noted above, it was of

interest to determine whether thyroid hormones increase enzyme activity in kidney tissue as well. Results of preliminary
experiments indicate that only in liver is there an increase
in aminotransferase activity after administration of T_3.
Radiothyroidectomy.

In addition to determining the effects of administering
T_3 and T_4 to normal animals, measurements were made of the
hepatic activity of L-triiodothyronine aminotransferase in
rats which had been rendered hypothyroid by ablation of the
thyroid gland with ^{131}I. This technique reliably produces
hypothyroidism (5), as documented by reduction or cessation
of weight gain and marked diminution in the uptake of a tracer
dose of ^{131}I by the thyroid gland.

The results of measuring hepatic L-triiodothyronine aminotransferase activity in radiothyroidectomised rats and in
age-matched controls is shown in Table 2. Enzyme activity was
reduced from control levels of 14.9 ± 0.5 to 12.4 ± 0.5 milli-
units/mg protein in livers of hypothyroid rats. This difference
was significant ($p < 0.01$).

In subsequent experiments it has been possible to demonstrate that the treatment of hypothyroid rats with daily
injections of T_3 in doses as low as 2.5 µg/ 100 grams body
weight for 8-9 days restores the decreased enzyme activity to
normal.

DISCUSSION

The results of the present study indicate that T_4 and T_3
administration to normal animals will significantly increase
the hepatic activity of L-triiodothyronine aminotransferase,
and that radiothyroidectomy will reduce enzyme activity. In
the two organs, liver and kidney, in which L-triiodothyronine

Table 2. *Hepatic Activity of L-Triiodothyronine Amino-*
transferase in Normal and Radiothyroidectomised
Adult Male Rats.

Treatment Group	Number of Animals	L-Triiodothyronine Aminotransferase Activity (milliunits/mg protein)
Control	16	14.9 ± 0.5 **
Radio - thyroidectomy*	9	12.4 ± 0.5 (p < 0.01)

* *300 μCi /100g of ^{131}I were given to weanling*
male rats after they had fed on a low iodine
diet for four weeks.

**'*Values are expressed as Mean ± S.E.M.*

(Data from reference 7).

aminotransferase activity is highest, thyroid hormones appear
to regulate the magnitude of enzyme activity only in liver.

In addition to being regulated by altered thyroid function, the hepatic activity of L-triiodothyronine aminotransferase is also influenced by age. Enzyme activity increases
steadily from birth to four months of age, at which time it
is 50% greater than at birth. It is recognised that information needs to be obtained about the pattern of development
of enzyme activity prior to birth, and its possible relation
to the onset of functioning of the fetal thyroid gland which
occurs late in gestation (8,9). In addition, it will be of
interest to determine whether the apparent decline in thyroid
function which occurs in elderly animals (10) is associated
with changes in the activity of L-triiodothyronine aminotransferase.

I

In attempting to define a physiological role for L-triiodothyronine aminotransferase, it may be useful to compare the tissue distribution of this enzyme with that of the nuclear receptor sites for T_3. It has been suggested that these binding sites may be involved in the initial event which leads to the eventual production of thyroid hormone effects (11). The number of binding sites per tissue weight is highest in the anterior pituitary gland, and is also high in kidney, liver and heart, organs in which increased oxygen consumption is produced after thyroid hormone administration (12,13). The number of binding sites per tissue weight is lower in those organs (spleen, brain and testes) in which no increase in oxygen consumption occurs after administration of T_3 (12,13). By contrast, L-triiodothyronine aminotransferase activity is almost undetectable in the pituitary gland, and is low in activity both in organs (heart) which exhibit increased oxygen consumption after T_3 administration, and in those which do not (spleen, brain, testes).

These findings suggest that L-triiodothyronine aminotransferase is probably not involved in the initiation of hormone action but may function instead as a degradative enzyme. Further support for the hypothesis that this enzyme is involved in the degradation or inactivation of T_3 is that the product of the reaction, L-3,5,3'-triiodothryopyruvic acid is only one-fifth as active as T_3 in stimulating tadpole metamorphosis (14), and that this compound is excreted in rat bile after the animals have been treated with T_3 (15). The present findings that T_3 and T_4 increase L- triiodothyronine aminotransferase activity make it likely that these hormones may regulate the rates of their own inactivation at least in part through transamination in liver.

Acknowledgements.

   The authors are indebted to Dr. Richard L. Soffer, Department of Molecular Biology, Albert Einstein College of Medicine, Bronx, New York, U.S.A. for numerous helpful discussions.

REFERENCES

1.   P. Hechtman, S.D. Schimmel and R.L. Soffer, *Biochem. Biophys. Res. Commun.* 43, 1395-1401 (1971).

2.   R.L. Soffer, P. Hechtman and M. Savage, *J. Biol. Chem.* 248, 1224-1230 (1973).

3.   M. Nakano, *Biochim. Biophys. Acta.* 92, 472-481 (1964).

4.   M. Nakano, *J. Biol. Chem.* 242, 73-81 (1967).

5.   R.S. Rivlin, C.E. Menendez and R.G. Langdon, *Endocrinology*, 83, 461-469 (1968).

6.   O.H. Lowry, N.J. Rosebrough, A.L. Farr and R.J. Randall, *J. Biol. Chem.* 193, 265-275 (1951).

7.   N. Fishman, D. Tergis and R.S. Rivlin, *Fed. Proc.* 33, 249 (1974).

8.   J.D. Feldman, J.J. Vazquez and S.M. Kurtz, *J. Biophys. Biochem. Cytol.* 11, 365-383 (1961).

9.   B. Nataf and M. Sfez, *C.R. Soc. Biol.* (Paris) 155, 1235-1238 (1961).

10. D.L. Wilansky, L.G. Newsham and M.M. Hoffman, *Endocrinology*, 61, 327-336 (1957).

11. J.H. Oppenheimer, H.L. Schwartz, D. Koerner and M.I. Surks, *J. Clin. Invest.* 53, 768-777 (1974).

12. J.H. Oppenheimer, M.I. Surks, H.L. Schwartz, D. Koerner and W. Dillman. *In* Proceedings of the International Conference on Thyroid Hormone Metabolism, (W.A. Harland and J.S. Orr, eds). (New York, Academic Press, in press).

13. L. Sokoloff, P.A. Roberts, M.M. Januska and J.E. Kline, *Proc. Nat. Acad. Sci.* (U.S.A.) 60, 652-659 (1968).

14. J. Roche, R. Michel, R. Truchot, W. Wolf and O. Michel, *Biochim. Biophys. Acta.* 20, 337-344 (1956).

15. R. Michel, R. Pitt-Rivers, J. Roche and S. Varrone, *Biochim. Biophys. Acta.* 57, 335-340 (1962).

14. The Metabolism of Tetraiodothyroacetic Acid and its Conversion to Triiodothyroacetic Acid in Man

A. BURGER AND M.B. VALLOTTON

Endocrine Division, Department of Medicine,
University of Geneva, Switzerland.

INTRODUCTION

The extent and importance of metabolic alteration of the amino acid side chain of the L-thyroxine molecule (T_4) have been studied to a minor extent only. The acetic acid derivatives of T_4 and 3,5,3' triiodo-L-thyronine (T_3), tetraiodothyroacetic acid or tetrac (TA_4) and triiodothyroacetic acid or triac (TA_3), respectively, have been found in muscle and kidney of rats and mice, and in the serum of dogs, injected with labelled T_4 (1-5). The formation of tetrac from labelled T_4 has been shown to occur in perfused rat liver and heart (6,7). In 1970 ^{125}I labelled tetrac derived from the peripheral metabolism of labelled T_4 was demonstrated in the blood of man and the following year studies with ^{14}C labelled T_4 revealed the presence of ^{14}C labelled thyroacetic acid derivatives in blood and urine (8,9).

In view of a better understanding of the physiological importance of tetrac and triac we developed a radioimmunoassay for the measurement of serum tetrac concentration (10) and report now on the metabolism of tetrac in hyper-and hypothy-

roid subjects. The study includes also data concerning the
conversion of tetrac to triac. They indicate the presence of
triac in human serum and give some preliminary indication on
the serum triac concentrations that can be expected.

M A T E R I A L   A N D   M E T H O D S

Studies of the metabolism of ^{125}I labelled tetrac were
carried out in 6 patients with primary hypothyroidism and 4
patients with hyperthyroid Graves' disease. Table 1 lists the
pertinent clinical and laboratory data. Tetrac was labelled
by the chloramine T method (specific activity 50-100 mCi/mg)
(11) and sterilised by filtration through millipore filter.
Each individual received an intravenous injection of 50 μCi
of tetrac in a 1% solution of human serum albumin. Thyroidal
recycling of inorganic iodide liberated by the degradation
of labelled tetrac was prevented in hypothyroid subjects by
10 drops of Lugol's solution twice daily. In hyperthyroid
patients, large doses of carbimazole (20 mg every 6 hours)
were administered. Throughout the study urine was collected
daily and samples of blood were taken every day or every other
day. Labelled iodide was determined after adsorption on an
anion exchanger (Iobeads, Technicon Inc.). Two ml serum were
enriched with 10 μl 2 *M* carrier iodide, then 300 mg of the
anion exchanger were added and the samples were agitated on
a whirl-mixer for one minute. The radioactivity in one millilitre of the supernatant was measured and the results used to
calculate the disappearance of tetrac. The non-extractable
iodine was estimated by extracting 2 ml of serum with 8 ml of
acidified butanol. The procedure was repeated five times. The
precipitate was then counted.

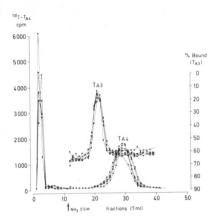

Fig. 1. *Adsorption of tetrac and triac on a Sephadex G 25 fine column. The first peak represents the fraction of labelled tetrac eluted with the proteins, the second peak was obtained by measuring the cold triac with a radioimmunoassay. The third peak is radioactive tetrac, which was adsorbed to Sephadex and later eluted with 0.5 N NH3.*

The *in vivo* conversion of tetrac to triac was estimated by adsorbing the thyroid hormones from 3 ml of serum on a Sephadex G-25 fine column (1.6 x 20 cm) equilibrated with 0.05 M. Tris buffer at pH 8.7 containing 0.005 M Sodiumdisulfite. The serum was enriched with 300 ng cold triac, 3.2 mg 8-anilino-1-naphthalene sulfonic acid (K & K Laboratories) and the pH adjusted to 12.0. When the serum had penetrated the column, the proteins were washed out with 60 ml buffer. The hormones were eluted with 0.5 N NH3. The triac peak was identified by a radioimmunoassay (to be published). It appeared in front of the labelled tetrac peak (Fig. 1). The eluate corresponding to the triac peak was lyophilised. The second chromatography was performed on a LH-Sephadex column (0.8 x 21 cm) in ethylacetate-methanol-2 N NH3 (20:5:2)(12). The sample was enriched with 100 ng cold tetrac. After the

Table 1. *Clinical and laboratory data obtained in the patients with primary hypothyroidism and with hyperthyroid Graves' Disease.*

Patient	Age	Sex	Clinical features	Treatment	T_4 ng/ml	T_3 ng/ml	TSH µU/ml
			Myxoedemas				
L.B.	86	M	B_{12} deficiency	Lugol's solution 25 µg T_4 daily	1.5	0.8	260
W.V.C.	35	M	Myxoedematous myopathy	Lugol's solution	9.3	0.3*	195
J.N.	53	F	Obesity	Lugol's solution 25 µg T_4 daily	8.0	0.3*	83
T.A.	82	F	Broncho-pneumonia	Lugol's solution, Ampicillin, digoxin	7	0.4*	134
A.A.	67	F		Lugol's solution	1.3	0 *	120
B.G.	74	F	B_{12} deficiency	Lugol's solution	25	1.0	78

Hyperthyroidism

P.T.	56	F	First episode diffuse goitre	80 mg Carbimazole	300	10.4**
B.B.	74	F	First episode multinodular goitre	80 mg Carbimazole	153	4.8**
C.S.	55	M	Relapse diffuse goitre exoph-thalmos	80 mg Carbimazole	200	2.4**
G.W.	47	F	Relapse diffuse goitre exoph-thalmos	80 mg Methimazole ***	260	3.5**

| | normal range 50-120 | 0.6 µU/ml |

Normal serum T_3 concentrations change with age and sex: the pathological values are therefore marked by asterisks : * below normal range, ** above normal range, *** this patient presented an allergic reaction to carbimazole.

chromatography the triac and tetrac peaks were identified by
specific radioimmunoassays (Fig. 2). At this point the recovery of the cold triac was quantitated by radioimmunoassay.

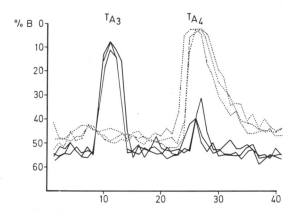

Fig. 2. *Chromatography of triac and tetrac on a LH-Sephadex
column in ethylacetate-methanol-2 N NH3 (20:5:2). Both peaks
were identified by radioimmunoassays. On the abcissa the
number of 3 ml fractions are indicated.*

Finally the triac peak enriched with 50 µg cold triac was
analysed on descending paper chromatography on Whatman 3MM
paper in hexane-tertiary amylalcohol-2 N NH3 (1:5:6). The
spots were localised by spraying with 2% aminoantipyrine in
2% sodium bicarbonate followed by 2% potassium ferrocyanate.
The area was cut out and its radioactivity counted. Sufficient counts were obtained to reduce the counting error to a
maximum of 5%. The measurement of the serum tetrac concentration was performed by radioimmunoassay (10).
Calculations : The serum radioactivity was plotted as a function of time. The regression coefficient for that part of the
curve which appeared to conform to a single exponential function was calculated by the method of the least squares. The

volume of distribution was obtained by extrapolation of the regression curve to zero time. The fractional turnover rate, the daily clearance and the daily degradation rate of tetrac were calculated by a method similar to that described by Ingbar and Freinkel (13).

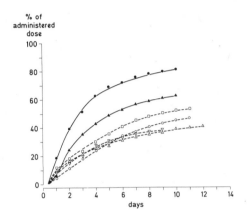

Fig. 3. *The cumulative urinary appearance of the injected radioactivity in four hypothyroid (dashed curves) and two hyperthyroid subjects (solid curves).*

R E S U L T S

In the hyper- and hypothyroid patients respectively the mean ± sem of the relative content of radioactive iodide was 13 ± 2.2% and 9.1 ± 3.4%. In hypothyroidism the relative content of the non-extractable iodine was insignificant (1.7 ± 1.3%). In hyperthyroidism it was 8.4 to 10.9% one day after injection and increased slightly five to eight days later to 16.1 and 17.1%. A large amount of the radioactivity was recovered in the urine (Fig. 3).

Kinetics of tetrac in hypothyroid patients : Two of the six

patients were treated with 25 µg-L-thyroxine daily. In all
patients, the individual disappearance curves drawn from the
data obtained during the period from 2 or 4 days to 10 or 13
days appeared to conform to a single exponential function
(Fig. 4). The results of the individual studies and the mean
± S.D. are shown in Table 2. The mean half life of the disappearance of labelled tetrac was 5.6 ± 1.1 days and fractional turnover rate was 12.7 ± 2.3% per day. The volume of
distribution was 18.9 litres. The daily clearance was 2.5 ±
0.4 litres. The serum concentration of tetrac was 1.70 ± 0.3
ng per millilitre. The values overlap with the euthyroid range
(0.75 to 2.9 ng per millilitre)..The daily degradation rate
was 4.2 ± 1.2 µg.

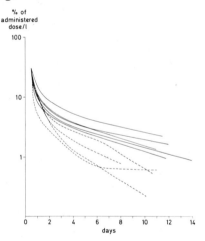

Fig. 4. *Disappearance from serum of labelled tetrac in five
hypothyroid (solid curves) and four hyperthyroid subjects
(dashed curves). The most recent study in one subject with
primary hypothyroidism is not shown. In one case of hyperthyroidism the terminal part of the disappearance curve is
nearly horizontal. This curve was not further analysed.*

Kinetics of tetrac in hyperthyroid patients : Three days

Table 2.   *Kinetic data on tetrac metabolism*

Patient	tetrac ng per ml	half-life days	Distribution volume litres	turnover rate per day (%)	clearance litre/day	degradation μg/day
			Hypothyroidism			
L.B.	2.05	5.05	19.6	13.7	2.7	5.5
W.V.C.	1.80	4.65	17.2	14.9	2.6	4.7
J.N.	1.80	5.12	19.6	13.5	2.6	4.7
T.A.	1.80	6.80	–	10.2	–	–
A.A.	1.45	4.85	19.7	14.3	2.8	4.1
B.G.	1.20	7.3	18.5	9.5	1.8	2.2
mean ± SD	1.70±0.3	5.6±1.1	18.9±1.1	12.7±2.3	2.5±0.4	4.20±1.2
			Hyperthyroidism			
P.T.	2.3	2.4	25	28.9	7.2	16.6
B.B.	3.1	2.9	16.7	23.5	3.9	12.1
C.S.	1.3	2.6	18.5	26.9	5	6.5
mean	2.2	2.6	20.0	26.4	5.4	11.7

after the injection an apparent equilibrium was attained.
Even then the individual disappearance curves did not strictly
follow a single exponential function. In one patient the disappearance of tetrac clearly declined according to a multi-
exponential function. This case was excluded. The individual
results of the three other cases are reported in Table 2. The
mean half life of the disappearance of tetrac was 2.6 days.
Compared to the values in hypothyroid patients the volume of
distribution was not different (20 versus 18.9 litres) but
the fractional turnover rate was greatly increased to 26.4%
per day. The mean serum concentration of tetrac was 2.2 ng
per millilitre; the normal range for 12 sera of hyperthyroid
patients was 0.7 to 4.45 ng per millilitre. The daily clearance was twice as large as in hypothyroidism. In consequence,
the degradation rate was 2.8 times higher than in hypothyroidism and was 11.7 µg per day.

In vivo conversion of ^{125}I *tetrac to triac* : To study *in vivo*
conversion it is crucial to eliminate artefactual conversion
of tetrac to triac occurring *in vitro*. Deiodination occurs
when thyroid hormones are extracted, chromatographed and dried
even when nitrogen is used. This artefact has to be avoided.
In addition a complete separation of triac from tetrac is necessary. We tested our extraction procedure in this respect
by adding highly purified cold or labelled tetrac to serum.
The proportion of tetrac found by radioimmunoassay in the
final triac spot was only 0.034% ± 0.0056 (n = 3). With labelled tetrac 0.07% ± 0.02 of labelled triac was found (n = 4).
The method can therefore be considered free of artefacts,
and this is probably due to the initial separation of triac
and tetrac before the drying step.

Table 3. *In vivo conversion of* ^{125}*I-triac from* ^{125}*I-tetrac. The labelled triac content is expressed as percent of the labelled tetrac.*

Patients	\multicolumn{9}{c}{days after injection of tetrac}
	1	2	3	4	5	6	7	8	9
Hypothyroidism									
J.N. *		0	0.3		3.7		5		4.9
T.A.		1.1		1.9					
A.A.	1.1					1.6			
Hyperthyroidism									
P.T.	0.2		0.48	1.3		1.35			
B.B.	0.2	0.67		0.74		1.4	0.37(?)		
C.S.					0.7	0.7			
G.W.	0.3		1.18				2.95		

* In this case, the LH-20 chromatography step was not performed and this may explain the higher values at day 5,7 and 9 of the study.

The *in vivo* conversion of tetrac to triac was measured
in the serum of four hyperthyroid and three hypothyroid subjects. The results are summarised in Table 3. The percent of
labelled triac formed increased over the first three to four
days. Later the values changed only slightly. The labelled
triac does rarely exceed 2.95% of the tetrac present. There
seems to be very little difference between the percent of
labelled triac formed in hyper- and hypothyroidism. Yet the
few cases studied preclude any conclusions on this subject.

D I S C U S S I O N

The interest in the peripheral metabolism of thyroid
hormones has been renewed by the recent recognition that T_3
is barely present in the human thyroid (14). It originates
mainly from the peripheral monodeiodination of T_4 to T_3.
Thirty to 40% of T_4 is transformed to T_3 (see review, ref.15).
It is assumed that the same percentage of T_4 is deiodinated
to reverse T_3 ($3,3',5'-T_3$) since deiodination seems to occur
randomly, (16,17). The fate of the 20 to 40% of the remaining
T_4 is not exactly known. But tetrac has long been known to be
another product of thyroxine metabolism. In this laboratory a
radioimmunoassay for the measurement of serum tetrac concentration was recently developed (10). The results indicated a
very small difference in its serum concentration in hypo-eu-
and hyperthyroidism. Further information was therefore needed
to see if the serum concentration reflected the actual turnover rate. The problem was approached by an appreciation of
the disposal rate by first order kinetics. This technique is
an approximation but seems sufficiently precise in the case
of both studies, in hypo- and hyperthyroidism, although the

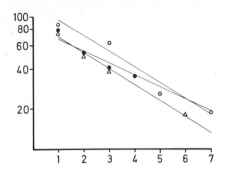

Fig. 5. *Disappearance curves of labelled tetrac in three*
hyperthyroid subjects. The values are expressed as a percent
of the 3 day value.

studies in the patients with hyperthyroidism were less satis-

factory. To justify the use of first order kinetics in the

case of hyperthyroidism the 4 to 7 day periods of the tetrac

disappearance were expressed as a percent of the 3 day value

(Fig. 5). In three cases the regression coefficients of the

curves were 0.95, 0.99 and 0.98.

In one case the regression coefficient was 0.75 which is

not compatible with a single exponential function. On the

basis of this result this case was excluded. The reasons for

the multicompartimental function of the tetrac disappearance

could be multiple. The non-extractable iodine was not sub-

tracted. Depletion of the intrathyroidal hormone reserves and

the decrease in serum T$_4$ from 26 to 18 μg per 100 ml could

have changed the equilibrium. In the other cases the decrease

in the serum T$_4$ concentration was less important.

There is ample evidence of deiodination being the major

metabolic pathway of thyroid hormones. Deiodination of tetrac

has been documented in man(18), the appearance of triac as

an intermediary step being therefore predictable. But the

kinetics of the two hormones are very different, triac having
a much faster turnover rate than tetrac. The serum concentration of labelled triac will therefore be much lower even
when a large part of tetrac were converted to triac. The
method of detection of triac has therefore to be reliable.
In particular *in vitro* conversion should be eliminated or has
to be measured concomitantly. There are two lines of evidence
indicating that the method described establishes true *in vivo*
conversion. First the *in vitro* conversion has been found to
be minimal and could be neglected. Second the measurement of
the *in vivo* conversion in serial blood samples shows a progressive rise of labelled triac, suggesting that the formation of triac was primarily due to metabolic events (Table 3).
Hence the occurence of triac as a metabolite of tetrac in
human serum appears certain. But no firm indications can be
given to the extent of this conversion. For any conclusions
two additional pieces of information would be necessary :
similar to reverse T_3, reverse triac (3,3',5'-triac) is probably produced to the same extent as triac. Yet no reverse
triac was available to us. Its localisation during the chro-
matrographic steps could therefore not be identified. Should
they be separated, the percentage of ^{125}I-triac would have to
be doubled. This conclusion rsults from the fact that triac
is probably randomly labelled in either one of the positions
of the outer ring, the 3' and 5' positions having an equal
chance. Hence only 50% of the deiodinated tetrac would still
be labelled. On the other side, if triac and reverse triac
migrated identically no corrections could be made without
knowing the metabolism of these hormones. Data are available
on the metaboliam of triac in the study of Green and Ingbar

(18). A half life of 19 hours was found, yet no corrections were made for the non-extractable iodine. Some preliminary data from our own laboratory indicate rather a half-life of approximately 10 hours and a volume of distribution of 40 litres. With these data a clearance of 60 to 70 litres per day could be estimated, compared to 3 or 4 litres in the case of tetrac. Hence the percentage of triac relative to tetrac would have to be multiplied 20 times to calculate the percentage that its production rate from tetrac would be, relative to the production rate of tetrac.

The data presented give some indication of the range of serum triac concentration that can be anticipated. The actual concentration must be very small, most likely less than 10 ng per 100 millilitre. This concentration could be slightly increased by the triac formed by decarboxylation and deamination of T_3, but the total concentration of triac must still be a small fraction of the serum T_3 concentration.

Currently the site of thyroid hormone action is being intensively studied (19,20). Nuclear receptors for thyroid hormones have been described and isolated. It is of interest that the affinity of these receptors is strongest for both T_3 and triac. Other hormones like T_4 and tetrac are bound less firmly (21). Yet triac differs from T_3. It dissociates more rapidly from the receptor (22). This could explain the much weaker *in vivo* action of triac when used for replacement therapy in myxoedematous patients (23). Its serum concentration seems to be very low. The physiological importance of this hormone is therefore not settled. Yet it may still have a function as a very short lived but active hormone.

Acknowledgements.

  The authors wish to express their acknowledgements to Miss M.Schilter for her technical assistance and to Miss. V. Nicolet for her outstanding secretarial help.

  This work was supported by the "Fonds National Suisse" grant No. 3.799.72.

R E F E R E N C E S

1. J. Roche, R. Michel and W. Wolf, *Endocrinology*, <u>59</u>, 425 (1956).

2. K. Tomita, H.A. Lardy, F.C. Larsen and E.C. Albright, *J. Biol. Chem.* <u>224</u>, 387 (1957).

3. J.R. Tata, J.E. Rall and R.W. Rawson, *Endocrinology*, <u>60</u>, 83 (1957).

4. E.V. Flock, J.L. Bollman, J.H. Grindlay and B.F. McKenzie, *Endocrinology*, <u>61</u>, 461 (1957).

5. V.A. Galton and R. Pitt-Rivers, *Biochem. J.*, <u>72</u>, 319 (1959).

6. E.V. Flock and Ch.A. Owen, *Endocrinology*, <u>77</u>, 475 (1965).

7. J.L. Rabinowitch and E.S. Hecker, *Science*, <u>173</u>, 1242 (1971).

8. L.E. Braverman, S.H. Ingbar and K. Sterling, *J. Clin. Invest.* <u>49</u>, 855 (1970).

9. C.S. Pittman, J.B. Chambers, Jr. and V.H. Read, *J. Clin. Invest.* <u>50</u>, 1187 (1971).

10. A. Burger, M. Schilter, C. Sakoloff, M.B. Vallotton and S.H. Ingbar, *Clin. Res.* <u>22</u>, 336 (1974).

11. A. Burger and S.H. Ingbar, *Endocrinology*, <u>94</u>, 1189 (1974).

12. A.D. Williams, D.E. Freeman and W.H. Florsheim, *J. Chromatog.* <u>45</u>, 371 (1969).

13. S.H. Ingbar and N. Freinkel, *J. Clin. Invest.* <u>34</u>, 808, (1955).

14. I.J. Chopra, D.A. Fisher, D.H. Solomon and G.N. Beall, *J. Clin. Endocr.* <u>36</u>, 311 (1973).

15. P.R. Larsen, *Metabolism*, <u>21</u>, 1073 (1972).

16. C.S. Pittman, T. Maruyama and J.B. Chambers, Jr. *Endocrinology,* 83, 489 (1968).

17. M.I. Surks and J.H. Oppenheimer, *J. Clin. Endocr.* 33, 612 (1971).

18. W.L. Green and S.H. Ingbar, *J. Clin. Endocr.* 21, 1548 (1961).

19. H.H. Samuels and J.S. Tsai, *J. Clin. Invest.* 53, 656 (1974).

20. J.H. Oppenheimer, H.L. Schwartz, D. Koerner and M.I. Surks, *J. Clin. Invest.* 53, 768 (1974).

21. J.H. Oppenheimer, H.L. Schwartz, W. Dillman and M.I. Surks, *Biochem.Biophys.Res. Comm.* 55, 544 (1973).

22. B. Goslings, H.L. Schwartz, W. Dillman, M.I. Surks and J.H. Oppenheimer (abstract), *Endocrinology,* 94, A95 (1974).

23. J. Lerman, *J. Clin. Endocr.* 21, 1044 (1961).

15.   The Day of the Dolphin: Thyroid Hormone Metabolism in Marine Mammals

KENNETH STERLING, PETER O. MILCH AND SAM H. RIDGWAY

Protein Research Laboratory, Bronx Veterans Administration Hospital and Department of Medicine, Columbia University College of Physicians and Surgeons, New York, N.Y. and Naval Undersea Center, San Diego, California.

We have undertaken to examine thyroid hormone metabolism in dolphin species because they are homeothermic mammals with a varied climatic distribution, which might yield information of value, and also because they are such engaging subjects to deal with.

Figure 1 illustrates some of the species whose blood serum was available for T_3 measurement, both by the original chemical procedure (1) and by the radioimmunoassay which entails thermal inactivation of TBG (2). The bottle-nosed dolphin (*Tursiops truncatus*) is the species widely known for its performance in water circuses where it has long entertained audiences. This dolphin lives close to the coast line and is confined to warm water. The individual bottle-nosed dolphins seen in New York or Seattle are sent south to winter quarters in Florida or Southern California because of their inability to withstand low temperatures. *Tursiops gilli* is a closely related coastal species which can cross-breed with *Tursiops*

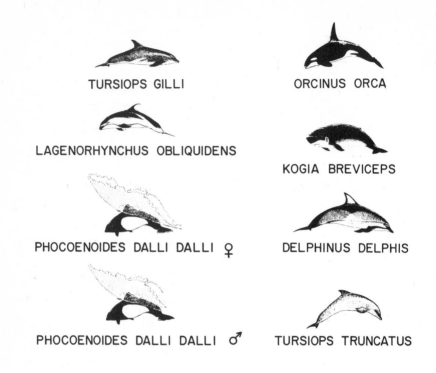

Fig. 1. *Species of sea mammals studied, as depicted in "Mammals of the Sea", Ed. Sam H. Ridgway, Charles C. Thomas, publisher.*

truncatus. The common dolphin (*Delphinus delphis*) is a deep sea form which frequently rides the bow waves of ocean-going vessels; this behavior, however, may also be exhibited by other dolphins. The Pacific white-striped or white-sided dolphin (*Lagenorhynchus obliquidens*) may enter cold water, but the outstanding example of cold water habitat is provided by the Dall porpoise (*Phocoenoides dalli*), which is often found as far north as the Aleutian Islands in the winter months and swims fast and dives deep in the frigid zone. The killer

whale (*Orcinus orca*) is the supreme predator of the ocean,
and it is very successful since most specimens captured in
nets by the Japanese have had a full stomach; some killer
whale stomachs have contained items as large as a 1500 lb.
intact walrus. The pygmy sperm whale (*Kogia breviceps*) is
represented by a single individual infant beached in Brooklyn,
N.Y. and kept alive for a few weeks at the New York Aquarium
at Coney Island. All other serum specimens were sent from the
Naval Undersea Center, San Diego, and at least seven of each
were provided with the exception of the Dall porpoise (*Phocoenoides dalli*) represented by samples from one male and one
female. The blood samples were obtained from the large veins
in the tail flukes.

Turnover studies were performed using simultaneous injections of $T_4-^{125}I$ and $T_3-^{131}I$. Plasma samples were counted
before and after precipitation with trichloroacetic acid (TCA).
The TCA precipitates were extracted for determination of the
non-hormonal (non-extractible) protein-bound iodine activity,
which was subtracted from the precipitate radioactivity. The
decay curves were analysed by non-compartmental kinetics, and
the results are given in Table 1. The results for *Tursiops
truncatus* represent the mean values of seven turnover studies
on six dolphins, whereas only a single *Lagenorhynchus obliquidens* was studied. The *Tursiops* serum T_4 concentration would
be slightly above the upper limit of normal for human serum
T_4, usually given as about 4.5 to 11.5 µg per 100 ml. The
serum T_3 concentration is well within our normal human range
by our method (mean ± S.D. = 189 ± 30 ng per 100 ml). The
biologic half-times of both hormones are shorter than the
human, presumably due to less serum protein binding. The pools

Table 1.

	Serum Concentration		$T\frac{1}{2}$ days		Pool (L)		MCR (L/day)		Removal rate (mg/day)	
	T_4 µg/ 100 ml	T_3 ng/ 100 ml	T_4	T_3	T_4	T_3	T_4	T_3	T_4	T_3
T. truncatus	12.9	161	2.0	0.7	18	80	8.78	70	1.23	0.11
L. obliquidens	2.6	60	1.4	1.1	52	137	11.22	41	0.29	0.02

and metabolic clearance rates are higher than the human. The calculated T_4 removal rate is 15 times the human mean, while T_3 removal is barely twice the human mean. On the other hand, *Lagenorhynchus obliquidens* had removal rates not so grossly different from the human : higher with respect to T_4 and lower with respect to T_3. The low serum concentrations of both T_4 and T_3 were in agreement with sera from other individuals of this species, which were not available for turnover studies.

The values for serum T_3 concentration are shown graphically in Fig. 2. With the exception of the Dall porpoise (*Phocoenoides dalli*), all other species had values similar to the human or else somewhat below. In contrast, the T_3 concentrations in the two Dall porpoise sera were markedly elevated to levels which would be compatible with frank thyrotoxicosis, if seen in human sera. Newly passed legislation protecting all cetacean species from capture in the U.S.A., without a federal permit, has obviated for the present the possibility of obtaining additional Dall porpoise sera, or carrying out turnover studies on them.

Since this species has the largest thyroid gland in relation to body weight, it seemed reasonable to infer in the

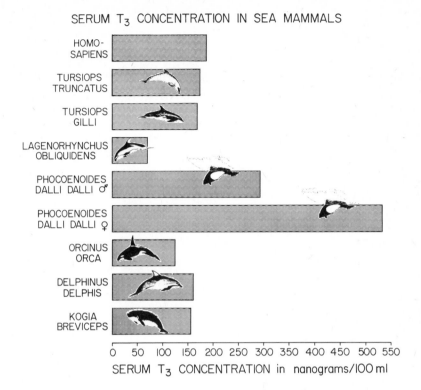

SERUM T₃ CONCENTRATION IN SEA MAMMALS

Fig. 2. *Serum T₃ concentration in sea mammals. The mean values follow.*

Species	Number of Sera	Mean T₃ Concentration in ng /100 ml
Homo sapiens	15	190
Tursiops truncatus	8	170
Tursiops gilli	3	170
Lagenorhunchus obliquidens	11	72
Phocoenoides dalli (male)	1	294
Phocoenoides dalli (female)	1	534
Orcinus orca	5	128
Delphinus delphis	8	159
Kogia breviceps	1	157

The coefficient of variation within each species did not exceed 15%.

absence of elevated T_4 concentrations that this gland might
be putting out T_3.

The speculation entertained by us is that T_3 hypersecretion in the Dall porpoise may be a physiological adapta-
tion to the cold. The conceptual schema is expressed in Fig.
3, in which the dotted lines depict the hypothetical occur-
rences during cold exposure. Other than some observations re-

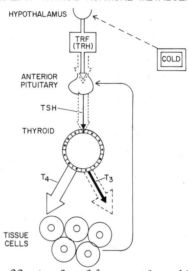

MAMMALIAN THYROID HORMONE METABOLISM

Fig. 3. *Postulated effect of cold upon thyroid hormone metabolism. The effects of cold are indicated by dotted lines,
showing a presumed effect upon the hypothalamus causing increased TRF, increased TSH, and increased T3 production from
the thyroid gland.*

garding increased TSH secretion in the rat, this might have
remained purely armchair speculation but for the recent intriguing findings of Jackson and Reichlin in the rat (3).
These workers have developed a radioimmunoassay for the tripeptide Thyrotropin Releasing Factor or Hormone (TRF or TRH)
which they have found in rat urine, apparently signifying the

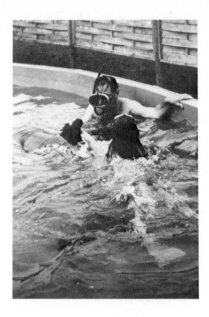

Fig. 4. *The senior author showing his daughter how to grasp the dorsal fin of a trained dolphin.*

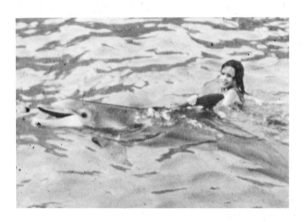

Fig. 5. *Donna and dolphin (Tursiops truncatus).*

portion of this hypothalamic hormone which escapes destruction in the circulating plasma. They have observed that the urine of cold-exposed rats contains five times the amount of tripeptide as the urine of control rats.

Such a mechanism of increased T_3 secretion should be sought especially in non-primate mammals, even if it is not operative in man and the primates.

The final figures (Figs 4 and 5) show the senior author demonstrating to his daughter how to hold the dorsal fin of a trained *Tursiops truncatus,* and the wee lass getting a ride.

R E F E R E N C E S

1.   K. Sterling, D. Bellabarba, E.S. Newman and M.A. Brenner, *J. Clin. Invest.* <u>48</u>, 1150 (1969).

2.   K. Sterling and P.O. Milch, *J. Clin. Endocrinol. Metab.* <u>38</u>, 866 (1974).

3.   I.M.D. Jackson and S. Reichlin, Program, Amer. Thyroid Assoc., Forty-Ninth Meeting, (1973).

16. Discussion of Binding and Metabolism

Papers 1 and 2

The first two papers, reviewing and introducing exciting new results on thyroid hormone binding proteins in serum, were discussed together.

The discussion on Paper 2 centred on the details of the way in which the T_4 molecule binds to the PA molecule. Ramsden suggested that it would be difficult for the T_4 molecule to penetrate the slot in the PA molecule from the phenol end and that this could account for the amino terminal part being hidden. Sterling asked if there was an explanation for the fact that although PA had two symmetrical binding sites for T_4, the binding of the second molecule was two orders of magnitude weaker than the binding of the first. Blake was not sure which end of the T_4 was deepest but suggested that if it was the amino end, then there might be repulsion resulting in negative co-operativity.

Robbins asked where the RBP binding occurred and pointed out that there was no competition between RBP and T_4. Blake suggested that the RBP sites might be in the large B-C loops (see Fig. 1 of Paper 2). Ingbar asked if there was any difference in the binding of the D and L isomers of T_4, but Blake had used only L-T_4.

Leading towards discussion on Paper 1, Oppenheimer asked if the physical structure of the PA molecule and its binding

of T_4 were compatible with the dissociation rates, and if
there might be a change of structure on the release of T_4.
Blake replied that the PA molecule looked very rigid and stable
and that he would not expect any conformational changes.

Oppenheimer wondered whether a full quantitative consideration of the T_4 dissociation rates for TBG, PA, and albumin
would really lead to the equilibrium FT_4 values. Robbins
replied that each contribution to FT_4 was proportional to
the dissociation rate, but Ingbar felt that the physical
chemistry view of the more weakly binding protein making the
larger contribution to FT_4 was not compatible with the current
picture of the importance and control of FT_4, as this would
present a kind of Alice in Wonderland situation where less
and less became more and more till nothing became everything.
Papers 3 and 4

The third and fourth papers dealt principally with studies
on the identification of thyroid hormone binding proteins
in liver cytosol, and with their specificity. The discussion
of cellular binding, however, moved naturally towards effects
on cell function.

In response to some friendly provocation by Sterling,
Oppenheimer claimed that his group had in fact been aware of
and had been working on cytosol binding since about 1966,
but as he had not yet established that the binding was specific
he could not yet support the concept of specific binding.

Ingbar and Sterling explored some of the problems and
anomalies arising from the methodology of investigation.
Although in every tissue studied separable T_3 and T_4 binding
proteins had been found, paper electrophoresis and acrylamide
gel electrophoresis gave different results. Moreover, the

multiplicity of peaks in electrophoresis studies indicated heterogeneity, whereas Scatchard plots suggested a single binding protein.

To add to the problems of disentangling the functional importance of the binding in the cytosol and in the nucleus, Robbins suggested that there might also be specific binding to cell membranes. It was reported that Edelman had shown that membranes do bind thyroid hormones and that much of the increase in metabolic rate could be ascribed to effects on the sodium pump which could amount to 65% of the total increase in thermogenesis. There had been a difference in results between thyroidectomised and normal rats.

Ingbar pointed out that Edelman had used large doses (e.g. 50 µg in the rat) and that these may have been unphysiological. Oppenheimer, however, objected that single doses of 50 µg need not be unphysiological since saturation of binding sites could limit the effects to the maximum found during normal function. Pitt-Rivers retaliated by recalling that one of the first patients treated with T_3 at Johns Hopkins had been given 1 mg instead of 100 µg and that the effect was certainly not physiological.

Oppenheimer pointed out that the increase in thermogenesis was a late effect which suggested that the action of thyroid hormones on the sodium pump should not be ascribed to direct membrane binding but rather to increased enzyme synthesis. Edmonds described results supporting this. He had been studying Na and K ATP-ase. In hypothyroid rats there had been impairment of sodium transport. It had taken 16h for 1 µg of T_3 to repair the impairment, which suggested that the T_3 acted through the nucleus. Furthermore, the action was

K

blocked by a small dose of actinomycin.

Paper 5

Harland and Orr's paper dealt with the effects of clofibrate on the kinetics of T_4 distribution and metabolism, particularly dealing with the relationship between the liver and the plasma, thus linking the first four papers.

There was general agreement, expressed mainly by Robbins and Thorp, that T_4 and T_3 enter into the liver very much more rapidly than into extra-hepatic tissues. Thorp reported that he had also found that plasma had a reduced capacity for T_4 binding and that free T_4 levels were reduced following clofibrate administration. Harland pointed out that the finding of lowered FT_4 despite the increase in T_4 secretion rate was anomalous, being contrary to what would be expected according to current dogma. Ingbar suggested, however, that FT_4 may be only one element in control and not necessarily the over-riding one. FT_4 should not be made a global explanation.

The discussion then turned to the question of exchange of T_4 between extra-hepatic tissues and plasma, on the existence of which Harland had cast some doubt. Thorp stated that he believed that such exchange did occur. Irvine gave a preview of some of his results, showing that when T_4 was given by microinjection into muscle, it could later be detected in the lymphatics. He could not agree with Harland on whether or not the labelled T_4 injected in this way into muscle should be regarded as pharmacological. The reappearance of T_4 in the lymphatics was late and this agreed with Harland's results on the difference between the disappearance rates of muscle and plasma in showing that any exchange must be a slow process

The possibility of enter-hepatic recirculation was

briefly raised. Harland pointed out that Myant's original
experiments had used very large doses of T_4. There did not
now appear to be much evidence to support the concept that
entero-hepatic recirculation was normally significant.

Papers 6 and 7

These two papers covered binding of T_3 and T_4 by pituitary
cytosol fractions and introduced evidence of temperature
effects on binding involving the conversion of pituitary
bound T_4 to T_3. Malan, in his discussion, dealt with most of
the problems arising from his results very thoroughly, but
in reply to questions from Orr he re-emphasised his conclusions
that there was a temperature effect linking T_4 and its cytosol
binding proteins.

Evered pointed out that temperature had a similar effect
on the binding of T_4 by T_4-specific antibodies and that binding
was significantly reduced if incubation was carried out at
$20^{\circ}C$ or $35^{\circ}C$. (See also the paper by Premachandra). Premachandra asked if pituitary cytosol binding protein concentration had been shown to correlate in any way with physiological status. Neither Steinbach nor Malan had data on this
point.

Papers 8 and 9

The subject of attention of the Conference was then
broadened by Papers 8 and 9 to link tissue binding with the
role which it plays in acting on T_4 by deiodination or in
other ways, and with resultant physiological effects.

Oppenheimer started the discussion by suggesting that
the different responses of pituitary and liver to thyroid
hormone were due to differences in memory function. The pituitary may adapt more quickly to changes in thyroid hormone

concentration. The mode of presentation of hormone – whether acute or chronic– was therefore important. Frumess replied that they were aware of that, and that they had therefore divided the T_3 dose so that it was administered twice daily. The TSH values fell to their lowest level 4h after administration of the dose of T_3. Wenzel suggested that conversion of T_4 to T_3 in the pituitary might account for the different time course of inhibition of TRH responsiveness in man.

Hadden asked if other antithyroid drugs had a similar effect on the regulation of TSH secretion by thyroid hormone. Frumess replied that methimazole did not affect T_4 to T_3 conversion in the same way. Evered reported the administration of T_4 and T_3 separately with and without PTU to normal subjects. The degree of inhibition of TRH responsiveness to a given dose of either T_4 or T_3 was unaffected by PTU. The serum T_4 concentration for a given dose of T_4 was unaffected by PTU administration (400 mg daily) although serum T_3 concentrations were marginally lower. Larsen pointed out that Hershman had reported an effect of PTU in this situation in hypothyroid patients.

Ingbar asked the fate of T_4 which was not peripherally converted to T_3 in PTU treated rats. Larsen suggested that it was excreted in the bile. Sterling asked if the effects of PTU on peripheral conversion were dose dependent, and reported a study of three athyreotic patients on T_4 with different doses of T_4 who were given PTU. Only one had a significant drop in T_3. Nicoloff pointed out that it required a large dose of PTU to produce a change. Urinary iodide excretion was reduced in normals on PTU, but there was no change in serum T_4 or in its disappearance rate.

Leaving the chemically produced changes in peripheral
metabolism and turning to natural peripheral resistance to
thyroid hormones, Sterling reported a case similar to Lamberg's
of a 70 year old woman who had been previously treated for
Grave's disease and was euthyroid with raised thyroid hormone
concentrations. He did not have the results of a TRH test.
Harland asked the fate of the excess thyroid hormone and
speculated as to whether this was being lost through liver
or kidney or both. Lamberg, in reply to a question from
Nicoloff, stated that there was no fluctuation in the patient's
thyroid state. Hall asked if there could have been an additional
binding protein and Lamberg replied that none had been seen
on electrophoresis and scanning. Oppenheimer asked if the T_4
measurements had been checked by immunoassay and Evered
replied that the later samples had been. Thomson reported a
family with high TBG and high thyroid hormone levels. Robbins
reported that Weintraub had observed some similar cases.
Ingbar wondered if sensitivity to thyroid hormone varied from
tissue to tissue. Lamberg replied that hydroxyproline excretion
was abnormal in two subjects.
Paper 10

The complexity of whole body thyroid hormone kinetics
brought about by the very wide variations in rates of transfer
and in binding was made clear by the very nice results presented by Irvine. Nicoloff asked what proportion of T_4 went
to the liver. Irvine replied that it was 30-35% in man and
about half of this amount in sheep. He wondered if it was
possible to do simultaneous T_4 and T_3 compartment studies
and study conversion. Oppenheimer said that it was possible
to do shorter experiments but that one could take the equili-

brium time point in man. Pochin asked the standard error of
the time constants since the presence of 4 compartments suggested the clustering of rates for different tissues. Irvine
replied that the half time of the final slope in man was $2\frac{1}{2}$
days and that sampling was continued for 96 hours. Final
analysis was carried out using the "Simplex" system and there
were major differences between the exponents of the various
terms. Robbins asked the rate from interstitial fluid into
the cell. Irvine replied that this occurred very rapidly and
that the slow stage of transfer was at the capillary wall,
and he was unable to detect any difference at any cell membrane
except in the liver which has no effective capillary wall.
Hilditch asked how these values compared with those derived
from the single compartment model. Irvine replied that lower
values were obtained with a single compartment model.

Paper 11

In Paper 11 Oppenheimer returned to the role played by
tissue binding in the expression of the physiological effects
of thyroid hormones, providing evidence that limited capacity
nuclear protein binding sites for T_3 were a major determinant
of the effects produced.

Burger pointed out that by employing the GPD level as an
index of T_3 activity, Oppenheimer had assumed the protein
synthesis model. He asked about effects on O_2 consumption,
but Oppenheimer had no data on this. Burger also raised the
problem of the real meaning of "activity", and Oppenheimer
agreed that care must be taken in defining it. Account must
be taken of such things as the mode of presentation. For
example, triac and T_3 have the same effect when they occupy
the binding sites for the same length of time.

Hoffenberg commented that the organ studies used whole organs. He suggested that it would be more satisfactory to look at different cell types in, for example, the kidney and the brain. Oppenheimer replied that they had done some work on cellular fractionation of the brain but that this was very difficult and that they had not yet managed to do it satisfactorily. The alternative of autoradiography was also very difficult. The only feasible way was in tissue culture.

Sterling commented that the association constants for the binding of T_3 to the nuclear sites had about the same values both for responsive and for unresponsive tissues. How was this? Oppenheimer replied that the essence of the difference between responsive and unresponsive tissues was the number of sites, not the association constants.

Larsen suggested that if the difference between the effects of two doses of T_3 was due to greater saturation of the binding sites, there should be a maximum response if the T_3 level was kept high enough persistently, and asked if this or the effect of giving more frequent injections had been studied. Oppenheimer had found that 20 µg/100g/d for 7 or 8 days gave the maximum response, which remained the same even for doses of 200 µg/100g/d. The maximum activity was 9 or 10 times the euthyroid level. Larsen was surprised that although at physiological concentrations of T_3, the binding sites were 50% saturated, the amounts of T_3 required to reach full saturation seemed very high (e.g. 15 µg/100g/d for the remaining 50%). Was it possible that the turnover rate of T_3 increased as the amount bound increased? However, Oppenheimer explained that the T_3 kinetics were almost identical at different T_3 levels although there was a slight increase in the fractional turnover with increasing saturation. The half-life became 4h at saturation instead of the normal 6h.

Nicoloff asked how the effects of one dose per day and three doses per day were distinguished. Was it the area under the activity-time curve or the absolute level of activity which was taken as a measure of effect? Oppenheimer replied that they were dealing with a non-linear system and must integrate two different functions. It was more complex than just the area under the curve.

Thorp asked if there was any difference between species in GPD response. The only data Oppenheimer knew of were those of Samuels who demonstrated the existence of nuclear binding sites in humans.

Papers 12 and 13

The next two papers presented results on the effects of thyroid hormone on two other measures of thyroid hormone activity, the responses of urinary and plasma cyclic AMP, and L-triiodothyronine aminotransferase activity.

Guttler was asked for his views on the source of the cAMP. He felt that it probably came from widely diffused locations. Sterling interpreted the results as an increase of the amount of membrane bound AC in hyperthyroids, and a reduction in hypothyroids. Guttler agreed that this was likely. There was a difference between the response of ATPase and cAMP — cAMP had a shorter induction time (2h).

Hoffenberg could not understand why Guttler did not get a blunted response to glucagon in hypothyroid conditions. He had found lower levels. Lazarus described and illustrated results he had obtained on plasma cAMP response to i.v.

glucagon, in hyper-, hypo-, and euthyroid subjects. All
showed a peak at 20 min, but the hyperthyroid peak was twice
as high as the euthyroid peak, which itself was twice as
high as the hypothyroid peak. Lazarus also described results by
Campbell and Kane-Maguire showing that the exposure of cultures
of rat liver to glucagon for 15 min produced a much higher
content of cAMP if the liver cultures had previously been
incubated with T_3.

Rivlin was asked why he had looked at steroids, and
explained that he had been interested in thyroid adrenal
steroid relationships, and had done work on the effects of
adrenal steroids on other transaminases. Thorp commented
that the action of the enzyme was chemically reversible, and
asked if the reaction could go in the opposite direction,
but Rivlin thought that it probably only went in one direction.

Paper 14

Ramsden suggested that Burger's methodology caused an
underestimate of the conversion of TA_4 to TA_3. Gas chromatography showed that 30% was converted. Burger, however, felt
that Ramsden's figures gave too high a production rate for TA_3,
and explained that he had used a competitive protein binding
assay at first, but that there were too many binding inhibitors
present, and that therefore he had changed to a radio-immuno-
assay. Larsen asked how an antibody specific to the correct
end of the TA_3 molecule was obtained. Burger replied that
they did an initial separation by chromatography; they did
not have an antibody specific for TA_3.

17. A Routine Method for the Estimation of Thyroxine Binding Globulin in Human Serum

I.P. DRYSDALE, D.B. RAMSDEN AND R. HOFFENBERG

Division of Clinical Investigation,

Clinical Research Centre, Harrow

and Department of Medicine, University of Birmingham.

INTRODUCTION

There are two commonly used methods of estimating thyroxine binding globulin in serum :

a) based on saturation analysis (1,2)

b) indirectly by the T_3 uptake method (3) which reflects unoccupied binding sites.

Both measure hormone binding capacity not concentration. Within the past five years a few reports have described methods for the direct measurement of TBG concentration. First of these was that of Freeman and Pearson (4) who used a Laurell two dimensional immuno-electrophoretic method to precipitate the proteins in the form of Gaussian or near Gaussian peaks whose area was proportional to antigen concentration. TBG was identified by saturating the precipitate with radioactive T_4, washing off excess T_4, then submitting the plate to autoradiography. Whilst this method has the advantage of simultaneously allowing measurement of the concentration of many other serum proteins, it is too cumbersome and costly in antiserum and other reagents for routine assay of TBG alone.

Several variants of this technique have been published which use serum prelabelled with radioactive T_4 and Laurell "monorocket" immuno-electrophoresis in which the antigen is electrophoresed directly into the antiserum-containing gel (5,6).

Radioimmunoassay for TBG has been developed by Levy *et al.* (7) but their method requires stringently pure TBG and a monospecific anti-TBG, which are not easily prepared.

In view of the above points the most readily available and cheapest system would appear to be the modified monorocket technique, since this requires little specialist equipment and materials. In this paper therefore we describe the technical details and validation of such a method for estimation of TBG concentration in serum.

E X P E R I M E N T A L

Materials

The following materials were obtained from the sources indicated below :-

Agarose "Indubiose-A37", Industrie Biologique Francaise, from Micro-Bio Laboratories, Pembridge Road, London, W11.

Anti-whole human serum from either Wellcome Reagents Ltd., Beckenham, Kent or Dakopats, Mercia Ltd., Sandown Road, Watford.

^{125}I-Thyroxine from the Radiochemical Centre, Amersham, Bucks.

TEAE-Cellulose from Sigma Chemicals Ltd., Croydon, Surrey.

Kodirex from Kodak U.K. Ltd.

Glass plates from the Chance Glass Co. Ltd., Birmingham.

The reference sera were gifts from Blood Products Laboratories Lister Institute, Elstree, Herts. or National Institute for Biological Standards, Hampstead, London (Batch No. 68/449).

All other chemicals were obtained from either B.D.H. Ltd.
or Hopkins and Williams Ltd. and were of "Lab. reagent" or
"General purpose reagent" quality.

Methods

Purification of Agarose. To a hot solution (80°C) of agarose (2% w/v) was added TEAE-cellulose powder (10g/1). The
mixture was stirred vigorously for 60 min then filtered, the
temperature being maintained at 80°C throughout. The filtrate
was divided into 200 ml lots and stored at 4°C until required.

Laurel "Monorocket" immunoelectrophoresis. "Monorocket"
immunoelectrophoresis was performed as described by Laurell
(8) with a number of modifications. These were :-

(a) the buffer used was sodium phosphate (0.025 M with regard
to phosphate) of pH 7.4.

(b) Agarose purified as described above was used to reduce
excessive electroendosmosis which otherwise occurs at this
pH.

(c) Since no specific anti-TBG was available, antiwhole human
serum was employed instead.

(d) TBG was identified by prelabelling the sample with ^{125}I-
T_4 and submitting the immunoelectrophoretogram to autoradiography before staining.

(e) Antigen wells were not punched directly into the antiserum
containing gel but into an agarose strip (2.5 cm wide) containing only buffer. This strip will subsequently be referred
to as the "buffer gel".

The buffer gel was placed on one edge of a glass plate
and antiserum containing gel poured on to the remainder of
the plate and allowed to set. Antigen wells were then punched
into the buffer gel approximately 0.5 cm from the outer edge,

so that the antigens were electrophoresed through 1.5 to 2
cm of buffer gel before coming into contact with antibodies.
Normally glass plates (11 cm x 11 cm) were used and each
contained either 2.5 ml of Wellcome antiserum or 1.5 ml of
Dakopats allowing eight TBG estimations per plate, two of
which were always reference sera. With large plates a greater
number of samples could be run simultaneously and correspondingly larger amounts of antiserum were used. Before electrophoresis, serum (50 µl) was equilibrated with $^{125}I\text{-}T_4$ solution (200 µCi/ml and 4 µg/ml) for 1 hour at room temperature.
The amount of radioactive T_4 added was sufficient to bring
the T_4 concentration to about 5x physiological (arbitrarily
acceoted as 8 µg/100 ml). Equilibrated serum (2 µl) was added
to each antigen well. After electrophoresis excess antiserum
was removed by placing a damp filter paper onto the surface
of the gel. The plate and paper together were then dried in
a stream of warm air. When both were thoroughly dry the filter
paper was peeled off and discarded. A thin sheet of plastic
was placed between the X-ray film and the immunoelectrophoretogram which was submitted to autoradiography for 7 days.
After this the X-ray film was developed and the immunoelectrophoretogram stained for protein using amido black solution.

R E S U L T S

Figure 1 shows a typical autoradiograph of human serum
prelabelled with $^{125}I\text{-}T_4$ and submitted to quantitative monorocket immunoelectrophoresis. One precipitin peak, TBG,
clearly possesses bound $^{125}I\text{-}T_4$ although from the stained
plate many protein peaks are visible. Other serum proteins
are known to bind thyroxine but under the conditions described

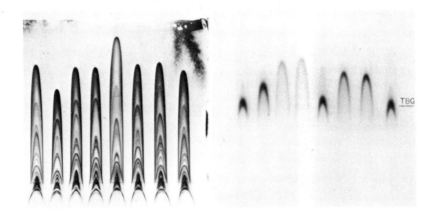

Fig. 1. *Typical "monorocket" immunoelectrophoretogram. Auto-radiograph shows one highly radioactive peak corresponding to TBG which is not visible on original plate when stained for protein with amido black, although many other serum proteins are visible. Broken line on autoradiograph indicates the position of buffer gel.*

either insufficient antiserum was used to precipitate them on the immunoelectrophoretogram or they bound too little ^{125}I-T_4 to cause an intense image to be formed on the X-ray film.

The advantage of using a buffer gel for consistent results is illustrated in Fig. 2. Here a wedge-shaped buffer gel was used so that some antigen wells are punched into antibody containing gel and others into the buffer gel at gradually increasing distances from the antiserum containing gel. Where the antigen well was directly surrounded by antiserum, ^{125}I-T_4 was displaced almost entirely from the sample, and where the antigen well was only partially surrounded by

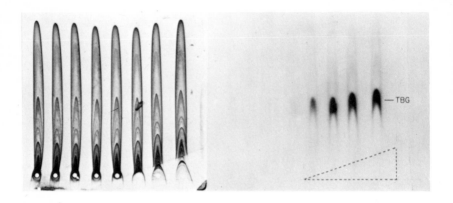

Fig. 2. *"Monorocket" immunoelectrophoretogram with wedge-shaped buffer gel. The autoradiograph shows that binding of ^{125}I-T_4 by sample serum was retained only when the antigen well was separated from antiserum-containing gel by the buffer-gel. Equal mounts of sample and radioactivity were placed in each antigen well. Broken line on autoradiograph indicates the position of buffer gel.*

antibody slightly more efficient binding occurred. Optimal binding was found when the antigen well was some distance from the antiserum. The factor in the antiserum responsible for the displacement of T_4 was not dialysable and was present in commercial preparations of purified sheep anti-human serum protein immunoglobulins. This factor was also present in specific rabbit or sheep antisera to a range of human serum proteins e.g. caeruloplasmin, transferrin, IgA, IgM, IgG, Albumin, α_1-antitrypsin.

Since no pure preparation of human TBG was available the

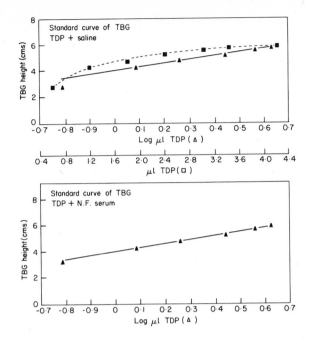

Fig. 3. *Upper graph shows a typical dilution curve when working standard serum (TDP) was diluted with saline. The broken
line is a plot of height of TBG in cm against sample volume
in µl. The solid line is a plot of height of TBG peak against
log sample volume. The lower graph is a dilution curve obtained when the working standard serum was diluted with a
serum with a very low TBG concentration. The parallelism of
the two solid lines indicates that the ratio of albumin to
TBG did not influence peak height of TBG.*

system was calibrated using a standard reference serum (Nat.
Institute for Biol. Standard Serum No. 68/449). Because only
limited quantities of this could be obtained a second standard
serum, which was part of a thousand donor pool (TDP) was
used throughout as an internal reference and working standard.
All results referred to in this communication are quoted in
terms of percentage of working standard which was diluted
with acid : citrate : dextrose at collection. All concent-

Table 1.   *Reproducibility Data*

	Number of Observations	Mean	S.D.	$\frac{\text{S.D.} \times 100}{\text{Mean}}$
Inter-assay Standard Serum	50	4.06 cm	0.12 cm	3.0
Normal Serum	50	113.6%	2.19%	1.9
Intra-assay Standard Serum	10	3.83 cm	0.026 cm	<1
Normal Serum	10	121 %	0.8%	<1

Units of Standard Serum = peak height in cm

Units of Normal serum = $\dfrac{\text{peak height of normal} \times 100}{\text{peak height of standard}}$

Reproducibility of measurement of the TBG concentration of a working standard serum and a normal serum.

rations of normal serum are therefore greater than 100%.
Inter-laboratory comparison may be made by reference to the
Standard Reference Serum (68/449, National Institute for
Biological Standards) which had a TBG concentration 1.21 times
greater than the working standard. Figure 3 shows a typical
calibration curve of the peak height of the TBG peak against
volume of working standard for the range 0.6 µl to 4.2 µl
serum. Although the plot of peak height v concentration is
not linear, probably because area under the precipitin peak
is a truer estimate of concentration, this proved to be the
most convenient way of expressing results. Linearity was
more nearly approached when peak height was plotted against
log volume. It has been suggested that TBG may undergo some
protein-protein interaction with albumin which may influence
its electrophoretic mobility (9). Whilst the above method
is relatively independent of mobility such interaction could
affect the precipitation by antibody. To test for this, a
serum from a subject with very low thyroxine binding globulin
concentration was diluted with increasing amounts of the
working standard serum. This had the effect of keeping albumin
and other serum proteins approximately constant with an increasing concentration of TBG. The results were compared with
those obtained when increasing amounts of working standard
were added to saline. The parallelism of the two lines indicated that any protein-protein interactions which did occur
did not affect this system.

An important feature of any assay is its reproducibility.
To test this a normal serum as well as the standard serum
was run on a number of plates. The results are shown in Table
1.

In the relatively short period of time that the assay
has been functioning, we have not collected serum from an adequate number of healthy euthyroid subjects to obtain a comp-
rehensive table of values of TBG concentration for ten year
age groupings. However the results obtained so far for both
males and females suggest that there is a noticeable increase
from the 20-29 age-group to the 30-39 group which then either
remains constant or increases slightly until the age of sixty.
Table 2 also shows the average TBG concentration expressed as
a percentage of the working standard for males and females
irrespective of age. There is a significant difference between
the means for males and for females (P < 0.05).

Table 2. *Serum TBG Concentration of Healthy Euthyroids*

	Male			Female		
	No.	S.D.	Mean	No.	S.D.	Mean
20 - 29	22	6.6	123	11	5.3	128
30 - 39	23	6.1	130	8	6.8	130
40 - 49	16	5.3	132	13	3.8	132
50 - 59	15	5.9	133	9	4.1	136
60 - 69	6	3.7	131	–	–	–
Total	82	6.9	129	41	5.5	132

Units = % TBG concentration of working standard serum.
Serum TBG concentration of normal males and females.

For a "normal" hospital population of patients with disorders other than those of the thyroid the mean TBG concentration was similar to healthy normals although the standard
deviation was greater (Table 3).

In both hyper- and hypothyroidism in females the mean
TBG concentration was not significantly different from the

Table 3. *Serum TBG Concentrations of Hospitalised Euthyroids*

	Hospitalised Euthyroid		Normal	
	Male	Female	Male	Female
Number	17	27	82	41
S.D.	9.5	7.8	6.9	5.5
Mean	130	135	129	132

Units = % TBG concentration working standard serum

Serum TBG concentration of hospitalised euthyroid subjects and healthy euthyroid subjects.

Table 4. *Serum TBG Concentration in Hypo- and Hyperthyroidism*

	Hypothyroid		Normal Euth.		Hyper.
	Female	Male	Male	Female	Female
Number	23	7	82	41	16
S.D.	11.9	16.7	6.9	5.5	9.7
Mean	132	145	129	132	130

Units = % TBG concentration of working standard serum

Serum TBG concentration of hypo- and hyperthyroid subjects and healthy euthyroid subjects.

mean for euthyroid females although the scatter as shown by the standard deviation was somewhat greater perhaps because of the wider age-range (Table 4).

Sera from pregnant females had a mean value some 30% higher than the normal, whilst the mean for cord serum was approximately mid-way between these two values (Table 5).

The sensitivity and highly reproducible nature of the assay allowed detection of relatively small changes in TBG concentration. Figure 4a shows the values of TBG concentration

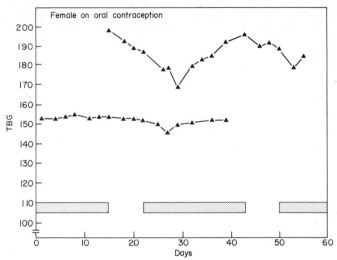

Fig. 4a

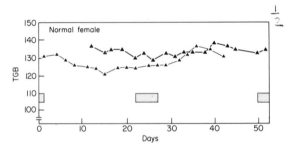

Fig. 4b

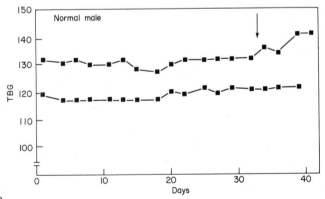

Fig. 4c

of sera taken at 2 or 3 day intervals through one cycle for two females taking oral contraceptives, two normal females (Fig. 4b) and over a similar time course two normal males of similar age (Fig. 4c).

The initial effect of oestrogen and its continuing effect after cessation of administration on TBG concentration is shown in Fig. 5. In one subject who had been taking a low oestrogen dose for more than three years the TBG level did not return to normal value until thirty days after stopping the pills. In a second subject on a two-month course of a high oestrogen dose the TBG level began to rise after an initial period of 3 days.

Thirteen patients were investigated before and after minor or medium surgery. In 12, within three days there was a mean decrease in TBG concentration of 6.8%, with a standard deviation of 3% of the preoperative level. After this the TBG either returned to the preoperative level or in some cases where the patient continued to be unwell remained low. In only one case did the TBG level rise immediately after surgery. A typical result for one patient is shown in Fig. 6.

DISCUSSION

The estimation of thyroxine binding globulin is usually made by measurement of binding capacity rather than actual

Fig. 4. *Plot of serum TBG concentration against time. (a) for two females taking low oestrogen oral contraceptives, cross-hatched bars indicate times during which contraceptive was administered; (b) for two normal females, here cross-hatched bars indicate menstrual periods; (c) for two normal males, the arrow indicates the time at which one of the males developed a common cold.*

Table 5.   *Serum TBG Concentration in Neonates (Cord) and*
Pregnant Females.

	Pregnant Females	Cord Serum	Normal Female
Number	34	66	41
S.D.	15.3	14.8	5.5
Mean	158	146	132

Units = % TBG concentration of working standard serum.
TBG concentration of serum from pregnant females,
healthy euthyroid females and neonates (cord).

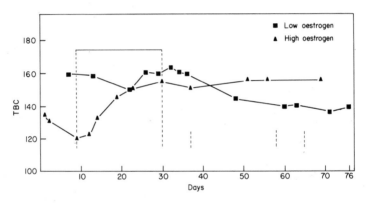

Fig. 5. *Plot of TBG concentration against time for two females
taking oral contraceptives. One female was on a high oestrogen
contraceptive for two months only, the other had been on a
low oestrogen contraceptive for more than three years, the
last one month being studied. The extended broken lines joined
by a solid horizontal line indicate time when concraceptive
was taken by both subjects. The smaller vertical broken lines
indicate alternating 21 and 7 day intervals. Only the subject
on the high oestrogen dose was taking the contraceptives
during the second 21 day period.*

concentration of protein and therefore any conclusion from

such measurements regarding concentration always possesses a

degree of uncertainty. In this communication a method has

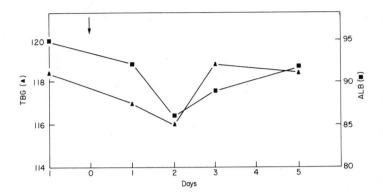

Fig. 6. *A graph of TBG and albumin concentration against time for a typical patient immediately pre-operatively and for five days post-operatively. The arrow indicates approximate time of operation.*

been described for the estimation of TBG concentration using a modified form of the Laurell "monorocket" immunoelectrophoretic technique combined with autoradiography. For consistently successful autoradiography in the method it was found necessary to ensure that the antigen well was punched into a strip of agarose gel which contained no antiserum. Why this buffer gel was essential is obscure but it is possible that the excess of animal TBG within the antiserum stripped the human proteins of T_4 if the two were allowed to come into contact. However when a buffer gel was used this appeared to allow sufficient physical separation for the animal TBG to be electrophoresed off the plate as the human migrated into the antiserum and competitive binding of T_4 was obviated.

It has been suggested that human TBG and albumin undergo some form of protein-protein interaction which is sufficiently

strong to influence the electrophoretic mobility of TBG (9).
Although the assay method employed here is theoretically independent of electrophoretic mobility such interaction may
affect the ability of antibodies to precipitate TBG. However
the parallelism of the curves when standard human serum was
diluted with either saline or serum from a patient with a very
low concentration of thyroxine binding globulin suggests that
if such interactions occur they are either disrupted by the
conditions employed or have no significant interfering effect
on precipitation by antibodies.

The results obtained using this method show a small but
significant difference between the TBG concentration of a
euthyroid male and female population. Comparison of hospitalised euthyroids with normal healthy euthyroid subjects showed
no significant difference which is in agreement with previous
workers using capacity measurements (10). For both hyper- and
hypothyroid females there appeared to be no significant difference between the mean values and that for euthyroid females
although the scatter as shown by the standard deviation was
greater. Most workers using capacity measurements have suggested that there is no significant difference between hyperthyroid and euthyroid subjects (10,11,12) and that TBG is
raised in hypothyroidism (13). Using radioimmunoassay Levy
et al. (7) have shown a significant decrease in TBG concentration in hyperthyroid subjects and no significant difference
in hypothyroidism when compared to euthyroid levels. The elevation in TBG concentration found in pregnancy and cord blood
is well recognised and in agreement with the results of capacity measurements (14, 15).

The effect of oestrogens in raising TBG concentration

are clearly demonstrated and in agreement with previous observations using capacity measurements (16,17). The results
obtained for normal females through one complete menstrual
cycle show raised TBG concentration at about the time of
ovulation when oestrogen values are known to be high, followed
by a decline to a minimum before the onset of menstrual blee-
ding. In two females who were taking an oral contraceptive
pill this picture was altered and the mean values were higher.
Here the TBG level appeared to be regulated by exogenous
oestrogen. Cessation was followed by a slow decline in TBG
concentration reaching a minimum value only 14-16 days later,
reflecting a continued action of oestrogen either on synthesis
or breakdown of TBG. Whether the very different mean values
in these two are due to differing normal response to oestrogen
or the different composition of the contraceptives used is
unclear since only two subjects were studied.

The continuing effect of oestrogens after cessation of
administration was clearly demonstrated in one subject. The
fact that even on a high oestrogen dose the lag period before
a rise in TBG was observed was 3 days after commencement of
administration in one person, would support the observation
that in females taking low oestrogen oral contraceptives
over a long period, the minimum TBG level occurs some while
after the start of a fresh cycle.

A recent paper has claimed that the major thyroxine
binding protein response to surgery is an interruption of
TBPA synthesis, with no alteration in TBG levels, but this
observation was based on the results of capacity measurements
(18). Using the modified "monorocket" technique described
here, consistent reduction in serum TBG concentration was

observed within 2 to 3 days of surgery. Whether this is due
to a decrease in synthesis, increase in catabolism or a shift
from an intra- to extra-vascular compartment is unknown. Since
most circulating thyroxine is bound to TBG, relatively smaller
alterations in TBG concentration could significantly affect
free hormone values, which have been shown to rise after
surgery, to an extent equal to the effects of larger alterations in TBPA concentration.

CONCLUSIONS

A method for the measurement of thyroxine binding globulin concentration in serum which involves immunoelectrophoresis combined with autoradiography is described. The method
requires little specialised equipment and materials and is
highly reproducible. The results obtained for a variety of
pathological conditions are consistent with those of previous
workers using techniques for estimation of thyroxine binding
capacity.

Acknowledgements
    *We wish to thank Dr. R.L. Himsworth, Division of Clinical
Investigation, Clinical Research Centre and Dr. B. Lewis,
Foyal Postgraduate Medical School for helpful advice and dis-
cussions.*

REFERENCES

1.   J. Robbins, *Arch. Biochem. Biophys.* **63**, 461-469 (1956).

2.   J. Robbins, *In* "Evaluation of Thyroid and Parathyroid
     Functions", (F.W. Sunderman and F.W. Sunderman, Jr.eds)
     Lippincott, Philadelphia, (1963).

3.   M.W. Hamolsky, M. Stern and A.S. Freedberg, *J. Clin.
     Endocrinol. and Metab.* **17**, 33-44 (1957).

4.   T. Freeman and D.J. Pearson, *Clin. Chim. Acta* **26**, 365-
     368 (1969).

5.   H.G. Nielson, O. Buus and B. Weeke, *Clin. Chim. Acta*
     36, 133-138 (1972).

6. T. Kranz, A. Trantwein and A. Sieber, *Z. Klin. Chem. Klin. Biochem.* 12, 124-127 (1974).

7. R.P. Levy, J.S. Marshall and N.L. Velago, *J. Clin. Endocrinol. and Metab.* 32, 372-381 (1971).

8. C.B. Laurell, *Anal. Biochem.* 15, 45-52 (1966).

9. M. Inada and K. Sterling, *J. Clin. Endocrinol. and Metab.* 31, 417-421 (1970).

10. J.H. Oppenheimer, R. Squef, M.I. Surks and H. Hauer, *J. Clin. Invest.* 42, 1769-1782 (1963).

11. J. Robbins and J.E. Rall, *Recent Progr. in Hormone Research,* 13, 161-208 (1957).

12. J. Robbins and J.E. Rall, *Physiol. Rev.* 40, Suppl. 4, 415-489 (1960).

13. M. Inada and K. Sterling, *J. Clin. Invest.* 46, 1442-1450 (1967).

14. J.T. Dowling, N. Freinkel and S.H. Ingbar, *J. Clin. Invest.* 35, 1263-1276 (1956).

15. J. Robbins and J.H. Nelson, *J. Clin. Invest.* 37, 153-159 (1958).

16. J.T. Dowling, N. Freinkel and S.H. Ingbar, *J. Clin. Endocrinol. and Metab.* 16, 1491-1506 (1956).

17. N.H. Engbring and W.W. Engstrom, *J. Clin. Endocrinol. and Metab.* 19, 783-796 (1959).

18. I.D.A. Johnston, *Advances in Clin. Chem.* 15, 255-285 (1972).

18. Thyroxine Antibody vs. Serum Protein Binding of T_4 in the Cold; Differential Charcoal Adsorption of T_4 from Immuno and Conventional T_4 Binding Sites

B.N. PREMACHANDRA AND I.I. IBRAHIM.

Veterans Admin. Hospital, Jefferson Barracks and Washington University, St. Louis, Missouri, U.S.A.

A radioimmunoassay (RIA) for thyroxine in unextracted serum was recently reported from this laboratory (1). The procedure basically consisted in denaturing T_4 binding proteins in serum by tricholoroacetic acid - sodium hydroxide mixture and T_4 released was allowed to react with $^{125}I\text{-}T_4$ labelled T_4 antiserum; the displaced $^{125}I\text{-}T_4$ was taken up by the resin sponge and this uptake was linearly related to T_4 present in serum or standards. In the course of these investigations it was noted that standard curve values obtained with T, antiserum freshly labelled with $^{125}I\text{-}T_4$ (30 min equilibration at room temperature) were invariably higher than those obtained with over-night refrigerated $^{125}I\text{-}T_4$ labelled anti-serum. To further investigate T_4 - T_4 antibody interaction, binding of radio-thyroxine ($^{125}I\text{-}T_4$) in T_4 antiserum at equilibrium was systematically examined in the cold, and for comparison binding of $^{125}I\text{-}T_4$ in normal human serum was studied in an identical manner. As activated charcoal was used to adsorb ("strip")

*
Investigations supported in part by Abbott Laboratories, North Chicago, Ill.

thyronines from serum to provide hormone free serum in the
preparation of T_4 standards for T_4-RIA, the "stripping" procedure was also used to examine the strength of the bond between
T_4 and T_4 binding proteins in normal human serum as well as
in rabbit T_4 antiserum.

Equilibration of tracer concentrations of radiothyroxine
was considerably delayed in T_4 antiserum and furthermore,
unlike in human serum, marked resistance to charcoal "stripping"
of T_4 was noted in thyroxine immune serum.

MATERIALS AND METHODS

T_4 RIA

The details of T_4-RIA procedure have been described in
detail elsewhere (1). T_4 antiserum used in this assay was generated in rabbits immunised against porcine thyroglobulin emul-
sified in Freund's adjuvant.

Equilibration Binding of ^{125}I-T_4 in T_4 Antiserum:

Binding of radiothyroxine (^{125}I-T_4) in thyroxine antiserum
was studied at a temperature of between $0^{\circ}C$ and $1^{\circ}C$. Antiserum
was labelled with ^{125}I-T_4 (5 μg/100 ml) and 80-fold dilution
(as used in T_4-RIA) was made in phosphate buffer. The vial of
diluted antibody solution was placed immediately in an ice
bath (0-1$^{\circ}C$). One ml aliquots of diluted labelled antiserum
were dispensed rapidly (within 2 min) into a series of tubes
which were then transferred to the ice bath. At 10, 15, 30
and 60 min after radiothyroxine labelling, and at hourly intervals thereafter up to 10 h, 5 anionic resin sponges were
introduced into the tubes and 5 min sponge ^{125}I-T_4 uptake in
quintuplicate were determined. Resin uptake of ^{125}I-T_4 represented a measure of unbound thyroxine and when this uptake

became constant, equilibration between ^{125}I-T_4 tracer and T_4 antiserum was considered complete. Binding of ^{125}I-T_4 in 1:80 diluted human serum was also studied in an identical manner.

^{125}I-T_4 and ^{131}I-T_4 Extraction Efficiency:
    Tracer amounts of ^{125}I-T_4 or ^{131}I-T_4 (2µg/100ml) were added to individual serum samples and allowed to bind for 30 min. Radioactivity in 1 ml labelled serum represented initial activity. One ml labelled serum was added dropwise to 2 ml 95% ethanol or any of the other extracting solvents (see results) and the contents of the tube were vigorously mixed in a Vortex mixer for 30 sec and left at room temperature for 30 min. Samples were then centrifuged at 3000 rpm for 5 min and supernatant radioactivity per ml determined. Radiothyroxine extraction

recovery (%) = $\dfrac{\text{Supernatant radioactivity x 3}}{\text{Initial radioactivity}}$ x 100.   95%

ethanol was chosen for T_4 extraction in most of the investig-ations as the coefficient of variance in extraction efficiency noted was the least (see results).

Charcoal "Stripping" of Normal Human Sera and Rabbit T_4 Anti-Sera.

    Endogenous T_4 in sera was "stripped" by treatment with activated charcoal (NoritA, Sigma Chemical Co.). Charcoal (20g) was added to 100 ml of Millipore filtered human serum. Unless noted otherwise, the slurry was stirred gently for 1 h at room temperature and left in the cold room (48-50°F) for 24 h; it was centrifuged 3 to 5 times at 10,000 rpm and subjected to serial filtration through Millipore filters (1.2 µ-0.22µ). In concurrent investigations, aliquots of serum labelled with ^{125}I-T_4 were also treated with charcoal as just described. The

L

radioactivity in 1 ml Millipore filtered charcoal treated serum
was compared with radioactivity in 1 ml prior to charcoal pro-
cessing. T_4 extraction was also confirmed by actual T_4 determinations in untreated and charcoal treated serum.

Immunoassayable TBG :

These estimations were performed by the Nichols Laboratory
(Wilmington, California).

TBG, TBPA and Antibody T_4 Binding Capacity :

The procedures for determining TBG and TBPA T_4 binding
capacity have been described in detail elsewhere (2). Similar
procedures were used to determine maximum T_4 antibody binding
capacity.

Total Protein :

Protein analysis was carried out by the biuret method.

R E S U L T S   A N D   C O M M E N T S

T_4-RIA Standard Curves :

Standard curves obtained with T_4 antiserum equilibrated
with ^{125}I-T_4 in the cold (0-4°C) for 30 min, 8h or 24 h are
shown in Fig. 1. A downward displacement of standard curves
was consistently noted when T_4 antiserum used in T_4-RIA was
allowed to equilibrate for increasingly longer intervals with
^{125}I-T_4. T_4 dose response curves generally became steady when
antiserum was equilibrated with ^{125}I-T_4 tracer at least overnight in cold. Standard curve values obtained with 30 min
equilibrated ^{125}I-T_4 antiserum were higher than the values obtained with the same T_4 antiserum but equilibrated for 8h with
^{125}I-T_4 by 3.1, 2.6, 2.3 and 1.8% respectively, corresponding
to 0, 5, 10 and 15 µg/100 ml T_4 standards. These differences
could not be attributed to the decrease in the sensitivity of
the assay with increased duration of equilibration of T_4 anti-

serum with radiothyroxine tracer since the differences in assay
response between 0 and 15 µg T_4 standards (29.7 graphical units)
were virtually the same whether or not $^{125}I-T_4-$ T_4 antiserum
equilibration was carried out for 30 min, 8h or 24h.

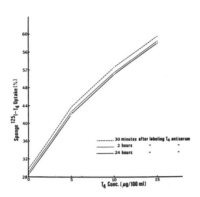

Fig. 1. *T_4 standard curves obtained in the RIA procedure
using T_4 antiserum equilibrated for 30 min, 2h or 24h with
thyroxine tracer. The values for standard curves stabilised
generally after an overnight equilibration in cold of $^{125}I-T_4$
tracer with T_4 antiserum.*

The differences in standard curve response became much
smaller when comparisons were made between values obtained
with 8h and 24h $^{125}I-T_4$ equilibrated antiserum. There was also
some indication that the differences in standard curve values
obtained with T_4 antiserum incompletely equilibrated with $^{125}I-T_4$ were more pronounced in a disequilibrated antigen–antibody
system (in contract to the completely equilibrated antigen–
antibody system as used in our T_4-RIA procedure) (3). That
the difference in standard curve values as noted in these
studies were largely due to incomplete equilibration of T_4
antiserum with $^{125}I-T_4$ tracer was also shown in more direct

Table 1. *Binding of* $^{125}I\text{-}T_4$ *in diluted (1:80)* T_4 *antiserum and pooled human serum as studied at a low temperature* (1^oC) *using resin sponges.*

Duration of Equilibration of $^{125}I\text{-}T_4$ with	Sponge $^{125}I\text{-}T_4$ Uptake [a]	
T_4 Antiserum or Human Serum	T_4 Anti- Serum	Pooled Human Serum
10 minutes	4.00	14.77
15 minutes	3.73	12.91
30 minutes	3.40	11.65
1 hour	3.19	11.01
2 hours	2.98	10.82
3 hours	2.73	10.86
4 hours	2.80	10.92
6 hours	2.60	10.89
7 hours	2.68	10.87
8 hours	2.53	–
9 hours	2.55	–
10 hours	2.54	–
24 hours	2.53	10.88

a *At the end of various equilibration periods, sponges were incubated with labelled serum for 5min and* ^{125}I *T_4 uptake was measured in quintuplicate samples.*

experiments as noted below.

Equilibration Binding of $^{125}I\text{-}T_4$ *in Normal Human Serum and Rabbit* T_4 *Antiserum :*

With increasing time interval up to 8h after radiothyroxine labelling 5-minute-sponge $^{125}I\text{-}T_4$ uptake showed a progressive decline after which no further decrease in uptake was noted (Table 1); this indicated that at 8h equilibrium had been attained in the interaction between ^{125}I-T$_4$ tracer and T$_4$ antiserum. Between 10 min and 8h after tracer labelling there was a 37% decrease in sponge ^{125}I-T$_4$ uptake. In human serum (diluted 80-fold) equilibrium binding was evident 2h after ^{125}I-T$_4$ labelling of human serum (Table 1). Between 10 min and at equilibrium there was a 27% decrease in sponge ^{125}I-T$_4$ uptake.

"Stripping" of T$_4$ from Human Sera and Rabbit T$_4$ Antisera :

When the strength of the bond between T$_4$ and T$_4$ antiserum and between T$_4$ and TBG was examined in the presence of a large excess of low affinity T$_4$ binding sites as provided in charcoal, some interesting differences were noted. In all human sera more than 80% of endogenous[*] T$_4$ could be "stripped" in about 2h (indeed in a matter of minutes) using 20% charcoal (Table 2). With occasional exceptions where slightly lower values were noted, approximately 95% of endogenous T$_4$ could be removed in all human sera by 6 h. regardless of TBG concentration, as shown by the results with genetically low TBG and pregnancy sera. After 6 h, only slight increases in "stripping" were noted (see 24h and 48h value, Table 2).

In contrast, marked resistance to T$_4$ "stripping" was noted in several T$_4$ antisera (Table 2). There was a gross inverse correlation between T$_4$ antibody titre (also ethanol T$_4$ extraction recovery) and the amount of ^{125}I-T$_4$ that could be "stripped". In high titre T$_4$ antiserum (antiserum 3, Table 2)

---

[*] As ^{125}I-T$_4$ tracer was used to determine the magnitude of T$_4$ "stripping", use of the term "endogenous" might seem inappropriate. However, in concurrent investigations the magnitude of endogenous "stripping" as determined by actual T$_4$ determinations in sera prior to and after charcoal extraction were in virtual agreement with the values obtained using ^{125}I-T$_4$ tracer.

Table 2. "Stripping" of $^{125}I\text{-}T_4$ from $^{125}I\text{-}T_4$ equilibrated human sera and rabbit T_4 antisera

	Ethanol $^{125}I\text{-}T_4$ Extraction Recovery (%)	"Stripping" (%) at Various Intervals After Addition of Charcoal to Sera				
		2 h	6 h	24 h	48 h	144 h
Normal Human Sera						
Pool 1	87.7	83.4	91.9	96.9	97.5	
Pool 2	86.7	93.9	95.4	95.9	96.0	
Pool 3	86.6	95.9	96.8	96.7	96.9	
Pregnancy Sera (pooled)	–	–	95.6	–	–	
Genetically low TBG serum	–	–	97.5	–	–	
T_4 Antisera						
1	70.0	2.5	28.9	49.4	57.8	
2	74.5	72.7	83.4	86.7	87.5	
3	34.0	1.5	12.0	22.0	36.7	94.0

ethanol $^{125}I\text{-}T_4$ extraction recovery was 34% and in this antiserum only 1.5% of endogenous T_4 could be "stripped" in 2h
(compare human serum where 80–95% could be "stripped in this
interval). With increased duration of contact of antiserum
with charcoal there was a slow gradual increase in the amount
of T_4 that could be adsorbed and even at 48h only 36.7% of
endogenous T_4 could be "stripped" from the immune serum. To
obtain the degree of T_4 "stripping" noted in human serum
(approximately 95%), continuous charcoal extraction for 6 days
was required in this antiserum. Similarly, in T_4 immune serum
with a moderately high antibody titre (antiserum 1, Table 2)
2.5% of endogenous T_4 could be "stripped" in 2 h and at 48h
only 57.8% "stripping" was noted. Even in a relatively low
titre T_4 antiserum (antiserum 2) prolonged extraction with
charcoal for 48h removed only 87% of endogenous T_4.

T_4 Binding Capacity of TBG, TBPA and T_4 Antibody :

Whether or not marked differences in T_4 "stripping" noted
in human and T_4 immune sera may be related to the charcoal
adsorption of T_4 binding proteins themselves was examined by
determining maximum T_4 binding capacities of TBPA and TBG in
human sera and antibody binding capacity of T_4 in T_4 antisera
prior to and after charcoal extraction. Results are shown in
Tables 3 and 4. Charcoal extraction of human sera did not
affect the TBG binding capacity and these data were consistent
with TBG–RIAs which also showed no differences in immunoassayable TBG in pre- and post-charcoal treated human sera.

However, marked decreases in TBPA binding capacity were
noted in charcoal "stripped" human sera. In 3 pooled serum
specimens mean TBPA binding capacity prior to charcoal extraction was 175 µg/100 ml which decreased to 93µg/100 ml or a

Table 3. T_4 *Binding Capacity$^\alpha$of TBG and TBPA and Immunoassay-*

Sera	Protein Conc. (gm/100ml)	TBG Capacity (μg/100ml)	TBPA capacity (μg/100ml)
		Before "Stripping"	
Pooled Human 1	6.1	31	160
Pooled Human 2	6.8	40	185
Pooled Human 3	8.1	36	180

α Glycine-acetate buffer (pH 9.0)

decrease of 46.9% after charcoal treatment (Table 3). These
data suggest that the speed withwhich endogenous T_4 could be
"stripped" from human serum may partly be attributable to the
charcoal adsorption of prealbumin and the consistently lower
protein concentration* noted in charcoal treated sera seems
consistent with this interpretation. The decrease in TBPA
binding capacity in charcoal treated serum could not be attributed to the antecedent local pH changes during the extraction
phase as solution of Norat A charcoal in water tends to increas
the pH and TBPA binding capacity increases with pH (4). Also,
the ready "stripping" of T_4 in human serum could not be attributed to the denaturing effects brought about by extreme change
in pH (5) since the pH of the charcoal extracted serum was
only 9.5 and at this pH spontaneous release of T_4 is not normally noted,

* *There is some indication that biuret protein estimations in*
charcoal treated serum may not be wholly satisfactory and this
aspect is under investigation. Values for protein concentration
are therefore considered tentative.

able TBG in Human Sera Before and After Charcoal "Stripping"

Immuno-assayable TBG (mg/100ml)	Protein Conc. (gm/100ml)	After "Stripping"		Immuno-assayable TBG (mg/100ml)
		TBG Capacity (μg/100ml)	TBPA Capacity (μg/100ml)	
3.5	5.8	30	98	4.0
2.9	6.1	41	91	2.7
3.8	7.4	38	89	4.4

Changes in maximum T_4 binding capacity of T_4 antibody were not noted in T_4 antisera, findings also in consonance with lack of changes in protein concentration in pre- and post-charcoal treated T_4 antisera (Table 4).

Ethanol T_4 Extraction Recovery in Pre- and Post-Charcoal Treated Human and T_4 Antisera.:

In light of the fact that maximum binding capacity in charcoal treated human serum was lower than in untreated serum (due to a partial loss in TBPA binding capacity as noted previously), it was expected that the T_4 extraction recovery in charcoal treated serum would be greater; no changes in T_4 extraction recovery were expected in T_4 antisera since differences in T_4 binding capacity were not noted in pre- and post-charcoal treated immune sera.

Several lower alcohols either alone or in combination were first tested in regard to their ability to extract ^{131}I-T_4 from ^{131}I-T_4 equilibrated serum to determine the best solvent for these investigations. The various solvents used are noted

Table 4. *Maximum T_4 Binding Capacity$^\alpha$ of T_4 Antibodies*

Sera	Before "Stripping"		After "Stripping"	
	Protein Conc. (gm/100ml)	T_4 Binding Capacity (μg/100ml)	Protein Conc. (gm/100ml)	T_4 Binding Capacity (μg/100ml)
Antiserum 1	6.4	92	6.8	118
Antiserum 2	6.6	68	7.2	66
Antiserum 3	7.3	130	7.6	140

$^\alpha$Glycine-acetate buffer (pH 9.0).

in Table 5. In general, use of the combination of ethanol and butanol increased T_4 extraction when compared with either ethanol or butanol alone. A slight increase in T_4 extraction recovery was also noted with butanol when compared against ethanol. While the combination of ethanol and butanol was the most efficient in extracting ^{131}I-T_4, the co-efficient of variance noted in 15 trials using the same serum specimen was also correspondingly larger. Similar results were also noted with 95% ethanol and 1-butanol. On the other hand, the variation within the same sample noted was the least with 95% ethanol (coefficient of variance 1.1) from Publicker Industries Inc. Hence this solvent was routinely used for studies on serum T_4 extraction. Significantly, when the same solvent from different companies was used, considerable variation in ^{131}I-T_4 extraction was noted; e.g. ^{131}I-T_4 extraction efficiency noted with 95% ethanol from Fisher Scientific Co. was 78.1% (CV 4.4%) in contrast to 72.9% (CV 1.1%) obtained with the same solvent but supplied from a different company (Pulb. Ind.). Such observation have also been noted by Murphy (6).

Table 5. $^{131}I\text{-}T_4$ *Extraction from* $^{131}I\text{-}T_4$ *Labeled Human Serum Effected by various Alcoholic Solvents used in* T_4 *(D) Procedure.*

Solvent	No. of * Deter- minations	Mean Recovery (%)	C.V. ** (%)
Ethanol (Publ. Ind.)	15	72.9	3.7
Ethanol (F)	15	77.4	3.1
95% Ethanol (Publ. Ind.)	15	72.9	1.1
95% Ethanol (F)	15	78.1	4.4
1-butanol (F)	6	82.0	3.5
iso-butanol (F)	6	81.6	2.6
Ethanol (F) + 1-butanol (F)	15	87.6	4.0
Ethanol (F) + 1-butanol (Merck)	15	85.9	2.9
Ethanol (F) + iso-butanol (F)	15	83.8	2.6
95% Ethanol (F) + 1-butanol (F)	15	86.6	3.2
95% Ethanol (F) + 1-butanol (Merck)	15	86.3	2.4
95% Ethanol (F) + iso-butanol (F)	15	82.5	6.5
Ethanol (F) + sec-butanol (East Org.)	15	80.0	3.7

(Publ. Ind.) = Publicker Industries Inc.

(F) - Fisher Scientific Company

(East Org.) = Eastman Organic Chemicals

* Number of determinations using the same serum specimen

** Co-efficient of variance

T_4 extraction recovery values using 95% ethanol in human

and T_4 antisera are noted in Table 6.

Table 6. *Ethanol Extraction of $^{125}I\text{-}T_4$ from $^{125}I\text{-}T_4$ Labeled*
    Human or T_4 Antisera prior to and after Charcoal
                      "Stripping"

	Before "Stripping"		After "Stripping"	
	Protein Conc. (gm/100ml)	^{125}I T_4 Extraction (%)	Protein Conc. (gm/100ml)	^{125}I T_4 Extraction (%)
Normal Human sera (Pool 1)	8.2	87.7	6.5	96.5[a]
Normal Human sera (Pool 2)	7.5	86.7	6.6	99.0[a]
Normal Human sera (pool 3)	7.9	86.6	7.0	98.3[a]
T_4 antiserum (1)	7.3	70.0	7.1	61.2[b]
T_4 antiserum (2)	7.3	74.5	7.4	65.5[b]
T_4 antiserum (4)	7.4	69.0	7.5	63.9[b]

a In all human sera endogenous T_4 was virtually completely "stripped".

b In all T_4 antisera endogenous T_4 was only partially "stripped." (50-60%).

Treatment of human sera with charcoal produced a consistent increase in ethanol $^{125}I\text{-}T_4$ extraction recovery. The mean ethanol $^{125}I\text{-}T_4$ recovery in 3 human serum pools prior to "stripping" was 87.0% whereas after charcoal adsorption the mean value was 97.9% or a 12.5% increase. These results are in accord with the expectations based on differences in TBPA binding

capacity in pre- and post-charcoal treated human serum as noted
previously.

On the other hand, in all three T_4 antisera tested, ethanol ^{125}I-T_4 extraction recovery decreased slightly after charcoal "stripping". The mean ^{125}I-T_4 recovery prior to extraction
was 71.2% whereas after "stripping" it was 63.5% or a decrease of 10.8%.

"Scatchard Plot"

Interaction of T_4 with T_4 antiserum was studed by means
of the "Scatchard plot" (Fig. 2).

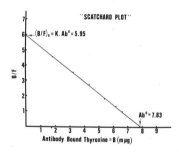

Fig. 2. *Interaction of thyroxine with T_4 antibody ("Scatchard
Plot"). Phosphate buffer (pH 7.2). Temperature = 37°C.*
$$K_a = 5.95 \times 10^{10} \text{ liters/mole.}$$

The affinity constant K_a was found by mass action law computations as derived by Scatchard (7) viz.,

$$B/F = K (Ab^o - B),$$

where K is the affinity constant, Ab^o is the binding capacity
of the antibody, and B is the total amount of hormone bound.
The intercepts on the X (B) and the Y Axes (K. Ab^o) have been
noted in Fig. 2. Substituting these values K_a was computed as
5.9×10^{10} liters(mole, a value slightly higher than that described for TBG at 37° (1.7×10^{10}) by Green *et al.* (8). It
should be pointed out that K_a for T_4 antibody is probably

underestimated by some orders of magnitude due to the limit-
ations inherent in the procedure used; e.g. although sponge
^{125}I-T$_4$ uptake within the interval selected (15 min) in T$_4$-RIA
procedure is a measure largely of unbound T$_4$, it is realistic
to expect some dissocation of bound T$_4$ as well within this
interval. On the other hand, the secondary or tertiary low
affinity interaction between T$_4$ and albumin present in T$_4$ antiserum has been ignored in antibody affinity constant computations. The fact that the "Scatchard plot" function representin
interaction between T$_4$ and T$_4$ antibody described a straight
line is suggestive of a univalent homogenous antigen–antibody
interaction. Although this observation may be rather surprising
in view of a variety of antibodies attendant on thyroglobulin
immunisation, the "Scatchard plot" reflects interaction only
between T$_4$ and T$_4$ antibodies, and only T$_4$-linked determinants
in thyroglobulin are responsible for T$_4$ antibody formation.
While it may be reasonable to suppose that the "Scatchard plot"
function should consist of at least 2 different slopes in view
of the interaction between T$_4$ and T$_4$ antibodies, and between
T$_4$ and T$_3$ specific antibodies, anti-T$_3$ antibodies are not
always elicited in response to thyroglobulin immunisation.

Concluding Remarks

The investigations described clearly show that (1) tracer
^{125}I-T$_4$ equilibration is attained considerably faster in normal
human serum than in T$_4$ antiserum; (2) charcoal "strips" T$_4$
bound in human serum faster than T$_4$ bount to T$_4$ antibody.
Furthermore, it was also noted that ready "stripping" of T$_4$
from human sera could not solely be explained on the basis of
charcoal adsoprtion of T$_4$ binding protein themselves since
the charcoal extraction procedure removed only part of the

prealbumin T_4 binding sites and TBG was not affected.

REFERENCES

1. B.N. Premachandra and I.I. Ibrahim, IAEA Symposium on Radioimmunoassay and Related Procedures in Clinical Medicine and Research, Istanbul, Turkey, 1973.

2. B.N. Premachandra, I.B. Perlstein and H.T. Blumenthal, *J. Clin. Endocrinol. Metab.* 30, 572 (1970).

3. B.N. Premachandra and I.I. Ibrahim, *J. Clin. Endocrinol. Metab.* (Submitted).

4. J.H. Oppenheimer, M. Martinez and G. Bernstein, *J. Lab. Clin. Med.* 67, 500 (1966).

5. L.E. Braverman, A.G. Vagenakis, A.E. Foster and S.H. Ingbar, *J. Clin. Endocrinol. Metab.* 32, 497 (1971).

6. B.E.P. Murphy, *J. Lab. Clin. Med.* 66, 161 (1965).

7. G. Scatchard, *Annals N.Y. Acad. Sci.*, 51, 660 (1948).

8. A.M. Green, J.S. Marshall, J. Pensky and J.B. Stanbury, *Biochim. Biophys. Acta.* 278, 117 (1972).

19. Alternative Approaches to *in vitro* Study of Thyroid Status

D. HUCKLE,

The Radiochemical Centre, Amersham.

A gradual replacement of *in vivo* procedures for the estimation of thyroid status by *in vitro* methods has taken place, supported by the reliability of methods for assay of T_4 and the indirect measurement of TBG-level by the radioactive T_3-uptake tests. The combination of these two parameters into an index, FTI, as suggested by Clark and Horn (1) is probably the most widely used combination at present. The advantages of this combination are evident from the scatter diagrams (Fig. 1) where, for example, raised T_4-levels due to raised TBG-levels, as in pregnancy, are compensated.

However, many borderline cases and other more complex thyroid-metabolic conditions are not fully assessed by use of an index alone. Of particular importance is the status of sick euthyroid patients who may have TBG or protein abnormalities. This loss of clinical information has led to the development of mapping techniques which allow quick visual assimilation of the two parameters and the index. The extent of deviation from the normal can be gauged quickly for each of the factors involved (Fig. 2 and Fig. 3).

The Normalised Thyroxine Ratio test developed by Mincey (2) and his fellow workers in Vancouver is designed to lay

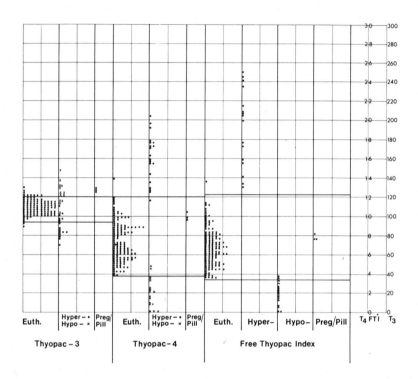

Fig. 1. *Scatter diagrams.*

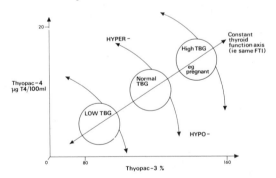

Fig. 2. *The significance of different areas of maps.*

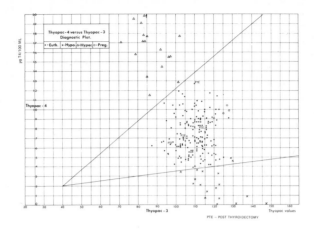

Fig. 3. *The data shown in Fig. 1 reproduced in map form.*
(PTE is Post-Thyroidectomy).

emphasis on the total T_4 level with an allowance for TBG
binding capacity to yield a single answer. The typical example
is the normalisation of pregnancy sera to give values, relative to a normal pooled serum standard, similar to euthyroid
sera. This approach has been shown to be useful as a screening test but can give false indications which might be expected since it is a simplification of a complex metabolic
situation. The area of defining hypothyroid conditions is
the most important of these.

The theoretical basis of the test is not clear. It uses
non-reversible ion exchange resin as the bound-free separation
system to which serum ethanol-extract containing T_4 and a
sample of patient serum are added. However, the development
of such a test using a reversible adsorbent system allows an
explanation of the steps involved with the consequent effects
upon the radioactive count rate of the assay tube. The explanation can be put in the form of a table.

Vial	Added	Serum	Super-nate Counts	Added	Bind-ing Capa-city	Super-nate Counts
Ref. TBG and radio-active T_4	$+ \chi\mu g.T_4$	Normal	Medium	Patient $-TBG$	Normal	Medium
	$+<<\chi\mu g.T_4$	Hypo	High	"	High	Very High
	$+>>\chi\mu g.T_4$	Hyper	Low	"	Low	Very Low
	$+>\chi\mu g.T_4$	Preg-nancy	Medium -Low	"	High	Medium

The clearest example of likely false diagnosis is in hypothyroidism when the TBG binding capacity is that normally associated with euthyroidism. Then

Vial	Added	Serum	Super-nate Counts	Added	Bind-ing Capa-city	Super-nate Counts
Ref. TBG and radio-active T_4	$+<<\chi\mu g$	Hypo	High	Patient $-TBG$	Normal	Medium -High

This example is more common than is often realised and is a major reason for the relatively low diagnostic efficiency of T_3-binding capacity tests when used alone.

The addition of the sample of neat patient serum, either at the same time as the serum-ethanol extract or in a sub-sequent step after determination of the T_4-value amounts to a T_4 binding capacity determination which has lower discrimination than a corresponding T_3-binding capacity determination. This disadvantage can be overcome by the combination of an NTR value with the total T_4-value using a mapping technique (Fig. 4). The overlap between euthyroid and pregnant groups

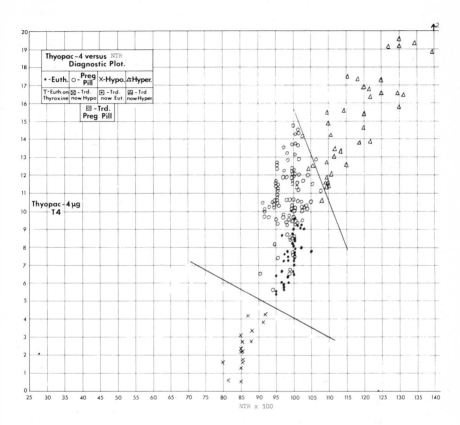

Fig. 4. *Map of* T_4 *and NTR values*

illustrates the lower discrimination of NTR tests as indicators
of binding capacity.

The hypothyroid group, where difficulty in distinguishing
some of the group from low value euthyroids is experienced,
is worth further comment. During the clinical trial of Thyopac-
5 the number of hypothyroid patients with low T_4 values but
low normal range NTR values was unexpectedly large. Parallel
studies with Thyopac-3 showed that nearly all of these had

Table. *Results from the Clinical Trial of Thyopac-5*

Centre	Thyopac-3 µg T_4/100ml	Thyopac-4	Thyopac-5, NTR 1 Step	2 Step	ETR
1	109	2.4	0.94	0.93	0.97
	106	2.8	–	0.90	0.87
	109	2.4	–	0.92	0.73
NR *	(97–120)	(4.0–12.9)	(0.89–1.08)		(0.84–1.11)
2	–	1.1	–	1.0	–
	–	1.1	–	0.90	–
	–	1.9	–	0.93	–
NR	–	(3.3–11.8)	(0.89–1.11)		–
3	119.9	2.9	–	0.89	–
	122.7	6.3	–	0.89	–
	119.6	3.5	–	0.91	–
NR	(96–120)	(3.8–10.5)	(0.89–1.10)		–
4	100	2.3	–	0.93	–
	106	2.9	–	0.97	–
NR	(98–124)	(3.5–11.5)	(0.88–1.11)		–
5	107.1	2.9	0.91	0.91	0.88
	110.0	0.5	0.85	0.89	0.87
	120.5	4.5	–	0.90	0.92
	112.4	3.2	0.86	0.87	0.84
	113.3	2.9	–	0.85	0.86
NR	(3.4–12.6 as FTI)		(0.88–1.12)		(0.86–1.05)
6	–	3.9	–	0.92	0.86
	–	4.2	–	0.93	0.87
NR		(3.5–12.0)	(0.89–1.09)		(0.86–1.10)
7	116	4.6	0.94	–	–
	95	3.0	0.92	–	–
	99	3.6	0.94	–	–
	115	4.6	0.98	–	–
NR	(91–119)	(3.0–12.3)	(0.87–1.11)		–

* NR is Normal Range

T_3-binding capacity values in the normal range. In other cases the combination of low T_4 and normal NTR value was confirmed by other normalised test methods – as in the Table. The incidence of such cases averaged about 20% of the hypothyroid populations studied.

    These comments are intended to illustrate the need for a two parameter regimen for the initial thyroid status screen.

R E F E R E N C E S

1.   F. Clark and D.B. Horne, *J. Clin. Endocrinology and Metab.* **25**, 39-45 (1965).

2.   Mincey *et al. J. Nucl. Med.* **13**, 165 (1971).

20. Kinetics of Renal Uptake of L-Triiodothyronine in Man

RALPH R. CAVALIERI, CHARLES MOSER, PETER MARTIN,
DAVID SHAMES AND VICTOR PEREZ-MENDEZ.

*Nuclear Medicine Service, Veterans Administration Hospital,
and Departments of Medicine and Radiology,
University of California, San Francisco, California, U.S.A.*

INTRODUCTION

3,5,3'triiodo-L-thyronine (T_3) is largely an intracellular hormone. In experimental animals, the liver and kidneys are the organs which contain the highest concentrations of tracer following injection of labeled T_3(1,2,3). Intracellular binding substances, specific for T_3, have been detected both in the cytosol and in the nuclear fractions of liver and kidney (4,5).

On the basis of previous work in our laboratory (6), it has been estimated that in normal humans approximately 5% of the total extravascular pool of T_3 is in the liver. Data are lacking, however, in regard to the renal content of exchangeable T_3 and kinetics of T_3 uptake by kidneys of living humans. We have adapted the method employed in our previous study of hepatic T_3 kinetics (6) in order to determine the uptake-rate and content of T_3 in the kidney of human subjects. This report will describe the method and present results in a small series of individuals with normal and abnormal thyroid function

M E T H O D S

The experimental approach involves the quantitative monitoring of radioactivity accumulated within the region of the
kidney during the intravenous administration of a sustaining
infusion of ^{131}I-labeled T_3. A total dose of 200–250 µCi ^{131}I-
T_3 is given during a period of from 50 to 90 min. Following
an initial "priming" dose, the infusion rate is adjusted at
frequent intervals in order to maintain a constant level of
^{131}I in the plasma. The details of the technique and its
rationale have been described(6).

Subjects

The subjects of the study were adult men with normal renal
function. Each gave informed consent. Five individuals served
as controls, having no history of thyroid disease and having
normal thyroid function by clinical and laboratory assessment.
Three patients with untreated hyperthyroid Graves' disease
and three cases previously treated with ^{131}I for hyperthyroidism were studied. Of the latter group, two were eumetabolic,
while receiving L-thyroxine as replacement therapy, and one
was hypothyroid at the time of the study.

Collection of Data

Quantitative monitoring of renal radioactivity was performed using a gamma camera (Anger-type) equipped with a small
computer. From two to four hours prior to the start of the
^{131}I-T_3 infusion, a standard dose (1 mCi) of ^{99m}Tc-labeled
dimercapto-succinate was injected i.v. This agent is taken
up with high efficiency in the renal cortex, providing a means
of localising the kidneys (7). The subject was seated with

his back resting against the collimator (1000-hole) of the
camera. At the energy setting for ^{99m}Tc (140 kev peak), two
areas-of-interest (AOI), equal in size, were placed, one
containing virtually the entire left kidney and the other, in
an adjacent background region away from both kidneys and liver.
During infusion of ^{131}I-T$_3$, one-minute counts (cpm) in each
AOI were recorded continuously in the ^{131}I-energy setting
(364 kev peak). Samples of blood were collected from a vein
in the contralateral arm at 10-15 min intervals.

The quantity of ^{131}I accumulated within the left kidney,
in terms of the plasma concentration of ^{131}I-T$_3$ was estimated
as follows : A hollow plastic model ("phantom") of human
kidney (capacity = 140 ml) was filled with a solution of ^{131}I
and positioned within a water-filled model of a human torso.
The entire model assembly was placed before the scintillation
camera. The counting rate was determined with the phantom
kidney positioned within the same AOI as that used for the
subject. The proper depth at which the phantom was to be
placed within the torso was determined from a lateral scinti-
photograph of the ^{99m}Tc-labeled left kidney in each subject.
A phantom-calibration factor, F, was calculated as the ratio
of the total ^{131}I cpm contained within the phantom (deter-
minèd by counting an aliquot in a well-type gamma counter)
to the cpm obtained with the phantom in the AOI of the camera.

Analysis of Data

The time-course of radioactivity in the kidney during
the infusion of ^{131}I may be described as a single-exponential
function :

$$R_{net}(t) = A (1 - e^{-kt}) + B$$

where R_{net} is the background-corrected cpm in the renal AOI, at time t during the infusion, k is a rate-constant in min^{-1}, A is a coefficient proportional to the quantity of $^{131}I\text{-}T_3$ taken up by the kidney following completion of isotopic exchange between plasma and the extravascular compartment of the kidney, and B is the time zero value of Rnet, a linear function of the renal vascular "background", which remains constant during the infusion.

The observed values for R_{net} (0-60 min) were fit by the method of least-squares to the above function in order to obtain estimates of A, B, and k. The extravascular renal T_3 distribution volume or plasma-equivalent volume, V_k, in ml was computed from :

$$V_k = A/P \times F$$

where A is in cpm (camera), P is the concentration of ^{131}I in plasma averaged during the period of infusion, in cpm/ml (well-counter), and F is the calibration factor, already defined. In all subjects, values of V_k were corrected to a body-surface area of $1.73 \ m^2$.

Renal content of T_3 (Q_k) was calculated as the product of V_k and the plasma T_3 concentration, determined by radioimmunoassay. Unidirectional (one-way) plasma-to-kidney clearance of T_3, C, in ml/min, was given by $C = V_k k$, where k is in min^{-1}. Absolute T_3 flux (unidirectional renal T_3 uptake rate) was given by C multiplied by plasma T_3 concentration, in ng/ml.

The proportion of unbound (free) T_3 in plasma was estimated by a modification (8) of a method employed for measurement of per cent free T_4, employing Sephadex uptake of labeled

T_3 from diluted plasma (9).

R E S U L T S

Figure 1 illustrates the results of a typical kinetics study. The background-corrected time-activity curve R_{net}, is approximated by a single-exponential build-up function with constant, k. This function represents the equilibration of ^{131}I T_3 between the plasma (constant during the study) and the extravascular compartment of the kidney.

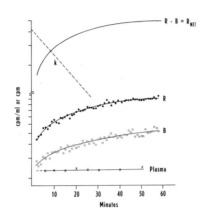

Fig. 1. *The time-course of radioactivity recorded within the renal area-of-interest, R, in the background area-of-interest, B, and the concentration of ^{131}I in the plasma, during the infusion of ^{131}I-T_3 into a control subject. The upper, solid line depicts the time-course of the background-corrected renal curve, R_{net}, the data having been smoothed. R_{net} approaches a final value asymptotically at a constant fractional rate, k, the slope of which is shown as a broken line. Note that the ordinate is a logarithmic scale.*

The values for renal distribution volume, calculated from the kinetics parameters, are shown graphically in Fig. 2. In the control subjects, V_k averaged 224 ml per kidney ± 37 ml (S.D.). Compared to the results in the controls, values

for V_k varied widely in the Graves' disease group being higher
in the toxic patients and lower in the hypothyroid individual.
Q_k averaged 220 ng T_3 (one kidney) and displayed a narrow
range (195–256) in the control group. All three of the toxic
patients yielded values higher than normal, in one case
nearly nine times the normal mean. The hypothyroid patient
showed the lowest Q_k, 114 ng.

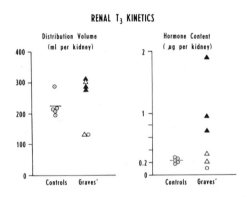

Fig. 2. *Renal T3 kinetics. Individual values for T3 distribution volume, Vk, shown at left, and renal T3 content, Qk,
at right, in five euthyroid control subjects, three thyrotoxic patients (solid triangles), two euthyroid Graves'
disease cases (open triangles), and one hypothyroid Graves'
disease patient (open circle). The same symbols are used in
Figs. 3 and 4. All values are given for one kidney, corrected
to 1.73 m² body-surface area.*

Values for k varied widely among the subjects studied.
The half-time($T_{\frac{1}{2}}$) of equilibration of labeled T_3 between
plasma and kidney, computed from the expression $T_{\frac{1}{2}} = ln2/k$,
ranged from 7 to 27 min. $T_{\frac{1}{2}}$ tended to be shorter in the toxic
cases than in the euthyroid subjects, but there was consider-

able overlap.

Unidirectional clearance, C, ranged from 7.4 to 16.6 ml /min (mean = 11.2 ml/min) in the control group and was significantly higher in the toxic patients (mean = 21.8 ml/min). The hypothyroid subject exhibited the lowest value, 3.8 ml/ min (Fig. 3).

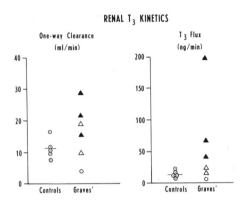

Fig. 3. *Renal T₃ kinetics. Unidirectional plasma-to-kidney T₃ clearance, C, at left, and absolute renal T₃ uptake (flux), at right, given for one kidney*

The absolute rate of renal uptake of T_3 ranged from 5.0 to 19.6 ng/min (mean = 11.5) in the controls, ranged from 37 to 196 ng/min (mean = 132) in the three toxic patients, was within the normal range in the euthyroid Graves' disease cases, and was lowest (3.3 ng/min) in the hypothyroid patient (Fig.3).

DISCUSSION

The assumptions underlying the analysis of kinetics data in the present study are similar to those employed in the previous investigation of hepatic T_3 kinetics and will not be discussed here, except to point out that in this type of tracer study the estimates of space and pool size apply only to exchangeable hormone. To the extent that a separate pool of T_3 exists which is not in rapid exchange with T_3 in the plasma, our values for renal T_3 pool size (Q_k) are under-estimates of the total renal T_3 content. Evidence for such compartmentation of T_3 in tissues has not been presented.

From the present estimates of V_k, it is possible to calculate the renal cell/plasma T_3 concentration ratio in the human. Given a normal renal parenchymal cellular mass of 77 g (55% of 140 g) (10) and neglecting any T_3 in the small interstitial space of the kidney, the mean value for V_k in our control subjects (224 ml) yields a renal cell/plasma T_3 concentration ratio of 224/77 = 2.9 /1. This is higher than the corresponding figure for hepatic cell/plasma ratio of 1.7/1, based upon previous work (6), indicating a higher intrinsic (cellular) T_3 binding activity in the kidney than in the liver. This is in general agreement with the data in rats (3).

The relatively narrow range of values for Q_k among the control subjects is noteworthy and suggests that the tissue content (or concentration) of T_3 may be under rigid homeo-static control in the euthyroid individual.

A report has appeared, in abstract form, describing results of measurements by radioimmunoassay of T_3 levels in extracts of human tissues obtained at post-mortem(11). The concentration of T_3 in the kidneys of individuals who died after brief illness averaged 6.8 ng/g ± 3.2, while the value obtained from cases dying after more prolonged (non-thyroid-a1) illness was much lower, 0.9 ng/g ± 0.6. Calculations based on our present *in vivo* data, assuming all of the extravascular renal T$_3$ to be cellular T$_3$, yield a T$_3$ concentration in the kidney of 220 ng/77 g = 2.8 ng/g. It is, however, premature to attempt a meaningful comparison of such an estimate with the data of Sullivan *et al.* (11), based upon assays of T$_3$ in tissue extracts.

The results of this study shed some light on the question of which form of the hormone, free or protein-bound, is taken up by the kidney. One-way clearance, as estimated from the kinetic data, may be considered a measure of the probability that a given molecule of T$_3$ in the plasma (without specifying bound or free) will be taken up by the kidney in a unit time. In each subject the value for C was compared to the proportion of free T$_3$ in plasma, determined *in vitro*. As shown in fig. 4, a good linear correlation was obtained over a wide range of thyroid function. This observation indicates that the free rather than the protein-bound form of T$_3$ is available for renal uptake. The same conclusion was reached from the previous studies of the hepatic uptake of thyroxine (12, 13) and of T$_3$ (6).

The one-way plasma-to-kidney T$_3$ clearance is undoubtedly influenced by factors other than the level of free *vs* bound T$_3$ in the plasma. One such factor may be renal plasma flow, which is known to be affected by alterations in thyroid metabolic function. A thorough investigation of the mechanism of hormonal uptake by the kidney should include observations made in euthyroid subjects with primary increases or decreases in plasma binding of thyroid hormone. Such studies are planned.

M

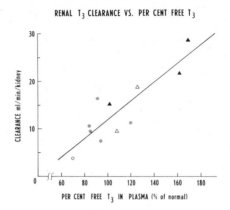

RENAL T$_3$ CLEARANCE VS. PER CENT FREE T$_3$

Fig. 4. *A comparison between the unidirectional renal T$_3$ clearance, C, and the proportion of free T$_3$ in plasma, in each of the subjects studied. The proportion of free T$_3$ is expressed as % of the value obtained in a pool of plasma samples from euthyroid individuals (more than 100) with no abnormality in thyroid hormone binding. The regression line was calculated by the method of least squares. The correlation coefficient is ± 0.76*

Measurements of the urinary excretion of T$_4$ and T$_3$ have been made using sensitive radioimmunoassays (14,15). According to one report, the rate of T$_3$ excretion in the urine of normal humans is approximately 30 ng/h (15). The absolute rate of T$_3$ uptake by the kidneys obtained in the present study averaged 23 ng/min (1,380 per hour). This implies that, of the T$_3$ taken up by the kidney from the circulation, only about 2% appears in the urine, the remainder being degraded within the kidney or returned to the plasma as unchanged hormone.

We have recently established the feasibility of conducting a complete T$_3$ kinetics study in humans with a single pulse-injection of labeled T$_3$ and without the need for a continuous infusion of tracer. In this approach, plasma time-activity curves and external body monitoring data, collected as already described in this report, are analysed by means of a three-compartment model using a digital computer and the program SAAM (16). In preliminary experiments, data analysis using the compartmental model has yielded values for V_k and C which are quite similar to the results obtained by the infusion technique.

Until the values for renal T$_3$ content and uptake obtained in the present study are confirmed by a more direct approach, they ought to be regarded as estimates which are probably valid in a comparative sense. Nevertheless, the methodologic approach which we have described provides a means of studying the effects of drugs, hormones, and a variety of physiologic and pathologic states on the binding of this hormone by a specific tissue in living humans.

R E F E R E N C E S

1.   P. Van Arsdel, J.R. Hogness, R.H. Williams and N. Elgee *Endocrinology*, __55__, 332-343 (1954).

2.   R.W. Heninger, F.C. Larson and E.C. Albright, *J. Clin. Invest.* __42__, 1761-1768 (1963).

3.   J.H. Oppenheimer, H.L. Schwartz, H.C. Shapiro, G. Bernstein and M.I. Surks, *J. Clin. Invest.* __49__, 1016-1024 (1970).

4.   S. Hamada and S.H. Ingbar, Program of 53rd Meeting, Endocrine Society, 134 (1971).

5.   J.H. Oppenheimer, D. Koerner, H.L. Schwartz and M.I. Surks, *J. Clin. Endocrinol. Metab.* __35__, 330-333 (1972).

6. R.R. Cavalieri, M. Steinberg and G.L. Searle,
    J. Clin. Invest. <u>49</u>, 1041-1050 (1970)..

7. T.H. Lin, A. Khentigan and H.S. Winchell, *J. Nuclear Med.* <u>15</u>, 512 (1974).

8. S. Snyder, R.R. Cavalieri and S.H. Ingbar (submitted for publication).

9. R.R. Cavalieri, J.N. Castle and G.L. Searle,
    J. Nuclear Med. <u>10</u>, 565-570 (1969).

10. F.P. Chinard, R. Effros, W. Perl and M. Silverman,
    In "Compartments, Pools and Spaces," (P.E. Bergner and
    C.C. Lushbaugh, eds) U.S.A.E.C. Sympos. Series No. 11,
    pp. 381-422 (1967).

11. P.R.C. Sullivan, J.A. Bollinger and S. Reichlin,
    J. Clin. Invest. <u>52,</u> 83 a (1973).

12. R.R. Cavalieri and G.L. Searle, *J. Clin. Invest.*
    <u>45</u>, 939-949 (1966).

13. J.H. Oppenheimer, G. Bernstein and J. Hasen,
    J. Clin. Invest. <u>46</u>, 762-777 (1967).

14. V. Chan, J. Landon, G.M. Besser and R.P. Ekins,
    Lancet, <u>2</u>, 253-256 (1972).

15. C.W. Burke, R.A. Shakespear and T.R. Fraser, *Lancet,*
    <u>2</u>, 1177-1179 (1972).

16. M. Berman, *In* "Computers in Biomedical Research"
    (R. Stacy and B. Waxman, eds), Vol. 2, pp. 173-201
    (1965).

21. Renal Excretion of T_3 and T_4, and Diagnostic Value of Urinary T_3 and T_4 Assays

C.W. BURKE AND R.A. SHAKESPEAR

Endocrinology Service, Radcliffe Infirmary, Oxford.

INTRODUCTION

It is surprising that so little attention has been paid to the excretion of T_3 and T_4 in urine. Early work (1-3) was followed by a long gap until 1972, when quantitative studies were first published (4-7). There has been no systematic information on the renal handling of T_3 and T_4, nor on the applicability of urinary T_3 and T_4 assays to diagnosis of thyroid disorders.

However, it has long been known that T_4 and T_3 are conjugated with glucuronide or sulphate in liver and kidney (8-11). Metabolites of T_3 and T_4-transaminated, and with other side chain alterations - have also been found in urine (8, 12,13). We suggested (4,7) that in addition to these products of metabolism of T_3 and T_4, free T_3 and T_4 might be found in urine, and be derived from their serum unbound moieties.

METHODS

Urine was collected over 1 g sodium bicarbonate to stabilise pH, tested for protein by an indicator error method (14) and stored at -20°C. Urines containing detectable protein are considered separately. Collections were for 24 hours,

except where specified. For radioimmunoassay (RIA) 0.5 ml
urine was incubated overnight with 100 pg of ^{125}I T_3 or T_4
(Radiochemical Centre, Amersham) and appropriate rabbit antiserum (1/50,000 final dilution for T_3, 1/5,000 final dilution
for T_4) in a total incubation volume of 1.2 ml. Bound/free
separation was made by shaking for 5 min with Dowex AG1 x 2
(quantity optimised by the method of Binoux and Odell) (15).
After settling for 5 min, the supernatant was sampled for
counting. Urine T_4 was measured in unextracted urine, unless
otherwise specified, by a competitive protein-binding (CPB)
assay (7).

Recoveries of T_3 and T_4 added to myxoedema urine were :
T_3 RIA, 102 ± 10 (S.D.)%; T_4 RIA, 99.6 ± 10 (S.D.)%; T_4 CPB
assay, 107 ± 10 (S.D.)%. Inter-assay variation for urines
could not easily be assessed, as the apparent T_4 and T_3 content
rose or fell in different urines stored at -20°C. Urines
were therefore assayed within a week of receipt. Values for
T_4 by RIA and CPB were very similar, except in certain situations discussed below. For example, in 13 overnight urines,
T_4 by RIA was 51 ± 20 ng/hr, and by CPB 54 ± 22 ng/hr. T_3
cross reaction in the T_4 CPB assay depended on concentration;
but in urine concentration ratios were such that T_3 cross-
reaction accounted for 5–15% of the observed T_4 values.

The specificity of the antisera is given in Table 1.
The amount of T_4 or T_3 found was directly proportional to
the volume of urine assayed in all three assays. The following
alterations to urine had no effect on observed urinary T_4 or
T_3 levels: added urea (up to 100 g/litre); urine pH (4.0–10.0);
added K_2HPO_4 or NaCl (0.01–0.3 M). Our previously published
data (4) suggest that the assays measure unconjugated T_3 and T_4

Table 1. *Specificity of antisera. Effect relative to same weight of T$_3$ or T$_4$ at midpoint of standard curve (350pg for T$_3$, 400 pg for T$_4$).*

T$_3$ Antisera (using 25 pg of ^{125}I T$_3$)

1. D-triiodothyronine   0.40 (parallel)

2. L-trichlorothyronine   0.04 (non-parallel)

3. L-thyroxine,D-thyroxine,
   L-triiodothyroacetic acid,
   L-triiodothyroformic acid,   <0.01 (non-parallel)
   3,3',5'-triiodothyroproprionic acid,
   D-tetrachlorothyronine,
   D-3,5-diiodothyronine

T$_4$ Antisera (using 100 pg of ^{125}I T$_4$)

1. D-thyroxine   0.36 (parallel)

2. D-tetrachlorothyronine,
   L-triiodothyronine and   < 0.01 (non-parallel)
   others listed above

Serum total T$_3$ levels were measured by RIA on 100 µl of unextracted serum, with 100 µg of 8-anilino,1-naphthalene-sulphonic acid and 1 mg of thiomersal per tube, with bound/free separation by charcoal. Normal values were 1.0-2.2 µg/l (mean 1.4 µg/l) and recovery of stable T$_3$ added to myxoedema serum was 102 ± 9.0% throughout the range. Serum total T$_4$ levels were measured by CPB assay (16,17) (modified by reduction of Sephadex bed volume to 1.2 ml). Normal values were 50 - 120 µg/l (mean 81 µg/l) and recovery of added stable T$_4$ was 97 ± 5.2% throughout the range. Serum unbound T$_3$ and T$_4$

were derived from total levels by estimation of percentage unbound at $37^{\circ}C$ and pH 7.4 using steady-state gel filtration (18) of 5 ml samples on 12.5 x 0.9 cm columns of Sephadex G-50. Normal ranges were 4.7 ± 1.8 ng/l for T_3 and 39.7 ± 13 S.D. ng/l for T_4.

S U B J E C T S

"Normal subjects" were laboratory staff. "Euthyroid patients" were persons in or attending hospital who were investigated for exclusion of suspected thyroid disease but later shown to be euthyroid in respect of T_3 and T_4 levels, and/or ^{131}I tests and TSH levels. "Primary hypothyroid patients" had symptoms of hypothyroidism, and at least two of the following test results : low serum T_4, low serum T_3, low 48 hour ^{131}I neck uptake, raised TSH levels. "Secondary hypothyroidism" was found in patients with low serum T_4 or T_3 levels following hypophysectomy or high dose ^{90}Y pituitary implants. "Hyperthyroid patients" had symptoms of thyroxoticosis, and at least two of the following : raised serum T_3, raised serum T_4, raised neck uptake of ^{131}I or ^{99}Tc, impaired T_3 suppression. Patients with "abnormal percentage binding" had high TBG levels (pregnancy, oral contraceptives) or diminished binding (idiopathic low TBG, hypoproteinaemia, or salicylate ingestion). Pregnant subjects were studied between 34 and 38 weeks of normal pregnancy.

RENAL FACTORS AFFECTING OBSERVED URINE T_3 and T_4

Proteinuria

Urine protein was shown to interfere in the T_3 radioimmunoassay, leading to a false elevation of percent label bound. This effect was insignificant at physiological levels of proteinuria, but led to underestimation of T$_3$ with protein excretion rates greater than approximately 250 mg/day. Protein also interfered in the T$_4$ RIA, but the amount of T$_4$ carried into the urine by the protein was great enough to cause an apparent increase in T$_4$ excretion rate. With the CPB assay of urinary T$_4$,protein extracted and concentrated from normal urine interfered with the adsorption of urinary T$_4$ on to the Sephadex. This effect was significant when amounts of protein equivalent to a protein excretion rate of greater than approximately 150 mg/day were applied.

Twelve euthyroid patients had clinically detectable proteinuria (Albustix or salicylsulphonic acid). Mean T$_3$ excretion rate in these subjects was low at 28 ng/h, and in 7 of them virtually undetectable levels of T$_3$ were found. Urinary T$_4$ excretion rate in contrast was high at 226 ng/h, and in one case the apparent T$_4$ excretion rate by CPB assay was over 1,000 ng/h. There was no correlation between the degree of proteinuria and the apparent rate of urinary T$_3$ or T$_4$ excretion. It must be concluded that the assays are totally valueless in patients with anything more than physiological proteinuria.

Renal function

The renal clearances of T$_3$ and T$_4$ (see below) were poorly correlated with creatinine clearance (r = 0.31 and 0.44 respectively; P > 0.10). Generally, however, the lower was creatinine clearance, the lower were apparent T$_4$ and T$_3$ clearances; the latter were below the normal range in the majority of subjects with creatinine clearances of less than 50 ml/min. These relationships were not different in hyper- and hypothyroidism, with the exception of the elevated clearance of

T_4 in hypothyroidism mentioned below.

EXCRETION RATES OF T_4 AND T_3 IN EUTHYROID PERSONS

Euthyroid subjects

T_3 and T_4 excretion rates in ng/h are shown in Fig. 1.

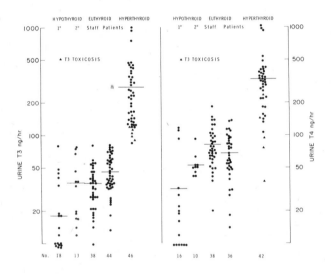

Fig. 1. *Excretion rates of T_3 (left) and T_4 (right) in euth-yroid, hypothyroid and hyperthyroid subjects. Lines denote arithmetic means; data plotted on logarithmic scale for clarity.*

In normal healthy subjects, a slight sex difference in T_3 ex-cretion rate (33.5 ± 14 ng/h in males, 37.4 ± 20 ng/h in

females) was not significant. In 44 euthyroid patients, the
mean T$_3$ excretion rate was 46.6 ±17 S.D. ng/h. There was no
significant difference in T$_3$ excretion rate between those
suspected of hyperthyroidism and those suspected of hypothyroidism.

T$_4$ excretion in the normal subjects was somewhat greater
being 87.9 ± 35 S.D. ng/h in males and 60.9 ± 19 ng/h in females. This sex difference was not statistically significant.
In 36 euthyroid patients, mean T$_4$ excretion was 69.0 ± 30
(S.D.) ng/h. These excretion rates are based on 24-hour
collections.

Neither urine T$_4$ nor T$_3$ excretion rates were normally
distributed, being skewed toward lower levels. The distribution was not normalised by taking logarithms. Therefore
while giving mean ± S.D. values, we have not used statistical
methods based on the differences between the arithmetic means.

In 18 normal subjects, urine was collected between 09.00
h and 21.00 h and between 21.00 h and 09.00 h during the
night. The mean urinary T$_4$ excretion by CPB assay was 89.5 ng
/h in the daytime, but only 55.5 ng/h at night; but this is
an artefact, for the day and night T$_4$ excretion rates found
by RIA on the same samples were more nearly equal (59.1 ng/h
day; 48.6 ng/h night). No day/night rhythm in urine T$_3$ excretion was found in 8 normal subjects (daytime mean 25 ng/h,
night-time mean 23 ng/h).

Seventeen patients taking thyroxine therapy for hypothyroidism were also studied. The T$_3$ excretion rate was 40
ng/h in those taking 0.1 mg T$_4$ daily, 50 ng/h in those taking
0.2, and 61 ng/h in those taking 0.3. The corresponding urinary T$_4$ excretion rates were 40 ng/h, 54 ng/h, and 61 ng/h.

The mean ratio of urine T_3 to urine T_4 in these subjects was thus approximately unity, whereas in normal subjects and euthyroid patients it was approximately 1 : 2.

Euthyroid patients with altered protein-binding

In 22 pregnant subjects, the mean T_3 excretion rate was 44 ± 19 ng/h. T_4 excretion rate could not be measured by the CPB assay because of interference present in pregnancy urine, which we have not characterised so far but may represent trace proteinuria. In subjects taking oral contraceptives, urine T_3 excretion was also normal (23 ± 13 ng/h) and so was urine T_4 excretion (67.3±33 S.D. ng/h). Five subjects with low percentage binding also had normal T_3 secretion rates (48.4±15 S.D. ng/h) and T_4 excretion rates (82±14 S.D. ng/h).

Neonates

Spot urine samples were collected from neonates between the first and seventh days of life. Expressed as μg hormone per g creatinine, T_3 levels were 0.82 ± 0.5 and T_4 levels 1.6 ± 0.5. (In euthyroid adults, urine T_3 was 0.73 ± 0.4 μg /g and T_4 1.3 ± 0.4 μg/g).

RENAL HANDLING OF T_3 AND T_4

Renal Clearances

These are shown in Table 2. It can be seen that in euthyroid persons the mean clearance of T_4 was approximately one-third of creatinine clearance, indicating tubular reabsorption of T_4 analagous to that of other low molecular weight hormones, such as cortisol (19).

With T_3, however, the clearance was consistently greater than creatinine clearance, though with a wide range. It is apparent that processes other than glomerular filtration of serum unbound T_3 are involved in the urinary excretion of T_3.

Table 2.   *Apparent Urinary Clearances of T₃ and T₄*

		Mean ± S.D. (No)	
		T_3 ml/min	T_4 ml/min
Euthyroid	Staff	164 ± 80 (12)	38 ± 21 (12)
	Patients	157 ± 36 (4)	43 ± 17 (4)
	Pregnant	177 ± 50 (7)	– – – – –
Hyperthyroid		221 ± 80 (10)	48 ± 22 (11)
Primary Hypothyroid		174 ± 72 (17)	138 ± 71 (7)

In euthyroid group : Mean Ratio of T_3 Clearance

to T_4 Clearance = 4.6 : 1

In hyperthyroidism, small increases in T_4 and T_3 clearances were statistically insignificant.

In hypothyroidism, the apparent clearance of T_3 was similar to that of the euthyroid group; but the apparent clearance of T_4 was extremely variable, ranging from 55 to 270 ml/min. The mean was considerably increased compared with that of euthyroid or hyperthyroid persons.

Relationship of urine T₄ and T₃ to serum unbound levels

Figure 2 shows a clear relationship between unbound T_3 and T_4 and the urinary excretion rate, maintained over a wide range of T_3 and T_4 concentrations. This relationship was sustained in the subjects who had an abnormal percentage binding. In these subjects, urine T_4 and T_3 excretion were more nearly related to the serum unbound level than to the serum total level. For example, in pregnancy where total T_3 levels were elevated, but unbound levels normal, T_3 excretion rate was close to that predicted from the unbound level. Conversely, in patients with low percentage binding, T_3 and T_4 excretion rates were normal despite low total levels of T_4 and T_3.

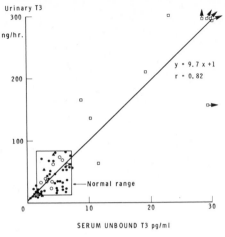

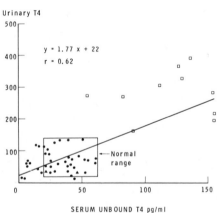

Fig. 2. *Relationship between serum unbound levels and urine excretion rates of T_3 (a) and T_4 (b). ● = euthyroid and hypothyroid; □ = thyrotoxicosis; O = 3rd trimester of pregnancy; ▲ = subjects with low percentage binding.*

DIAGNOSTIC VALUE OF URINE T_4 AND T_3 ASSAYS

Figure 1 shows results in hyper- and hypothyroid subjects, compared with the euthyroid group. Mean urine T_3 excretion in thyrotoxicosis was 281 ± 212 (S.D.) ng/h, 8.2 times the mean in normal subjects. Urine T$_4$ excretion was, however, only increased to 337 ± 226 ng/h, 4.1 times that found in normal subjects. This is in line with the greater increase in T$_3$ compared with T$_4$ levels in thyrotoxicosis generally (20). It can be seen from the figure that urine T$_3$ excretion gives good diagnostic separation between thyrotoxicosis and the euthyroid state, even taking into account patients with T$_3$ toxicosis in whom T$_3$ excretion rate is more modestly elevated. Urine T$_4$ however gives misleading results overlapping with the normal range in over 15% of cases of thyrotoxicosis. The ratio of urine T$_3$ to urine T$_4$ was similar in T$_3$ toxicosis and in patients with more obvious thyrotoxicosis (21). Of 46 patients studied, none had elevated T$_4$ levels in serum or urine with normal T$_3$ levels in both.

In hypothyroidism, however, the diagnostic discrimination of the urinary assays was very low. This was particularly true in secondary hypothyroidism, in which mean urinary T$_3$ and T$_4$ excretion rates were close to those found in normal subjects. In primary hypothyroidism, normal values were not uncommon except in obvious and gross cases of myxoedema which can be seen clustered towards the bottom of the figure in each case. Urine T$_3$ fell slightly more than urine T$_4$ in primary hypothyroidism (39% of the mean in euthyroid subjects compared with 53% respectively) but it is not possible to exclude significant hypothyroidism by urinary T$_4$ or T$_3$ assays alone.

D I S C U S S I O N

Our data (4) suggest that the glucuronide and sulphate conjugates of T$_3$ and T$_4$ are present in amounts roughly equal to that of the free hormone. We are not able to state the origin of these urinary conjugates; they are known to be

formed in liver and excreted in bile, where T_4 and T_3 undergo
a degree of entero-hepatic circulation (9,10,11) but T_4 and
T_3 conjugates in urine are also likely to have been formed
in kidney (10, 22). Our data suggest that our assays detect
mainly unconjugated T_4 and T_3. The specificity also seems to
be adequate in terms of tested metabolites and analogues of
T_3 and T_4, with the exception of the dextro-isomers. A variety
of side-chain alterations completely abolished immuno-react-
ivity in our systems and we are not aware of any metabolites
of T_3 or T_4 known to be in urine which interfere in the assay.

Our measured T_4 and T_3 excretion rates in all situations
are considerably less than those found by Chan and co-workers
(5,6). We believe this to be due to methodological differences. Our data agree with those of Hufner and Hesch (23) for
T_3 excretion rate; and with those of Black *et al.* (24) who
showed that the ethyl acetate extraction procedure adopted
by Chan and her colleagues introduces an artefact which increases the observed values of T_4. We have found, too, that
the handling of the urine prior to assay considerably alters
observed values of T_4 and T_3. For example, alkaline chromatography of the urine markedly increases the observed T_4 and
T_3 excretion rates.

While it is clear that excretion in urine occurs by
glomerular filtration of unbound serum T_4 and tubular reabsorption, we are not able to indicate the fate of the reabsorbed thyroxine from our data. We have found no evidence
of a tubular maximum reabsorption rate of thyroxine, even
at rates of excretion up to 10 times physiological or more.
It would seem likely that the reabsorbed T_4 will be deiodin-

ated, as enzymes capable of doing this are known to be present in kidney (25,26). T_3 excretion appears to be somewhat different; there must be tubular excretion of T_3 since the clearance exceeds glomerular filtration rate in the majority of subjects studied. This T_3 excreted by the tubules might be derived from reabsorbed and deiodinated T_4; or alternatively may represent T_3 arriving at the tubules via the blood stream. We have studied three athyreotic subjects taking 20 µg/day of T_3 by mouth; their urine T_3 excretion was normal at 0.5 – 0.7 µg/g creatinine, although their serum levels of T_4 were sub-normal. This suggests that reabsorption and deiodination of thyroxine do not contribute to the high clearance of T_3. We feel that this question can only be resolved by renal perfusion experiments. Again, we found no evidence of a tubular maximum for T_3.

We are still studying the effects of renal function changes on the excretion of T_3 and T_4, but our data show that T_4 clearance is systematically altered in only two clinical situations; firstly when creatinine clearance is significantly reduced, and secondly in hypothyroidism. We do not yet know the mechanism for the apparent increase in T_4 clearance when plasma levels are low; two alternative explanations might be an increase in proteinuria in hypothyroidism (we found it often necessary to exclude hypothyroid urines from study because of clinically detectable proteinuria), or alternatively hypothyroidism of the kidney with partial failure of the reabsorbing mechanism for T_4. We would have expected apparent T_3 clearance to be changed if proteinuria was the cause, but since the mechanism of T_3 excretion is different from that of T_4 we would not necessarily expect failure of the reabsorbing mechanism to alter T_3 clearance.

We have been disappointed in the clinical applicability
of these assays. It is perfectly true that urine T_3 is an
excellent diagnostic test for hyperthyroidism and also that
it is a useful measure of serum unbound T_3 levels in patients
taking thyroxine and is therefore useful for assessing the
adequacy of thyroxine replacement therapy. However, for neither of these purposes is it any more sensitive than the
measurement of serum T_3 and it suffers from technical and
practical disadvantages compared with this. In hypothyroidism,
the measurement of urinary T_3 and T_4 is a much less sensitive
diagnostic discriminator than is serum T_4 estimation; this is
partly because of the technical drawbacks referred to, partly
due to the fact that the lower limit of T_4 and T_3 excretion
in normal subjects is very low, and partly due to the increase
in apparent T_4 clearance in hypothyroidism which increases
the overlap with the euthyroid range. Three major practical
disadvantages of T_4 and T_3 assay in urine are their dependence
on renal function, the need for timed urine collections or
alternatively measurement of creatinine simultaneously; and
the unpredictable effects of quite small amounts of proteinuria. These disadvantages make the estimation of urinary thyroid hormones practically useless in the elderly, which is
unfortunate for this is one situation in which conventional
thyroid function tests and measurement of serum levels may
be misleading due to alterations in TBG level and other cir-
cumstances. The misleading effect of proteinuria may explain
the apparent day/night variation of T_4, as physiological proteinuria is greater in the daytime than at night.

It would seem that the main clinical application of

urinary T_4 and T_3 assays will be in patients with abnormal protein binding of T_4 and T_3, where they represent a simple indirect method of measuring serum unbound levels; and possibly also in children where they may avoid the need for venepuncture. One condition in which urinary T_3 is of great use is in the management of thyrotoxicosis of pregnancy, especially during carbimazole treatment; it is an easy matter using this assay to detect the earliest signs of a fall in circulating unbound T_3 levels which may be detrimental to the foetus. However, it appears that only in such defined situations are urine T_4 and T_3 assays of greater value than thyroid function tests available hitherto.

Acknowledgements

The authors are in receipt of a Medical Research Council Grant. Grateful thanks are due to all those who referred patients; to our many colleagues and volunteers for collaborating in this study; and to Mrs. H. Faulkes, Miss L. Graves and Miss R. Ames for skilled technical assistance.

R E F E R E N C E S

1. J. Roche, S. Lissitzky and R. Michel, *Compt. rend. Soc. Biol.* **146**, 1474–1477 (1952).

2. J. Roche, R. Michel and J. Tata, *Compt. rend. Soc. Biol.* **146**, 1003–1005 (1952).

3. J. Roche, R. Michel and J. Tata, *Biochim. Biophys. Acta.* **15**, 500–507 (1954).

4. C.W. Burke, R.A. Shakespear and T.R. Fraser, *Lancet*, **2**, 1177–1179 (1972).

5. V. Chan and J. Landon, *Lancet*, **1**, 4–6 (1972).

6. V. Chan, B.M. Besser, J. Landon and R.P. Ekins, *Lancet*, **2**, 253–256 (1972).

7. C.W. Burke and C.J. Eastman, *Brit. Med. Bull.* **30**, 93–99 (1974).

8. J. Roche, O. Michel, R. Michel and J. Tata, *Biochim. Biophys. Acta.* 13, 471-479 (1954).

9. J. Roche, R. Michel, J. Cleson and O. Michel, *Biochim. Biophys. Acta.* 33, 461-469 (1959).

10. A. Taurog, F.N. Briggs and I.L. Chaikoff, *J. Biol. Chem.* 194, 655-668 (1952).

11. E.V. Flock, J. Bollman and J.M. Grindlay, *Endocrinology,* 67, 419-429 (1960).

12. J. Roche, R. Michel and J. Tata, *Biochim. Biophys. Acta.* 15, 500-507 (1954).

13. J. Roche, R. Michel, P. Jouan and W. Wolf, *Endocrinology,* 59, 425-432 (1956).

14. F. Fiegle, Spot tests in organic analysis. Trans. E. Oesper, Elsevier, Amsterdam, p. 40 (1966).

15. M.A. Binoux and W.D. Odell, *J. Clin. Endocr.* 36, 303-310 (1973).

16. L.E. Braverman, A.G. Vagenakis, A.E. Foster and S.H. Ingbar, *J. Clin. Endocr.* 32, 497-502 (1971).

17. H. Seligson and D. Seligson, *Clin. Chim. Acta.* 38, 199-205 (1972).

18. C.W. Burke, *Biochim. Biophys. Acta.* 176, 403-413 (1969).

19. C.W. Burke and C.G. Beardwell, *Quart.J. Med. NS.,* 42, 175-204 (1973).

20. R. Hoffenberg, *Clin. Endocrinol.* 2, 75-87 (1973).

21. C.W. Burke, *J.Roy.Coll.Phys. Lond.* 8, 335-354 (1974).

22. N. Etling and S.B. Barker, *Endocrinology,* 64, 753 (1959).

23. M. Hufner and R-D. Hesch, *Lancet* 1, 101-102 (1973).

24. E. Black, S. Griffeths, R. Hoffenberg and B. Leather-dale, *Lancet* 1, 152-153 (1973).

25. W.E. Sprott and N.F. Machagan, *Biochem.J.* 59, 288-294 (1955).

26. J.B. Stanbury, M.L. Morris, H.J. Corrigan and W.E. Lassiter, *Endocrinology,* 67, 353-362 (1960).

22. The Interrelationship between Triiodothyronine and Thyroxine in Thyroid Disease

DAVID EVERED,

*The Royal Victoria Infirmary and the Department of Medicine,
University of Newcastle upon Tyne.*

INTRODUCTION

The major fraction of the organic iodine present in the circulation is in the form of L-thyroxine (T_4), and the demonstration that thyroid extract or synthetic T_4 was effective in the treatment of thyroid failure indicated that this was an active thyroid hormone (1). A quarter of a century was to elapse before Gross and Pitt-Rivers (2) described the second major thyroid hormone , 3,5,3' triiodo-L-thyronine (T_3). The relative importance of these two hormones in normal physiology, however, remains uncertain. It is known that there is conversion of administered T_4 to T_3 (3,4) and recently a number of workers have demonstrated the extrathyroidal conversion of endogenous T_4 to T_3 (5-7). The data suggest that 30-40% of the endogenous T_3 pool is derived from the extrathyroidal conversion of T_4 to T_3. This transformation can occur in a number of tissues (8) but little is known of the factors which control the rate of conversion.

T_4 and T_3 circulate in the plasma in association with specific thyroid hormone binding proteins. It is generally accepted that T_4 is bound by TBG, TBPA and albumin (9) and

recent work has demonstrated that this is also true for T_3
(10). The major thyroid hormone binding protein (TBG) has a
much lower affinity for T_3 than T_4. A small fraction of T_4
($\sim 0.05\%$) and T_3 ($\sim 0.3\%$) remains free in the plasma and it is
thought that this fraction determines the thyroid status of
the patient. The ratio of total T_4 to T_3 is 66:1(11),but the
ratio of free T_4 to free T_3 is of the order of 8:1, and turnover rate of T_4 is only three times greater than that of T_3.
It is known that T_3 is about five times more potent than T_4
when given on a pharmacological basis, and it therefore seems
probable from the kinetic data available that T_3 makes a significant contribution to maintaining the euthyroid state in
normal subjects.

The paucity of information relating to the relative roles
of T_4 and T_3 in normal physiology and thyroid disease has resulted from the lack of a suitable tissue test to assess the functional significance of any change in circulating thyroid hormone
concentration. The development of sensitive radioimmunoassay
techniques for T_3 (12) and TSH (13) together with the availability of synthetic thyrotrophin-releasing hormone (TRH) (14,
15) have solved many of these problems. Studies of serum TSH
and its response to TRH coupled with measurements of circulating T_4 and T_3 have made it apparent that there is a spectrum
of thyroid function between normality and overt thyroid disease (16). The pattern of TSH response to TRH depends upon
the thyroid hormone concentration. An increase in thyroid hormone level depresses the basal TSH and reduces the response
to TRH, whereas a decrease in thyroid hormone level leads to
an increased basal TSH and an exaggerated response to TRH.
Minor changes in thyroid hormone concentration, which are not

associated with symptoms, and do not fall without the generally
accepted normal range, are associated with alterations in basal
TSH and TRH responsiveness (17,18). It is apparent,therefore,
that the range of serum T_4 and T_3 concentrations in which the
TSH response to TRH is normal is very narrow. This range varies
from individual to individual and is much narrower than the
normal range for the general population (19).

The pattern of thyroid hormone concentrations seen in
subjects with thyroid disease is described and related to
changes in basal TSH and TRH responsiveness.

NORMAL SUBJECTS

T_4 values

Serum T_4 is commonly measured by a competitive protein
binding technique. The original technique (20) has now been
modified and a number of kits, based upon this method, are
available commercially. Serum T_4 concentrations show a normal
distribution in the general population and the normal range
quoted for serum T_4 is generally 4-12 µg/100 ml.

T_3 values

There is general agreement that the mean serum T_3 concentration in European and North American populations lies between
1.1 and 1.5 ng/ml - when measured by radioimmunoassay with a
range from 0.75 - 1.75 ng/ml (21-24).

TSH values

Serum TSH concentration may be measured by precise and
specific radioimmunoassay techniques (25). The normal ranges
published by various workers vary substantially. Normal TSH
levels in many subjects are below the lower limit of sensitivity of most assays. Normal TSH values in the general popul-

ation range from undetectable to 5 μU/ml in one assay (26) and show a non-normal distribution (27).

Relation between T_4, T_3 and TSH values

There is, in general, a good correlation between T_4 and T_3 levels over a wide range of thyroid hormone concentrations (r =+0.68) (28) although there are clinical situations in which these factors vary independently. It can also be shown that there is a significant inverse relationship between $\log_{10} T_4$ and $\log_{10} TSH$ (r= −0.71) and also between $\log_{10} T_3$ and $\log_{10} TSH$ (r= −0.56) (28). This correlation is not improved in the generality of patients with thyroid disease by using the product of T_4 and T_3 since the normal $T_4 : T_3$ ratio is altered in many subjects with disturbed thyroid function.

THYROID DISEASE

Low T_4 and T_3 concentrations

Subnormal T_4 and T_3 concentrations in the absence of a reduced thyroid hormone binding capacity, are only seen in patients with symptomatic hypothyroidism. The converse, however, is not true and significant thyroid failure may be present in subjects with circulating thyroid hormone concentrations within the normal range (17).

Low T_4, normal T_3 concentrations

The serum T_4 tends to fall before the T_3 in subjects developing thyroid failure (17,29) and this probably reflects a compensatory mechanism whereby smaller amounts of iodine are utilised to produce a metabolically more potent thyroid hormone. There is no direct evidence at present to establish whether the altered $T_4 : T_3$ ratio is the result of TSH action on the thyroid (30) or increased peripheral conversion of T_4

to T_3 (5-7). These subjects have an elevated serum TSH and their
symptoms resolve on replacement therapy (17).

Normal T_4 and T_3 concentrations

Normal T_4 and T_3 concentrations are found in many subjects
with subclinical thyroid failure (17). This condition is defined as the presence of a raised serum TSH in an asymptomatic
subject. A study of 72 subjects with this condition revealed
a range of serum TSH concentrations from 5.0 to 51 μU/ml. The
mean serum T_4 concentration in this group was 6.5 (SD ± 1.88)
μg/100ml and although 73% of values were within the "normal"
range the T_4 concentrations were significantly lower (p<0.001)
than in a group of control subjects. The serum T_3 concentration (1.37 ± 0.41 ng/ml) was not significantly different from
that in a control group (1.29 ± 0.29 ng/ml) although a wider
scatter was noted. It is concluded that the euthyroid state is
maintained in the early stages of thyroid failure by a relative increase in T_3 production. It seems probable that the
maintenance of T_3 production is dependent upon an increase in
TSH secretion engendered by a reduction in serum T_4. These
findings imply that T_3 cannot be the sole regulator of pituitary TSH release.

Normal T_4, high T_3 concentrations

An elevated serum T_3 concentration in the presence of a
normal T_4 may be seen in a number of clinical situations.
Hyperthyroid states.

Hyperthyroid states may be the result of an increased T_3
concentration alone. T_3 thyrotoxicosis (30) has been described
in patients with diffuse goitre, multinodular goitre and thyroid nodules (31). The criteria for diagnosis are :
(a) Clinical features of hyperthyroidism; (b) Raised serum T_3

concentration; (c) Normal total and free T_4 concentration;
(d) Normal TBG capacity; (e) Other evidence of thyroid over-
activity or autonomy; (f) Normal iodine uptake.

Thyrotoxicosis due to T_3 alone is more common in areas
where iodine deficiency is endemic (32). It is not clear at
the present time whether T_3 toxicosis represents a fundament-
ally different form of hyperthyroidism in areas where iodine
deficiency is not endemic.

Thyroid autonomy with euthyroidism.

1. *Ophthalmic Graves' disease.* A wide range of thyroid function
may be observed in this condition ranging from hypothyroidism
to subclinical hyperthyroidism. It has been shown that the TSH
response to exogenous TRH may be absent, impaired, normal or
exaggerated (18). The changes in TRH responsiveness reflect to
a certain extent the changes in serum T_4, but show a much better
correlation with the serum T_3 concentration (Table 1). Serum
T_3 values were elevated in those subjects with an impaired or
absent response to TRH. The changes in thyroid hormone concentration were insufficient to induce symptoms of hyperthyroidism, and it would appear that the TSH response is largely
modulated by T_3 in this clinical situation (18).

2. *Autonomous thyroid nodules.* Normal T_4 and raised T_3 levels
are found in euthyroid subjects with autonomous thyroid nodules. These subjects are identified by the following criteria:
(a) Clinically euthyroid; (b) Selective uptake of ^{131}I in a
well-defined nodule; (c) Absent suppression by T_3; (d) Responsiveness of resting parenchyma to TSH; (e) Normal conventional
tests of thyroid function.

A group of these subjects have been shown recently to have
an absent or impaired TSH response to TRH and elevated serum

Table 1. *Thyroid hormone concentrations in ophthalmic Graves' disease and in normal controls*

	T_3 ng/ml		FTI	
Normal TSH response to TRH	1.26 ±0.23		6.17 ±1.24	
Impaired TSH response to TRH	2.04 ±0.23	p < 0.001	6.80 ±1.10	NS
Absent TRH response to TRH	1.75 ±0.25	p < 0.001	6.45 ±1.27	NS

T_3 levels (1.89–3.07 ng/ml) (33). It is, therefore, concluded that autonomous nodules in euthyroid subjects are associated with elevated T_3 levels sufficient to produce pituitary suppression – but insufficiently high to be associated with the clinical manifestations of hyperthyroidism.

3. *Precursor of relapse of hyperthyroidism.* Raised T_3 levels have been observed in euthyroid patients as a precursor of relapse of hyperthyroidism (34). The recurrence of the clinical features is generally associated with an increase in serum T_4 and T_3.

Compensatory elevation of serum T_3.

1. *Subclinical hypothyroidism.* The serum T_4 tends to fall before the T_3 level in subjects with developing thyroid failure. The serum T_3 level is generally normal in the asymptomatic state but may be significantly elevated (V.S.) The association of a marginally raised serum T_3 with a raised TSH emphasises that T_3 cannot be the sole regulator of pituitary TSH release.

2. *Endemic goitre.* Studies on subjects with endemic goitre have demonstrated that there is a significant negative corr-

elation between goitre size and serum T_4, and a significant
positive correlation between goitre size and serum TSH. The
T_3 levels are, however, uniformly elevated and independent
of thyroid size (Table 2) (25).

Table 2.   *Endemic Goitre.*

Variable	Grade of goitre		
	1	2	3
Serum T_4 µg/100 ml	8.7	6.8	5.0
Serum TSH µU/ml	3.5	4.1	14.1
Serum T_3 ng/ml	1.75	2.01	1.73

These findings suggest that developing thyroid failure
(secondary to iodine deficiency) is largely reflected in a
reduced serum T_4. This results in an increase in TSH production
leading to an increase in thyroid size and serum T_3 concentration. Those subjects with the more advanced degrees of thyroid failure (and the lowest T_4 values), therefore, require
a higher TSH response and greater thyroid size to maintain the
euthyroid state by an increased T_3 level. The TSH drive is
maintained despite the absolute increase in T_3 concentration.
3. *Pendred's syndrome.* A single family with this disorder has
been studied. These subjects show an exaggerated TSH response
to TRH (increment at 20 min : 27-43 µU/ml), serum T_4 in the
lower part of the normal range (3.7-6.9 µg/100 ml) and a minor
elevation of serum T_3 (1.91-2.14 ng/ml) (36).

A compensatory rise in T_3 is found in response to an increased TSH drive in a number of clinical situations which are
characterised by a reduced intrathyroidal iodine pool. The
euthyroid state is maintained by the increase in serum T_3 concentration, and these studies confirm that T_3 is not the sole

regulator of pituitary TSH release.

High T_4 and T_3 concentrations

Elevated T_4 and T_3 concentrations, in the absence of an increase in thyroid hormone binding protein capacity, are almost invariably associated with the clinical features of hyperthyroidism (21). Asymptomatic subjects with an elevated T_4 and T_3 are occasionally encountered and have an absent TSH response to TRH and may, therefore, be considered to have subclinical hyperthyroidism. Elevated T_4 and T_3 levels are found in subjects treated with conventional replacement doses of T_4 and it has been shown that these doses are unphysiological and associated with an absent TSH response to TRH (37).

CONCLUSIONS

The relative importance of T_4 and T_3 in normal physiology and in many pathological states remains uncertain.

Low serum T_4 and T_3 concentrations are associated with hypothyroidism, while low serum T_4 and normal T_3 concentrations are associated with mild thyroid failure. Normal T_4 and T_3 concentrations are generally found in subclinical thyroid failure (asymptomatic but raised TSH).

Normal T_4 and elevated T_3 concentrations are found in : (a) Some hyperthyroid states; (b) Thyroid autonomy with euthyroidism; (c) Compensated euthyroidism. Raised T_4 and T_3 concentrations are found in hyperthyroidism.

REFERENCES

1. G. Barger and C.R. Harrington, *Biochem. J.* 21, 169–181, (1927).

2. J. Gross and R. Pitt-Rivers, *Lancet,* 1, 439, (1952).

3. R. Pitt-Rivers, J.B. Stanbury and B. Rapp, *J. Clin. Endocr.* 15, 616 (1955)..

4. L.E. Braverman, S.H. Ingbar and K. Sterling, *J. Clin. Invest.* <u>49</u>, 855 (1970).

5. K. Sterling, M.A. Brenner and E.S. Newman, *Science,* <u>169</u>, 1099, (1970).

6. C.S. Pittman, J.B. Chambers and V.H. Read, *J. Clin. Invest.* <u>50</u>, 1187, (1971).

7. H.L. Schwartz, M.I. Surks and J.H. Oppenheimer, *J. Clin. Invest.* <u>50</u>, 1274, (1971).

8. R. Hoffenberg, *Clin. Endocr.* <u>2</u>, 75 (1973).

9. J.H. Oppenheimer, *New. Eng. J. Med.* <u>278</u>, 1153, (1968).

10. P.J. Davis, B.S. Handwerger and R.I. Gregerman, *J. Clin. Invest.* <u>51</u>, 515, (1972).

11. D.C. Evered, *Schilddruse* 1973, In Press.

12. B.L. Brown, R.P. Ekins, S.M. Ellis and W.S. Reith, *Nature,* <u>226</u>, 359, (1970).

13. R. Hall, J. Amos and B.J. Ormston, *Brit. Med. J.* <u>1</u>, 582, (1971).

14. R. Hall, J. Amos, R. Garry and R.L. Buxton, *Brit. Med. J.* <u>2</u>, 274, (1970).

15. B.J. Ormston, R. Garry, R.J. Cryer, B.M. Besser and R. Hall, *Lancet,* <u>2</u>, 10, (1971).

16. P.J. Snyder and R.D. Utiger, *J. Clin. Invest.* <u>51</u>, 2077, (1972).

17. D.C. Evered, B.J. Ormston, P.A. Smith, R. Hall and T. Bird. *Brit. Med. J.* <u>1</u>, 657, (1973).

18. B.J. Ormston, L. Alexander, D.C. Evered, F. Clark, T. Bird, D.A. Appleton and R. Hall, *Clin. Endocr.* <u>2</u>, 369, (1973).

19. R. Hall, D.C. Evered and W.M.G. Tunbridge, Ninth Symposium on Advanced Medicine (Ed. G. Walker, Pitman Medical (1973).

20. B.P. Murphy, *J.Lab.Clin.Med.* <u>66</u>, 161, (1965).

21. R-D Hesch and D.C. Evered, *Brit. Med. J.* <u>1</u>, 645, (1973).

22. P.R. Larsen, *J. Clin. Invest.* <u>51</u>, 1939, (1972).

23. T. Mitsuma, N. Gershengorn, J. Colucci and C.S. Hollander, *J. Clin. Endocr.* 33, 364, (1971).

24. J.M. Lieblich and R.D. Utiger, *J. Clin. Invest.* 50, 60a (1971).

25. R. Hall, *Clin. Endocr.* 1, 115 (1972).

26. W.M.G. Tunbridge, R. Hall and D.C. Evered, In preparation.

27. D.C. Evered and R. Hall, *Brit. Med. J.* 3, 695, (1973).

28. R. McDougall, W.R. Greig, D.C. Evered and R. Hall, In Preparation.

29. H.W. Wahner and C.A. Gorman, *New Eng. J. Med.* 284, 225 (1971).

30. K. Sterling, S. Refetoff and H.A. Selenkow, *J. Amer. Med. Ass.* 213, 571 (1970).

31. C.S. Hollander, T. Mitsuma, N. Nihei, L. Shenkman, S.Z. Burdaz and M. Blum, *Lancet*, 1, 609 (1972).

32. C.S. Hollander, C. Stevenson, T. Mitsuma, G. Pineda, L. Shankman and E. Silva, *Lancet*, 2, 1276 (1972).

33. D.C. Evered, F. Clark and V.B. Peterson, *Clin. Endocr.* 3, 149 (1974).

34. C.S. Hollander, L. Shankman, T. Mitsuma, M. Blum, A.J. Kastin and D.G. Anderson, *Lancet*, 2, 731 (1971).

35. N. Kochupillai, M.G. Deo, M.G. Karmarker, M. McKendrick, D. Weightman, D.C. Evered, R. Hall amd V. Ramalingaswami, *Lancet*, 1, 1021 (1973).

36. A. Gomez-Pan, D.C. Evered and R. Hall, *Brit. Med. J.* 2, 152 (1974).

37. D.C. Evered, E.T. Young, B.J. Ormston, R. Menzies, P.A. Smith and R. Hall, *Brit. Med. J.* 3, 131 (1973).

23. Radioimmunoassay of T_3 and T_4 in Serum and Urine

E.G. BLACK, R.S. GRIFFITHS, J. FINUCANE AND R. HOFFENBERG

Department of Medicine, University of Birmingham.

INTRODUCTION

The publication of a chemical method for assay of T_3 and demonstration of its biological significance is man (1) has stimulated the development of a radioimmunoassay for this thyroid hormone and for T_4. A number of different radioimmunoassays have been reported during the past five years with many variations in technique. These variations mainly concern

(1) Methods of extraction of hormones from serum (2,3) or the use of unextracted serum (4,5).

(2) Techniques to inhibit hormone binding by serum proteins. 8-anilino-1-naphthalene sulphonic acid (ANS) has proved the most popular blocking agent (4) but salicylates (6), diphenylhydantoin (7), tetrachlorothyronine (8), and heat-inactivation (9) have all had proponents.

(3) Temperature at which incubation takes place, ranging from 4°C (10) to 60°C, (9) and duration of incubation, which ranges from 40 min (11) to three days (10).

(4) Methods for final separation of free and antibody-bound hormone. Double antibody methods are most popular (10) but dextran-coated charcoal (4) and non-specific

N

protein precipitants, e.g. polyethylene glycol (PEG)
(9) have also been used.

In this paper we present a simple, quick, cheap and reliable method for radioimmunoassay of T_3 and T_4 in unextracted serum and urine based on the use of ANS and PEG. The
assay is carried out at room temperature and is complete
within five hours excluding counting time. It compares fav-
ourably with those based on the use of double antibody or
heat inactivation. A comparison has been carried out of T_4
measured in urine and serum by this method and by a competitive protein binding method using Sephadex columns (CPB).

M A T E R I A L S   A N D   M E T H O D S

Radioimmunoassay

(1) ^{125}I-T_3 ($\sim$500 mCi/mg) was obtained from Abbott Laboratories, North Chicago, Illinois; ^{125}I-T_4 and ^{131}I-T_4
($\sim$30 mCi/mg) from the Radiochemical Centre, Amersham,
Bucks., England.

(2) Non-radioactive standards of T_3 and T_4 (Sigma Chemical Corp.) were in the free-acid form and were made up at
a concentration of 1 mg/ml in NH_3. They were diluted for
use with hormone-free serum or buffer.

(3) Rabbit antiserum to T_3 was kindly donated by Dr. K.
Sterling and Prof. H. Schleusener and antiserum to T_4 by
Prof. Schleusener.

(4) Second antibody was swine anti-rabbit IgG obtained
from Mercia Diagnostics.

(5) Serum free of T_3 and T_4 (hormone-free serum) was prepared by incubating pooled human serum with untreated
charcoal (10 g charcoal/100 ml serum) for 18h. Tracer
amounts of ^{125}I-T_3 and ^{131}I-T_4 were added to check rem-

oval of hormone from the serum. Charcoal was removed by
centrifugation at 30,000x*g* for 30 min. The resulting serum
contained less than 2% of the added T_3 and 5% of T_4. Hormone free serum was diluted 1 in 2 with Tris/HCl buffer
for serum T_3 assay, and 1 in 4 with barbital buffer for
serum T_4.

(6) ANS was obtained from Sigma Chemical Corp. A stock
solution of 175mg/100ml buffer was diluted 1 in 7 immediately before assay to give 175 µg of ANS in each assay
tube (ANS-buffer).

(7) Buffer used for the T_3 assay was Tris/HCl (pH 7.9,
0.1 M); for T_4 assay the buffer was barbital (pH 8.6,
0.05 M).

(8) A solution of 30g of polyethylene glycol 6000 (Koch-
Light) in 100 ml of appropriate buffer was used.

(9) Bovine gamma globulin (Sigma) was used at a concentration of 10 mg/ml.

All chemicals were Analar grade. All solutions were made
up in, and sera diluted with, the appropriate buffer.

Serum standards were made up in hormone-free serum,
urine standards were diluted with the appropriate buffer.
Standard curves covered the range 0.05 - 10 ng/ml for serum
T_3, urine T_3 and urine T_4 and 0.5 - 100 ng/ml for serum T_4.
In later assays the use of the lowest standard was discontinued since most samples had hormone concentrations above 0.1
ng/ml for T_3 and 1 ng/ml for T_4.

Assays were carried out on serum and urine samples obtained from healthy normal volunteers, hospital patients with
no evidence of thyroid disease (euthyroid controls) and patients whose thyroid status was abnormal as judged by clinical

assessment and confirmed by routine thyroid function tests.

Competitive Protein Binding Assay

(1) Standards of T_4 were diluted from a stock solution
(1 mg/ml in NaOH) with 2% albumin (serum assay) or 1%
urea (urine assay). Standard curves for serum covered the
range 0-160 ng/ml, and for urine 0-8 ng/ml.

(2) Sephadex G25 (medium) was obtained from Pharmacia
Fine Chemicals.

(3) Bovine serum albumin (Sigma Chemical Corp.) was made
up in a 2% solution for serum assay.

(4) Late pregnancy serum was used as a source of TBG and
was diluted for the assay with barbital buffer (0.075M,
pH 8.6) (1 in 50 for serum, 1 in 300 for urine).

A S S A Y   P R O C E D U R E S

Radioimmunoassay

(1) *Serum*. All assays were performed in duplicate and
blank tubes were included in each assay (a) without added
antiserum but with buffer to keep a constant volume (non-
specific binding = 0%) and (b) without added non-radioactive T_3 (hormone blank = 100%).

To each tube was added in sequence :-

T_3 assay

(i)   100 µl of hormone-free serum

or   100 µl of standard

or   50 µl of unknown serum +

      50 µl of Tris/HCl buffer

(ii) 700 µl of ANS-buffer

(iii) 100 µl of antiserum to T_3

      (1:30,000 final dilution)

$$T_4 \text{ assay}$$

(i)   100 µl of hormone-free serum

or   100 µl of standard

or   25 µl of unknown serum +

       75 µl of barbital buffer

(ii) 700 µl of ANS-buffer

(iii) 100 µl of antiserum to T_4

       (1:3,000 final dilution)

Tubes were thoroughly mixed and incubated at room temperature for 2h. Then 100 µl of $^{125}I\text{-}T_3$ ($\sim$10 pg) or $^{125}I\text{-}T_4$ ($\sim$100 pg) was added and tubes again mixed and incubated at room temperature for a further 1½h. Tubes were then placed in a refrigerator at 4°C for 0.5h. Antigen/antibody complex was precipitated by addition of 1 ml of 30% PEG followed by 100 µl of hormone-free serum. It was subsequently found that 100 µl of bovine gamma globulin (10 mg/ml) adequately replaced the hormone-free serum as an aid to precipitation, so this was used in later assays. Centrifugation (2500 x g) was carried out for 20-30 min, the supernatant fluid poured off, tubes drained for at least one-half hour and the precipitate radioactivity assayed in an automatic gamma-counter (Tracer-lab Gammaset 500) to a counting accuracy of not less than 98%.

The T_3 assay system was compared with two variants :-

(i) all tubes were preincubated at 60°C for two hours in the presence of antiserum, but without ANS(9), $^{125}I\text{-}T_3$ was added and a further 1.5h incubation was carried out at the same temperature. After overnight standing at 4°C antibody-bound hormone was precipitated by addition of PEG or second antibody (see below).

(ii) Second antibody was used instead of PEG. 50 µl of

anti-IG and 50 µl of normal rabbit serum (1/100 dilution) was added to each tube after incubation with ^{125}I T$_3$. Further incubation was carried out for 24h at 4°C and tubes centrifuged for 15 min at 2500 x g, the supernatant fluid poured off, tubes drained for 30 min and the bound fraction assayed as above.

(2) *Urine*. The urine assay was essentially the same as that for serum, except that standards were made up in buffer and 100 µl of urine was used in the assay of both T$_3$ and T$_4$.

Calculations. True sample counts were expressed as percentages of 100% cpm (those to which no stable hormone was added) i.e.

$$^B/_{B_{100}} = (\frac{\text{sample cpm} - 0\% \text{ cpm}}{100\% \text{ cpm} - 0\% \text{cpm}} \times 100)$$

where 0% cpm represents non-specific binding of hormone (tubes to which no antiserum was added).

Standards were plotted on probability x 2-cycle log paper which gave a linear relationship between hormone concentration and bound hormonal radioactivity over the whole range. Unknown sample values were determined from this line, the values being corrected for dilution of the sample in each assay. Standard concentrations were 5, 10, 25, 50, 100, 250, 500 and 1000 pg/tube for serum T$_3$ and urine hormones, and 50 – 10,000 pg/tube for serum T$_4$, corresponding to 0.05 to 10 ng/ml for serum T$_3$ and urine and 0.5 to 100 ng/ml for serum T$_4$.

Two methods were used to validate each of the assay procedures :-

(i) Increasing amounts of non-radioactive hormone were

added to a sample of serum or urine which had a very low
initial hormone concentration.

(ii) A sample of serum or urine from a hyperthyroid patient
was serially diluted to cover the range of standards used.

In both these validations bound fraction plotted against
the calculated amount of hormone in each sample should fall
on a line parallel to the standard curve.

Competitive Protein Binding Assay

(1) *Serum*. Sephadex G25 (medium) was swelled for at least
three hours in 0.1 M NaOH. Columns were prepared by filling
2 ml disposable plastic syringes to the 2 ml mark with a
slurry of Sephadex. The gel was retained on the column by
a disc of course filter paper, and the outlet from the
column was covered by a removable plastic cap. Before use,
columns were washed with 12 ml of 0.1 M NaOH to ensure a
pH of 11-12.

Standards were made up in 2% bovine serum albumin.
200 µl of standard or sample was pipetted on to the column,
followed by 200 µl of ^{125}I T_4 (<0.5 ng/ml). This was added
with an automatic pipette which ensured adequate mixing.
The outlet cap was removed and the mixture allowed to run
into the column, which was then washed with 4 ml of barbital buffer, and the effluent discarded. TBG solution
(0.5 ml of 1/50 dilution) was then pipetted on to the column and allowed to equilibrate for 15 min – thereafter the
column was washed with 4 ml of barbital buffer, the effluent collected and assayed for radioactivity.

Duplicate columns were run for each sample, and counting
performed on a Tracerlab Gammaset 500 to an accuracy of at
least 98%.

Radioactivity was plotted directly against standard concentration giving a sigmoid curve, and sample concentrations
were read off this curve.

The columns were washed with 12 ml of 0.1 M NaOH and
could then be re-used in consecutive assays.

(2) *Urine*. The method for urine had only three differences

(i)   500 µl of standard or urine were used initially

(ii) Standards were made up in 1% urea

(iii) TBG solution was diluted 1/300.

R E S U L T S

Serum

Triiodothyronine. Figure 1 shows a standard curve for T_3,
plotted on log-probability graph paper to produce a straight
line throughout the range of 0.05 - 10 ng/ml. The lower limit
of sensitivity of this assay, taken as the value which gives
90% binding, is between 10 and 15 pg/tube, and the precision,
the smallest amount of stable hormone added to serum to give
a significant decrease in percentage binding, is 5 pg/tube.
Also plotted in Fig. 1 are the results of the two validation
methods. Mean recovery of T_3 added to serum was 98.8% with a
range of 84% - 111%, and it can be seen that the points fall
on the standard curve. Dilutions of serum from a hyperthyroid
patient also gave values on the standard curve. Intra-assay
variability was tested by repeating one serum sample 18 times
and the coefficient of variance was 5.1%. Inter-assay variability was 7.1%, the same sample being tested in 10 separate
assays.

Values for serum T_3 are shown in Table 1. Mean concentration
in normal subjects is 1.73 ± 0.33 ng/ml and in euthyroid

Table 1.   *Values for* T_3 *and* T_4 *in various thyroid states measured by radioimmunoassay*

	No.	Serum (ng/ml) T_3	T_4
Normal	48	1.73 ± 0.33	95 ± 20
Euthyroid control	20	1.50 ± 0.39	91 ± 27
Hypothyroid	34	<0.20 − 0.98	< 1 − 96
Hyperthyroid	48	2.65 −14.20	132 − 376

	No.	Urine (μg/24 h) T_3	T_4
Normal	24	0.95 ± 0.33 (0.59 − 1.73)	1.21 ± 0.49 (0.44 − 2.05)
Euthyroid control	15	0.84 ± 0.23 (0.55 − 1.25)	1.60 ± 0.98 (0.41 − 3.46)
Hypothyroid	5	0.18 − 0.53	0.20 − 0.78
Hyperthyroid	11	1.86 − 9.60	1.71 − 19.26

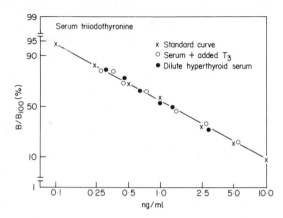

Fig. 1. *Serum T₃ - standard curve and validation. Standards represent 10, 25, 50, 100, 500 and 1,000 pg /tube. B /B₁₀₀ = bound fraction as percentage of hormone blank.*

controls 1.50 ± 0.39 ng/ml. The range in hyperthyroid patients is 2.65 - 14.2 ng/ml and in hypothyroid < 0.20 - 1.09 ng/ml. *Thyroxine.* A standard curve for T_4 is shown in Fig. 2, as are the results of the validation experiments. Standards range from 0.1 - 10 ng/tube and again it can be seen that a linear relationship is maintained throughout this range. Sensitivity is between 90 and 170 pg/tube, and precision is 50 pg/tube. Inter-assay variability was 4% on 8 replicates and 12 intra-assay replicates showed 5% variability.

The mean concentration of serum T_4 in normal subjects is 95 ± 20 ng/ml as shown on Table 1. Serum from hyperthyroid subjects ranges from 132 to 376 ng/ml and hypothyroid from <1 to 96 ng/ml. Euthyroid control subjects show a mean of 91 ± 27 ng/ml. The CPB assay gives a mean serum concentration of T_4 in normal subjects of 100 ± 17 ng/ml and a hyperthyroid range of 130 - 304 ng/ml.

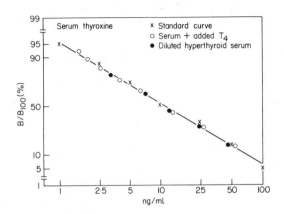

Fig. 2.*Serum* T_4 *– standard curve and validation. Standards epresent 0.1, 0.25, 0.5, 1, 2.5, 5 and 10 ng /tube.*

Comparison of Assays. Figures 3 and 4 show the comparison between this assay for T_3 and assays introducing two variables viz :-

(i) change of temperature,

(ii) change of final precipitating agent.

All assays were performed on the same day in order to reduce non-methodological variations. Figure 3 compares assays performed at room temperature and $60^{\circ}C$ using PEG as precipitant. The calculated regression line shows mean values of the $60^{\circ}C$ assay to be 0.28 ng/ml higher than those obtained at room temperature. Results of the comparison of second antibody and PEG precipitation, using room temperature for the assay, are shown in Fig. 4. There would appear to be no systematic difference between these two precipitants.

Urine.

Standard curves and validation experiments for urine T_3 and T_4 are shown in Figs 5 and 6 respectively. The range of

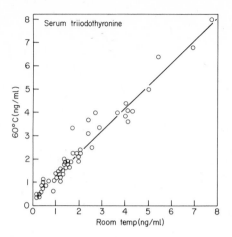

Fig. 3. *Comparison of serum T_3 assays incubated at $60^{\circ}C$ and room temperature, with PEG as precipitant. Equation of line: $y = 0.98x + 27.97$.*

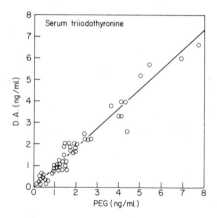

Fig. 4. *Comparison of PEG and second antibody (D.A.) as precipitant in serum T_3 assay incubated at room temperature. Equation of line : $y = 0.92x - 1.57$.*

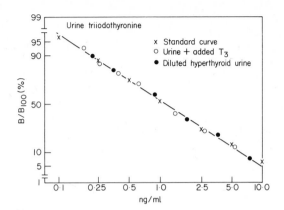

Fig. 5. *Urine* T_3 – *standard curve and validation. Standards as in Fig. 1.*

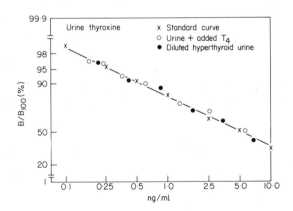

Fig. 6. *Urine* T_4 – *standard curve and validation. Standards as in Fig. 1.*

standards for both assays is 10-1000 pg/tube and again linearity is achieved throughout the range.

Sensitivity for T_3 is between 12 and 21 pg/tube and precision is 5 pg/tube. Intra- and inter-assay variability are
5% and 6% respectively. The mean normal T_3 excretion as shown
in Table 1 is 0.95 ± 0.33 µg/24 h, hyperthyroid urines range
from 1.86 to 9.60 µg/24 h and hypothyroid from 0.18 to 0.53
µg/24 h. Euthyroid controls have a mean value of 0.75 ± 0.28
µg/24 h.

Table 1 also shows the mean normal value for urinary
T_4 as 1.21 ± 0.49 µg/24 h and euthyroid controls as 1.60 ±
0.98 g/24 h. Hypothyroid urines range from 0.20 to 0.78 µg/24
h and hyperthyroid from 2.39 to 19.26 µg/24 h. Sensitivity and
precision are 60-100 pg/tube and 5 pg/tube respectively. The
intra-assay variability is 12% and interassay variability 8%.
The mean normal urine T_4 value by CPB assay is 2.00 ± 0.63 µg
/24 h.

Comparison of the two assays for T_4 performed on the same
samples are shown in Table 2. Serum values for both methods
are essentially the same, but CPB systematically gives higher
values for urine T_4 than those measured by RIA. (Fig. 7).

Figure 8 presents a comparison of T_3 and T_4 concentrations
in serum and urine taken from the same group of subjects. The
improved discriminatory power of the T_3 assay is clearly evident.

D I S C U S S I O N

The radioimmunoassay presented in this paper has several
advantages over those published by other workers. The total
time taken is 5 h and, although there are a few assays which
are accomplished in less time (1.5 h (4); 40 min (11)) these

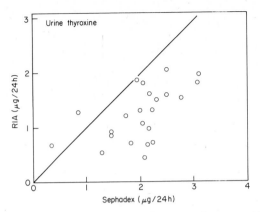

Fig. 7. *Comparison of urine T_4 measured by radioimmunoassay and competitive protein binding (Sephadex).*

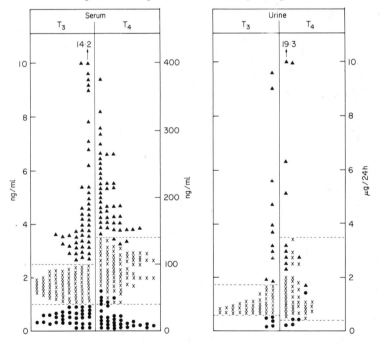

Fig. 8. *Comparison of hormones in serum and urine.*
x *Normal* ▲ *Hyperthyroid* ● *Hypothyroid.*

Table 2.   *Comparison of T_3 and T_4 using RIA and CPB assay (Sephadex)*

	Serum T_4 (ng/ml)	
	R.I.A.	Sephadex
Normal (24)	100 ± 20	100 ± 17
Hyperthyroid (12)	215 ± 48	217 ± 57

	Urine (μg/24 h)			
	R.I.A.			Sephadex
	T_3	T_4	$T_3 + T_4$	T_4
Normal (23)	1.00 ± 0.35	1.23 ± 0.49	2.23 ± 0.71	2.00 ± 0.63
Hyperthyroid (11)	4.51 ± 2.63	5.57 ± 5.39	10.1 ± 7.7	6.1 ± 3.5

require incubation at higher temperatures and a shaking water
bath. This assay needs no specialised equipment as it is performed at room temperature, and the minor variations of temperature experienced in the laboratory seem not to affect the
results. The assay of Sterling and Milch (9) uses incubation
at 60°C to inhibit binding of hormoen to serum proteins, but
overnight incubation at 4°C is required before addition of
PEG, which again lengthens the time of assay. Comparison of
incubation at 60°C with that at room temperature using ANS
shows a difference of about 0.30 ng/ml, with the 60°C assay
giving higher mean values. When ANS was added to tubes incubated at 60°C, levels of T_3 were similar to those found using
the room temperature assay. Methods which require incubation
at 4°C during the assay are of necessity longer since the
reaction is considerably slower at this temperature.

Polyethylene glycol is used by several workers as precipitant of the bound fraction (9,11), but use of dextran-
charcoal (4,12) or second antibody (5,10) is far more widespread. The former requires no incubation, but must be added
to the tube under strictly controlled conditions and the
latter, as well as requiring an additional 24 h incubation,
is far more costly than PEG. Comparative assays using PEG
and double antibody show no consistent difference between
the two. The cost of using commercially available second antibody is about £0.12 per tube (40 times that of PEG).

The normal values obtained for serum T_3 using this assay
are higher than those of some other workers (4,11,12) but
lower than those of earlier workers (9,13,14).

Serum T_4 levels are somewhat higher than those of Mitsuma *et al.* (4) and Dunn and Foster (15), but compare well

with those obtained by the competitive protein binding method
as performed in our laboratory.

Very little information has so far been published about
values of T_3 and T_4 in urine, but the figures obtained with
the present assay are similar to those published by Burke
and Eastman (16).

Comparison of results obtained by RIA and CPB in our
laboratory shows good agreement for serum T_4 and a slight
discrepancy for urine T_4 values. It is tempting to ascribe
this to measurement of T_3 by CPB, since its contribution is
negligible in serum and substantial in urine. But this is
not so. In hyperthyroid subjects urine T_4 by CPB is considerably less than the sum of T_3 and T_4 measured by RIA and
additions of graded amounts of T_3 to a standard urine barely
affects urine T_4 by CPB until extremely high concentrations
are reached. Thus artificial augmentation of urine T_3 concentration to 5 ng/ml results only in 0.3 ng/ml increase in
T_4 concentration measured by CPB; and even at 25 ng T_3 per
ml of urine, total T_4 by CPB increases by only 2.5 ng/ml.
It seems that about 10% of the urine T_3 concentration is
measured as T_4 by CPB.

Evaluation of the relative merits of T_3 and T_4 as an
effective test of thyroid status seems to show that overlap
between normal, hyper- and hypothyroid levels is somewhat
less with T_3 than with T_4, inferring that the former is a
better indicator of thyroid function.

The assay presented in this paper is quick, up to 70
sera or urines in duplicate can be processed within a working
day; it is reliable and reproducible - samples processed in
two separate assays differ by less than 5%; and it is simple -

no special equipment or expensive chemicals are required.

REFERENCES

1. K. Sterling, D. Bellabarba, E.S. Newman and M.A. Brenner, *J. Clin. Invest.* <u>48</u>, 1150 - 1158 (1969).

2. Y.C. Patel and H.G. Burger, *J. Clin. Endocrinol. Metab.* <u>36</u>, 187-190 (1973).

3. M. Hufner and R.D. Hesch, *Acta Endocrinol.* (Copenhagen) <u>72</u>, 464-474 (1973).

4. T. Mitsuma, J. Colucci, L. Shenkman and C.S. Hollander, *Biochem. Biophys. Res. Commun.* <u>46</u>, 2107-2113 (1972).

5. H. Meinhold and K.W. Wenzel, *Horm. Metab. Res.* <u>6</u>, 169-170 (1974).

6. P.R. Larsen, A.J. Atkinson, Jr., H.N. Wellman and R.E. Goldsmith, *J. Clin. Invest.* <u>49</u>, 1266-1279 (1970).

7. J.M. Lieblich and R.D. Utiger, *J. Clin. Invest.* <u>50</u>, 60a (1971).

8. T. Mitsuma, N. Nihei, M.C. Gershengorn and C.S. Hollander, *J. Clin. Invest.* <u>50</u>, 2679-2688 (1971).

9. K. Sterling and P.O. Milch, *J. Clin. Endocrinol. Metab.* <u>38</u>, 866-875 (1974).

10. C. Beckers, C. Cornette and M. Thalasso, *J. Nucl. Med. Biol.* <u>1</u>, 121-129 (1974).

11. C.B. Sekadde, W.R. Slaunwhite, Jr. and T. Aceto, Jr. *Clin. Chem.* <u>19</u>, 1016-1021 (1973).

12. R.-D. Hesch and D. Evered, *Br. Med. J.* <u>1</u>, 645-648 (1973).

13. H. Gharib, R.J. Ryan, W.E. Mayberry and T. Hockert, *J. Clin. Endocrinol. Metab.* <u>33</u>, 509-516 (1971).

14. J. Benotti, R. Grimaldi, S. Pino and F. Maloof, *In* "Further Advances in Thyroid Research" (K. Fellinger and R. Hofer, eds). Verlag der Wiener Medizinischen Akademie, Vienna. 1st Edition. <u>2</u>, 1121 (1971).

15. R.T. Dunn and L.B. Foster, *Clin. Chem.* <u>19</u>, 1063-1066 (1973).

16. C.W. Burke and C.J. Eastman, *Br. Med. Bull.* <u>30</u>, 93-99 (1974).

24. Serum Triiodothyronine and Thyroxine in Patients in Prolonged Clinical Remission after Treatment of Thyrotoxicosis and in Patients Receiving Triiodothyronine

M.J. HOOPER[1], J.G. RATCLIFFE, W.A. RATCLIFFE, C.A. SPENCER,

D.G. McLARTY AND W.D. ALEXANDER

Gardiner Institute, Western Infirmary and Radioimmunoassay Unit, Stobhill Hospital, Glasgow, Scotland.

Antithyroid drug therapy and destruction or removal of most of the thyroid gland with radioiodine or surgery remain the conventional forms of therapy for thyrotoxicosis. Rational choice of the most appropriate treatment requires, amongst other things, knowledge of thyroid function during and following each form of therapy.

This paper describes the changes in the levels of serum T_3, T_4, TSH and other indices of thyroid function in patients in prolonged clinical remission after treatment of thyrotoxicosis with antithyroid drugs and in patients receiving Triiodothyronine.

PATIENTS STUDIED

These were drawn from a group of 105 essentially unselected patients who had previously been included in a prospective study of the treatment of thyrotoxicosis with Carbimazole

1 *Dr. M.J. Hooper is supported in part by Searle Travel Grant in Endocrinology and Internal Medicine, and in part by a Thomas and Ethel Mary Ewing Scholarship in Medicine from the University of Sydney.*

and T_3 at the Western Infirmary, Glasgow (1,2). Patients who
were still attending the clinic and had not had destructive
therapy at the time of the study were investigated. These
patients havebeen followed for at least five years from presentation until the time of the study. The mean duration of
follow-up was seventy-five months.

A   Thirty-five patients had a prolonged remission after antithyroid drug therapy, were off all treatment, and could be
grouped as follows.

       1. Twenty-seven patients had a prolonged remission after
one course of Carbimazole and at the time of the study had
been off antithyroid drugs for a mean interval of 63.3 months.

       2. Eight patients had a prolonged remission after two
courses of Carbimazole and had been off drug therapy for a
mean interval of 36.8 months.

B   Thirty-five patients were studied while receiving T_3 20μg
q.i.d. after, or in conjunction with, antithyroid drugs and
fell into the following two groups.

       1. Seventeen clinically euthyroid patients who were re-
ceiving T_3 after antithyroid drug therapy. Eight of these
patients were in prolonged clinical remission after two courses
of drug therapy and nine patients had only had a brief clinical
remission after several courses of antithyroid drugs.

       2. Eighteen patients who were receiving both Carbimazole
and T_3. Patients were considered to be clinically euthyroid
if they had a normal Wayne Index (3) and had regained and
maintained their normal body weight.

                    M E T H O D S

       Total serum T_3, T_4, TSH, protein bound iodine (PBI), T_3
Resin Uptake (T_3RU), early radioiodine uptakes and clearance

rates, plasma inorganic iodine (PII) and absolute iodine uptake
(AIU) were measured in each patient.

Serum T$_3$, T$_4$ and TSH levels were measured by radioimmunoassay (RIA). In the T$_3$ and the T$_4$ assays, binding of thyroid
hormones to serum proteins was inhibited with 8-anilino-1-
naphthalene-sulphonic acid (ANS). Separation of bound and free
tracer was by methyl-cellulose-coated charcoal (4) in the T$_3$
assay and by double antibody on polyethylene glycol in the
T$_4$ assay (5,6). Charcoal stripped serum was employed to equal-
ise concentrations in tubes containing standards.

Serum TSH was measured by double antibody RIA. Each sample
was assayed with two different rabbit antisera; one raised to
porcine TSH and the other to human TSH (the latter was a gift
from the National Institutes of Health, U.S.A.). Purified
human TSH (DE 32, Dr. A.S. Hartree, Cambridge) was used for
iodination and a reference preparation of human TSH (MRC 68/38)
for standardisation of both assays. The interassay coefficient
of variation over the ranges of concentrations studied in each
assay were : T$_3$, 7.5%, T$_4$ 5.5% and TSH, 12%.

The PBI was measured by Technicon Autoanalyser (7). The
T$_3$RU was determined by the Trisorb-125 kit (Abbott Laboratories).
From the PBI and T$_3$RU a free thyroxine index (FTI) was calculated as an indirect estimation of free thyroid horm-ne (8).
The early radioiodine uptakes and clearance rates (9), and
the PII (10) and AIU (11) were measured using ^{132}I. LATS was
measured by the mouse bioassay described by McKenzie (12).
The TSH response to thyrotrophin releasing hormone (TRH) was
assessed by measuring TSH levels before, 20 and 60 min after
a 200 µg intravenous bolus of TRH.

R E S U L T S

Patients in prolonged remission after antithyroid drug therapy

In 33 of the 35 patients the radioiodine uptakes and clearance rates, the absolute iodine uptake, and the protein bound iodine were not significantly different from a control euthyroid population. This included 25 patients out of the 27 patients in group 1 and all 8 patients in group 2. The T_3 resin uptake and free thyroxine index were however, significantly elevated although falling within the respective normal ranges (Table 1).

The mean T_3 (Fig. 1) and T_4 levels (Fig. 2) were significantly elevated (P< .001) above the means obtained in a euthyroid control population. $T_4:T_3$ ratios tended to be lower than those in the control euthyroid population (P< .02) (Fig. 3).

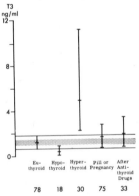

Fig. 1. *T_3 levels after Antithyroid Drugs : Means and observed ranges.*
Observed range (horizontal lines) and one standard deviation above and below the mean in the euthyroid control population (shaded area) are shown across the figure.

TSH levels measured with both antisera were within the respective normal ranges and near the limit of detection of the assay systems. (Table 1).

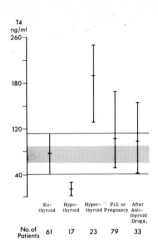

Fig. 2. *T_4 levels after Antithyroid' Drugs Means and observed ranges.*
Horizontal lines and shaded area shown across the figure are explained in Fig. 1.

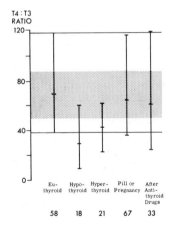

Fig. 3. *T_4 :T_3ratios after Antithyroid Drugs :Means and observed ranges.*
Horizontal lines and shaded area shown across the figure are explained in Fig. 1.

TRH Stimulation tests were performed on 9 patients. Five

Table 1.   *Indices of Thyroid Function in Control Euthyroid*

PARAMETERS

---

20 Min ^{132}I Uptake (% Dose)

2-20 Min ^{132} Thyroid Clearance (ml/min)

Plasma Inorganic Iodine (μg/100ml)

Absolute Iodine Uptake (μg/hr)

Protein Bound Iodine (μg/100 ml)

T_3 Resin Uptake Ratio

Free Thyroxine Index

Total Serum Thyroxine (ng/ml)

Total Serum Triiodothyronine (ng/ml)

T_4 : T_3 Ratio

Serum Thyrotropin (μU/ml)

     a) Antiporcine Antisera

     b) Antihuman Antisera

---

* Obtained in hospitalised patients with no clinical evidence of thyroid disease.

** Two patients who might be expected to have altered T_4:T_3 ratios excluded.

Patients and Patients Studied After Antithyroid Drugs

CONTROL EUTHYROID*				AFTER ANTITHYROID DRUGS			
Mean ± ISD	Range	No	Mean ± ISD	Range	No	P
3.4 ± 1.5	1.0 - 8.7	43	3.8 ± 1.9	1.2 - 9.3	29	<.4
21.7 ± 8.2	7.4 -46.4	41	21.1 ± 10.0	6.7 -48.2	28	<.9
0.3 ± 0.29	0.03-1.14	41	0.29 ± 0.55	0.05-3.08	29	<.95
3.6 ± 3.3	0.3 -15.2	40	2.6 ± 3.9	0.6 -21.6	29	<.3
5.3 ± 1.2	3.0 - 7.2	43	5.7 ± 1.1	3.6 - 7.6	33	<.1
0.90 ± 0.09	0.76- 1.1	43	0.96 ± 0.12	0.7 -1.26	32	<.025
4.8 ± 1.2	2.5 - 7.3	43	5.4 ± 1.1	3.7 - 8.1	32	<.05
77.4 ± 16	43 -112	61	99 ± 21	69 - 140	33**	<.001
1.23 ± 0.26	0.62- 1.8	78	1.75 ± 0.47	0.88-2.84	33**	<.001
68 ± 19	38 -118	58	57 ± 24	25 - 118	33**	<.02
2.7	<0.6 -9.9	169	3.3	<0.6- 9.3	34***	****
2.3	<0.6 -8.5	76	1.2	<0.6- 6.4	34***	****

*** Patients with a short-lived episode of thyrotoxicosis
   excluded

**** P value was not calculated because of non-Gaussian distribution of TSH values and because TSH was undetectable
   in many of the samples.

patients had a normal TSH response, 2 had an inadequate response and 2 an exaggerated response. There was no correlation
between the type of TSH response obtained and the levels of
T_4 or T_3 or the T_4 : T_3 ratio.

LATS was detected during the period of observation in
only 2 patients. The T_4 and T_3 levels and the T_4 : T_3 ratios
were 80 ng/ml, 1.68 ng/μl and 48 and 69 ng/ml, 1.84 ng/ml and
38 respectively.

No correlation was found between the total T_3, total T_4
or T_4 : T_3 ratio and either the radioiodine uptake or clearance
rates, PII, AIU,or serum TSH levels.

Serial measurements were performed over periods of 1-6
months in 17 patients while they remained euthyroid clinically.
In this period, T_3 and T_4 levels tended to fall to values
within the normal range although no obvious trend in T_4 : T_3
ratios occurred. Recurrence of thyrotoxicosis occurred in one
patient who had previously had two courses of antithyroid
drugs and had been euthyroid for 27 months. T_4 levels rose
first (T_4 136 ng/ml; T_3 1.3 ng/ml; T_4 : T_3 ratio 105) with
subsequent elevation of T_3 levels as well and development of
a low T_4 : T_3 ratio (T_4 192 ng/ml; T_3 4.8 ng/ml; T_4 ; T_3 ratio
40), (Fig. 4).

The remaining two patients will be considered separately.
One had a TSH level at the upper end of the TSH range with
both antisera (9.3 μU/ml and 6.4 μU/ml respectively), an exaggerated response to TRH, a T_4 level at the lower limit of
normal and a relative hypersecretion of T_3 (T_4 : T_3 ratio 42).
The other, although she was clinically euthyroid, had biochemical evidence of hyperthyroidism on conventional tests at
the time of the study, (serum T_4 and T_3 levels of 144 ng/ml

and 3.4 ng/ml respectively with a T$_4$: T$_3$ ratio of 43) but when seen before and after the study these parameters were normal.

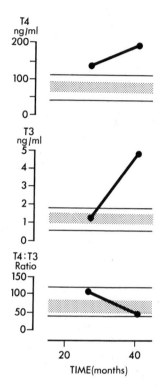

Fig. 4. *Recurrent Hyperthyroidism.*
Horizontal lines and shaded area shown across the figure are explained in Fig. 1.

Patients receiving triiodothyronine

Markedly elevated T$_3$ levels, within the thyrotoxic range, were found in patients receiving T$_3$. In patients on T$_3$ alone, levels ranged from 2.6 to 8 ng/ml, with a mean of 4.8 ± 1.6 ng/ml. The level of serum T$_3$ found did not appear to be related to the legnth of clinical remission. The patients receiving both Carbimazole and T$_3$ had slightly lower T$_3$ levels, mean 3.5 ± 1.1 ng/ml.(Fig. 5).

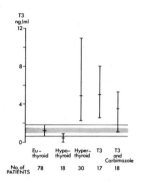

Fig. 5. *T₃ levels in patients receiving T₃ : Means and observed ranges.*
Horizontal lines and shaded area shown across the figure are explained in Fig. 1.

Studies of T$_3$ levels in four patients over a 24 h period showed no relationship to time of dose or meals although there were slight variations greater than the variation in the assay itself. (Fig. 6).

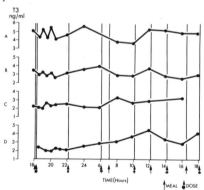

Fig. 6. *Relationship of T₃ levels to time of dose and meals in four patients receiving T₃ 20 μg q.i.d.*

Serum T$_4$ levels ranged from undetectable values to 248

ng/ml (Fig. 7). Patients who had had a prolonged clinical
remission after antithyroid drug therapy had serum T_4 levels
within or below the normal range while patients who had only
a short period of clinical remission after antithyroid drug
therapy or who were receiving Carbimazole as well as T_3, had
a wider range of T_4 values. In both groups of patients, serum
TSH levels were within the normal range and near the limit of
detection of the assay systems.

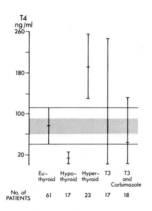

Fig. 7. *T_4 levels in patients receiving T_3 : Means and ob-*
served ranges.
Horizontal lines and shaded area shown across the figure are
explained in Fig. 1.

DISCUSSION

A small but significant increase in T_3 and T_4 levels
associated with a relative hypersecretion of T_3 has been shown
in clinically euthyroid patients many years after cessation of
treatment with Carbimazole for thyrotoxicosis. This change in
pattern of thyroid hormones has been found despite exclusion
of two patients who might be expected to have altered T_4 ; T_3
ratios. One had a TSH level at the upper limit of the normal
range and it is known that TSH stimulation of the thyroid may

alter the $T_4 : T_3$ ratio (13). The other presumably had a
short-lived episode of thyrotoxicosis of the kind that has
been previously described from this clinic (14).

T_3 concentrations, like T_4 concentrations, parallel
variations in TBG (4,13,15) and elevations in protein binding
could contribute to the elevation of T_3 and T_4. However mean
FTI was significantly higher than that found in the euthyroid
control population indicating that protein binding alone did
not completely account for the elevation of thyroid hormones.

The mechanism of these changes is not clearly established
but antithyroid drugs are known to cause an intrathyroidal
iodine deficiency (16) with preferential synthesis of MIT
rather than DIT (17,18) and T_3 rather than T_4 (19.20). Thyrotoxicosis itself is characterised by an absolute or relative
iodine deficiency with a low T_4 ; T_3 ratio which in the extreme
presents as T_3-toxicosis (21,22). Studies by Ermans and Camus
(23) and in this clinic (24) have shown that iodide therapy
may precipitate thyrotoxicosis in the presence of autonomous
thyroid function or following antithyroid drug therapy. Thus
it is suggested that iodine depletion persisting after antithyroid drug therapy may account for the relative hypersecretion
of T_3 and may protect the patient from overt recurrence of
thyrotoxicosis.

Despite the elevation of thyroid hormone levels, consistent
impairment of the TSH response to TRH was not found. If the
normal TSH values found in treated patients are confirmed with
more sensitive assays their inappropriateness in the presence
of elevated T_3 and T_4 levels may indicate that the normal
feedback control mechanism has been reset. This interpretation
might explain the pattern of thyroid hormones found, since

TSH stimulation of the thyroid gland leads to a greater fractional increase in T$_3$ than T$_4$ levels (17).

In previous studies of the relationship between LATS and
circulating thyroid hormone levels, Hollander *et al.* (25)
found higher serum T$_3$ levels in LATS positive than LATS negative
cases of Graves' disease. Enrich *et al.* (26) found no difference in the levels of labelled T$_3$ after the administration of
radioiodine between those two groups but had a significant
positive correlation between the percentage of labelled T$_3$
and corrected LATS values and Foldes *et al.* (27) found no
difference in the ratio of labelled T$_3$ and T$_4$ in the serum
after radioiodine in similar groups of patients. In the two
LATS positive patients in the present series the T$_3$ levels
were not significantly different from the mean level of the
total group studied but the T$_4$: T$_3$ ratios were lower than
the mean. Because of the small number with positive LATS
responses no conclusions can be drawn.

The evolution of hyperthyroidism in one patient whose
thyrotoxicosis recurred is unusual. The development through T$_3$-
toxicosis to T$_3$- plus T$_4$-toxicosis has been described by Hollander and the concept of T$_3$-toxicosis as a premonitory manifestation of classical thyrotoxicosis proposed (25). Shenkman
and his colleagues (1972) reported 10 cases of recurrent hyperthyroidism following each of the three conventional therapies
for hyperthyroidism presenting with hypertriiodothyroninaemia
(28). Whilst this situation with elevation of T$_3$ and T$_4$ levels
is now well established, our finding in one of our patients
of initial hyperthyroxinaemia with a high T$_4$; T$_3$ ratio and
normal T$_3$ levels, appears to be unusual (29). Subsequently,
in this patient, elevation of both T$_3$ and T$_4$ occurred with a

o

low T_4 ; T_3 ratio.

The present study emphasises the low incidence of hypothyroidism after antithyroid drug therapy (30, 31). No patients
were clinically hypothyroid but one patient had a high normal
TSH level with an exaggerated response to TRH.

In patients receiving T_3 (group B) markedly elevated
serum T_3 levels were found. Previous studies (32,33,34) have
reported similar results. Surks *et al.* showed a marked rise
in serum T_3 levels one to two and half hours after single
daily doses of T_3 with a fall to within the euthyroid range
before the next dose. Warner and Gorman showed a stepwise increase in the serum T_3 levels after the commencement of 100
µg T_3 daily by mouth. The maximum levels were two to three
times higher in two of the patients, than those found in euthyroid subjects. In the same study T_3 concentrations far above
those found in euthyroid subjects were produced by administration of doses of T_3 to myxedematous patients just sufficient
to suppress effectively TSH values. Lieblich and Utiger (34)
found a wide variation in serum T_3 levels in T_3 treated patients
and considered this could be explained by the fact that blood
sampling was not carried out at a fixed time after the previous
dose of T_3. However, in our patients there was no obvious
relationship of T_3 levels to the time of dose or meals. Patients
who had lack of suppression of T_4 levels clearly had persistent
thyroid autonomy. However levels in the thyrotoxic range were
found in many patients with lor or undetectable serum thyroxine
levels who were in prolonged clinical remission.

R E F E R E N C E S

1. W.D. Alexander, D.G. McLarty, P. Horton and A.D. Pharma-
   kiotis, *Clin. Endocrinol.* 2, 43 (1973).

2. D.G. McLarty and W.D. Alexander, *Clin. Endicrinol.* (In Press).

3. E.J. Wayne, *Brit. Med. J.* 1, 1 (1960).

4. C.J. Eastman, J.M. Corcoran, A. Jequier, R.P. Ekins and E.S. Williams, *Clin. Sci. Mol. Med.* 45, 251 (1973).

5. W.A. Ratcliffe, J.G. Ratcliffe, A.D. McBride, W.A. Harland, and T.W. Randall, *Clin. Endocrinol.* (In Press)

6. W.A. Ratcliffe, G.S. Challand and J.G. Ratcliffe, *Ann. Clin. Biochem.* (In Press).

7. M. Riley and N. Gochman, Technicon Symposium, 1964.

8. F. Clark and D.B. Horn, *J. Clin. Endocrinol. Metab.* 25, 39, (1965).

9. J. Shimmins, T. Hilditch, R.McG. Harden and W.D. Alexander *J. Clin. Endocrinol. Metab.* 28, 575 (1968).

10. R. McG. Harden, D.K. Mason and W.W. Buchanan, *J. Lab. Clin. Med.* 65, 500 (1965).

11. W.D. Alexander, D.A. Koutras, J. Crooks, W.W. Buchanan, E.M. MacDonald, M.H. Richmond and E.J. Wayne, *Quart. J. Med. (New Series)*, 31, 281 (1962).

12. J.M. McKenzie and A. Williamson, *J. Clin. Endocrinol. Metab.* 26, 518 (1966).

13. P.R. Larsen, *Metabolism* 21, 1073 (1972).

14. D.G. McLarty, W.D. Alexander, R.McG. Harden and J.W.K. Robertson, *Lancet* 1, 6 (1967).

15. P.O.D. Pharoah, N.F. Lawton, S.M. Ellis, E.S. Williams and R.P. Ekins, *Clin. Endocrinol.* 2, 193 (1973).

16. H. Studer and M.A. Greer, *Endocrinol.* 80, 52 (1967).

17. D.W. Slingerland, D.E. Graham, R.K. Joseph, P.F. Mulvey, A.P. Trakas and E. Yamazaki, *Endocrinol.* 65, 178 (1959).

18. J.B. Richards and S.H. Ingbar, *Endocrinol.* 65, 198 (1959).

19. D. Bellabarba, B. Bernard and M. Langlois, *Clin. Endocrinol.* 1, 345 (1972).

20. C.S. Hollander, L. Shenkman, T. Mitsuma and S.P. Asper, *Hopkins Med. J.* 131, 184 (1972).

21. W.D. Odell, D.A. Fisher, S.G. Korenman, D.H. Solomon, I.J. Chopra and R.S. Swerdloff, *Calif. Med.* <u>113</u>, 35 (1970).

22. M.A. Greer, Mayo Clin. Proc. <u>47</u>, 944 (1972).

23. A.M. Ermans and M. Camus, *Acta. Endocrinol.* <u>70</u>, 463 (1973).

24. W.D. Alexander, R.McG. Harden, D.A. Koutras and E.J. Wayne *Lancet,* II, 866 (1965).

25 C.S. Hollander, L. Shenkman, T. Mitsuma, M. Blum, A.S. Kastin and D.G. Anderson, *Lancet,* II 731 (1971).

26. D. Emrich, M. Albain and A. Muhlen, *Acta Endocrinol. (Kbh)* <u>68</u>, 445 (1971).

27. J. Foldes, G. Gyertyanfy, J. Tako, Cs. Banos and E. Gesztesi, *Endokrin.* <u>61</u>, 52 (1973).

28. L. Shenkman, T. Mitsuma, M. Blum and C.S. Hollander, *Ann Intern. Med.* <u>77</u>, 410 (1972).

29. Editorial, *Brit. Med. J.* <u>2</u>, 306 (1972).

30. J.G. Pittman and F. Maloof, *Am. J. Med. Sci.* <u>264</u>, 499, (1972).

31. J.M. Hershman, J.R. Givens, C.E. Cassidy and E.B. Astwood, *J. Clin. Endocrinol.* <u>26</u>, 803 (1966).

32. M.I. Surks, A.R. Schadlow and J.H. Oppenheimer, *J. Clin. Invest.* <u>51</u>, 3104 (1972).

33. J. Leidlich and R.D. Utiger, *J. Clin. Invest.* <u>51</u>, 157 (1972).

34. H.W. Warner and C.A. Gorman, *New Eng. J. Med.* <u>284</u>, 225 (1971).

25. TSH and Thyroid Hormone Levels after ^{131}I Therapy for Thyrotoxicosis

A.D. TOFT, W.J. IRVINE, W.M. HUNTER, J.G. RATCLIFFE
AND J. SETH.

*Department of Endocrinology, Royal Infirmary;
University Departments of Therapeutics and Clinical
Chemistry; M.R.C. Radioimmunoassay Team, Edinburgh;
and Radioimmunoassay Unit, Stobhill Hospital, Glasgow.*

INTRODUCTION

Radioiodine is widely used in the treatment of thyrotoxicosis in patients over 40 years of age. The subsequent
onset of hypothyroidism is a well recognised complication,
the highest incidence occurring in the first post-treatment
year at 7-22%, and continuing at 2-4% per year thereafter
(1), resulting in a cumulative incidence of 80% fifteen years
after therapy in some centres (2). Unfortunately, it has not
proved possible, using conventional tests of thyroid function
to predict when or in whom hypothyroidism will develop with
the result that the follow-up of large numbers of patients
is necessary. Since the serum thyrotrophin (TSH) is a sensitive index of thyroid failure, being elevated in both overt
and subclinical hypothyroidism (3,4), it was hoped that the
routine measurement of circulating TSH and thyroid hormones
might select those patients at risk of developing hypothyroidism after ^{131}I therapy. However, approximately 50% of all

patients who are euthyroid after radioiodine treatment for
thyrotoxicosis have a raised serum TSH (5-9) which may persist
for many months. An elevated TSH level in this group of patien
is not a sign of impending hypothyroidism. Furthermore from
a preliminary study (10) it would appear that the serum T_4
may be a more sensitive index of thyroid failure than TSH in
patients developing hypothyroidism in the early months after
radioiodine treatment.

The present paper describes TSH and thyroid hormone level
both in patients in the early months after ^{131}I therapy for
thyrotoxicosis, when the incidence of hypothyroidism is greatest, and in patients treated some years earlier in whom there
is a lower but significant annual incidence of thyroid failure
In the light of these results not only is a rational follow-
up policy presented for the ever increasing number of patients
who have been treated with ^{131}I for thyrotoxicosis, but also
further progress is made in the understanding of the homeo-
stasis of the brain-thyroid axis.

PATIENTS AND METHODS

Early follow-up after ^{131}I therapy for thyrotoxicosis :

Sixty-two female and 10 male patients were studied,
aged 37-74 years, who had been treated with ^{131}I (4-50 mCi:
mode 7 mCi) for thyrotoxicosis between August 1972 and October
1973 in the Royal Infirmary, Edinburgh. The thyroid status
of each patient was assessed clinically by one observer (A.
D.T.) at 1-2 monthly intervals after treatment and blood withdrawn for the estimation of serum T_4, T_3 and plasma TSH. The
prospective period of follow-up was 2-18 months.

Late follow-up after ^{131}I therapy for thyrotoxicosis :

In February, 1972, the plasma TSH and serum T_4 were
estimated in 233 euthyroid patients who had been treated with
^{131}I for thyrotoxicosis between 1954 and 1966 in the Royal
Infirmary, Edinburgh. A group of 69 of these euthyroid patients
with raised plasma TSH levels was studied again 15 and 24 months
later, and a further group of 61 euthyroid patients with normal
plasma TSH levels was restudied at 24 months. Each patient
was examined clinically by one observer (A.D.T.) and blood
was withdrawn for the estimation of serum T_4 and plasma TSH.

In both the early and late follow-up studies a diagnosis
of hypothyroidism was made on clinical grounds and on the
basis of a low serum T_4 (<4.5μg/100 ml) and a raised plasma
TSH (>7.4μU/ml). Serum T_4 was measured by competitive protein-
binding analysis (11) (normal range 4.5-11.5 μg/100 ml), serum
T_3 by radioimmunoassay (12) (normal range 0.6-1.8 ng/ml) and
plasma TSH by a sensitive double-antibody radioimmunoassay
(13).

R E S U L T S

Early follow-up after ^{131}I *therapy for thyrotoxicosis :*

Forty-one patients were clinically euthyroid at intervals
of 4-18 months after treatment, of whom 32 had a normal plasma
TSH and a normal serum T_4 level. In 3 of these 32 patients,
each followed up for over 12 months, a transient fall in serum
T_4 to below 4.5 μg/100 ml was observed in the early weeks
after treatment and was associated with plasma TSH levels of
1.7, <1.5 and 8.9 μU/ml. In the other 9 patients remaining
clinically euthyroid, normal serum T_4 levels were associated
with plasma TSH values in excess of 7.4 μU/ml.

Clinical hypothyroidism developed in 31 patients 2-8
months (mean 4.3 months) after treatment. In 17 of these

patients a low serum T_4 and a high plasma TSH preceded the
clinical features of hypothyroidism by 1-4 months, and in 6
patients both indices of thyroid function were normal at the
clinic visit 1-2 months before hypothyroidism was diagnosed.
A rise in plasma TSH preceded a fall in serum T_4 in only 1 of
the 31 patients and in 7 patients a low serum T_4 in the presence of a normal plasma TSH level was the first indication
of thyroid failure, suggesting that a low serum T_4 is a more
sensitive index of impending hypothyroidism than the plasma
TSH. Serial serum T_3 levels were estimated in the 7 patients
in whom a low serum T_4 was the first sign of developing hypothyroidism. In 3 of these patients the low serum T_4 and normal
plasma TSH were associated with serum T_3 levels of 2.24, 1.2
and 0.88 ng/ml, 1-2 months after therapy with [131]I. Pituitary
TSH secretion was presumably suppressed, albeit temporarily,
by the high or normal serum T_3 concentrations, but as the serum
T_3 fell in subsequent weeks, not necessarily into the hypothyroid range, the plasma TSH rose and clinical hypothyroidism
developed. In the remaining 4 patients a low serum T_3, low
serum T_4 and a normal plasma TSH were observed while the patient was clinically euthyroid. (Fig. 1). This phenomenon was
temporary and in each case not only was the plasma TSH elevated 1 month later but hypothyroidism had developed in 3 of
the 4 patients. The fourth patient remained clinically euthyroid despite low serum T_3 and T_4 levels and a high plasma TSH
for 2 months.

Late follow-up after [131]*I therapy for thyrotoxicosis:*

The plasma TSH level was raised in 136 (58%) of the 233
patients euthyroid after ^{131}I therapy for thyrotoxicosis between 1954 and 1966 and normal in 97 (42%) when estimated in
February 1972.

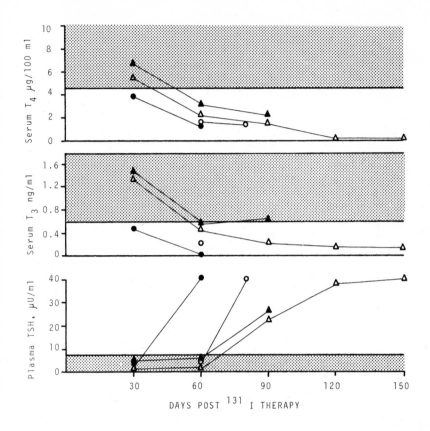

Fig. 1. *Serum T_4, T_3 and plasma TSH levels in the 4 patients in whom low serum T_4 and T_3 levels were observed in the presence of a normal plasma TSH prior to the development of hypothyroidism. (From Journal of Clinical Endocrinology and Metabolism, 39, 607 (1974).*

The mean (± S.E.) serum T_4 and plasma TSH levels in the 69 euthyroid patients with high plasma TSH levels in 1972 and in those remaining euthyroid in 1973 and 1974, 15 and 24 months later are shown in Table 1. Only 3 of the 69 patients developed hypothyroidism over the 15 month period; the plasma TSH had

Table 1.

	Serum T_4 (μg/100 ml)	Plasma TSH (μU/ml)
February 1972	6.8 ± 0.1	25.0 ± 2.0
May 1973	6.5 ± 0.1	22.6 ± 1.8
February 1974	6.5 ± 0.1	21.6 ± 2.0

Mean serum T_4 and plasma TSH levels (± S.E.) in 69
patients with high plasma TSH levels in 1972 and in
66 and 61 patients remaining euthyroid in 1973 and
1974. All were treated with 131I for thyrotoxicosis
between 1954 and 1966. (From reference 9).

Table 2.

	Serum T_4 (μg/100 ml)	Plasma TSH (μU/ml)
February 1972	8.7 ± 0.3	4.0 ± 0.2
February 1974	8.1 ± 0.2	4.1 ± 0.3

Mean serum T_4 and plasma TSH levels (± S.E.) in 61
patients with low plasma TSH levels in 1972 and 1974.
All were treated with 131I for thyrotoxicosis between
between 1954 and 1966. (From reference 9).

risen in one (from 34.6 to 67.3 μU/ml), had fallen in the
second (from 45.6 to 28.2 μU/ml), and had remained virtually
unchanged in the third (90.4 and 92.8 μU/ml). At 24 months
64 of the 66 patients remaining euthyroid in 1973 were available for study. Hypothyroidism had developed in a further 3
patients in whom the plasma TSH levels remained essentially
unchanged (32.8 and 32.0, 23.5 and 26.1, and 27.5 and 31.2
μU/ml).

All 61 euthyroid patients with normal plasma TSH levels
in 1972 remained euthyroid over a 24 month period and the

mean serum T_4 and plasma TSH levels in 1972 and 1974 are
shown in Table 2. In 3 of these 61 patients, however, the
plasma TSH became slightly raised to 9.4, 9.7 and 12.6 µU/ml
respectively. The mean serum T_4 level in the euthyroid patients
with a high plasma TSH was significantly lower than that in
the euthyroid patients with a normal plasma TSH both in 1972
(P<0.001) and in 1974 (P<0.001).

D I S C U S S I O N

Although a raised plasma TSH is a good index of thyroid
failure, the present study has shown that a low serum T_4 level
is more indicative of impending hypothyroidism in the early
months after radioiodine treatment of hyperthyroidism than
the plasma TSH. A low serum T_4 is a well recognised finding
in euthyroid patients many years after ^{131}I treatment, but is
invariably associated with high circulating levels of TSH and
normal or high levels of T_3 (14,15). In such patients the thyroid remnant presumably fails to meet secretory demands, pituitary TSH output is no longer suppressed and the resulting
rise in the level of TSH increases the T_3/T_4 ratio and the
euthyroid state may be maintained indefinitely.

In contract a low serum T_4, which may be associated with
a normal plasma TSH level, occurring in the early months after
^{131}I therapy for thyrotoxicosis usually indicates the onset
of clinical hypothyroidism within weeks. Of the 7 patients
in whom a low T_4 and a normal TSH level were found before the
onset of hypothyroidism a normal or high T_3 concentration was
observed in 3 patients which may simply reflect the ability
of the thyroid gland damaged by irradiation to maintain T_3
synthesis and secretion longer than that of T_4. The T_3 level

fell in subsequent weeks, not necessarily into the hypothyroid range, in these 3 patients, the plasma TSH rose and clinical hypothyroidism developed. In the other 4 patients the transient phenomenon of low serum T_4 and normal TSH was associated with a low serum T_3 level. The TSH level rose and hypothyroidism developed in the subsequent two months.

It is possible that the metabolic effects of T_3 and T_4 at the hypothalamic and/or thyrotroph level persist for some time after an alteration in circulating thyroid hormone concentration, and the plasma TSH is slow to rise despite low levels of serum T_3 and T_4. Indeed if T_3 replacement therapy is withdrawn from athyreotic patients plasma TSH levels remain suppressed for some days (16) and in humans administration of thyroid hormone for relatively short periods results in a marked decrease in pituitary TSH content (17). Furthermore, there is a reduced number of thyrotrophs in the pituitary glands of patients with thyrotoxicosis (18). The transient lack of TSH response to thyrotrophin-releasing hormone, for a period of 4 weeks in patients with normal or low serum T_3 and T_4 levels after partial thyroidectomy for thyrotoxicosis (19), suggests that the main site of suppression of the hypothalamo-pituitary -thyroid axis by excess circulating thyroid hormone occurs at the thyrotroph level. There may also be an element of suppression at the hypothalamic level, however, and a situation in thyrotoxicosis may exist which is analogous to the suppression of the hypothalamo-pituitary-adrenal axis in patients exposed to prolonged high levels of circulating cortico-steroids (20, 23). A sluggish response of the pituitary thyrotroph to the presence of low serum thyroid hormone levels in patients recently treated with ^{131}I for thyrotoxicosis might therefore be expected.

Since the early 1950's radioiodine has been widely used in the treatment of thyrotoxicosis, and in 1973 at least 3,000 patients were treated for the first time with ^{131}I in the United Kingdom. In most centres, since patients are seen frequently in the first post-therapy year when the incidence of hypothyroidism is highest, and at intervals of 6 to 12 months thereafter on a life-long basis or until hypothyroidism develops, the major out-patient commitment in an endocrine clinic is the follow-up of thyrotoxic patients treated with radio-iodine. Unfortunately, in the past no test of thyroid function has been of use in predicting the onset of hypothyroidism.

Following radioiodine some 50% of euthyroid patients have raised plasma TSH values which may persist for many months, implying that a high plasma TSH is of no more value than conventional tests of thyroid function in selecting patients at an increased risk of developing hypothyroidism. It is of interest, therefore, that no patient in the present study with a normal plasma TSH level after ^{131}I treatment 6–18 years earlier for thyrotoxicosis developed hypothyroidism over a 2 year period, whereas hypothyroidism developed at the rate of 5% per year in similarly treated euthyroid patients with raised TSH levels. On the assumption that plasma TSH levels are of the same significance in patients between 1–6 years after ^{131}I therapy for thyrotoxicosis, we would suggest that in addition to clinical examination at 2, 4 and 6 months after therapy the serum T_4 alone is estimated. At 12 months the circulating TSH level should be determined and if it is raised the patient should be seen again one year later, but if it is normal review need not be undertaken for at least a further

2 years.

One possible interpretation of the significantly lower mean serum T_4 levels in the euthyroid patients with high plasma TSH levels compared with the euthyroid patients with normal plasma TSH levels after ^{131}I therapy is that the serum T_4 levels in the former group were suboptimal. Any increase in morbidity such as ischaemic heart disease, in these patients will become apparent only in future years and at present no thyroxine replacement therapy has been instituted.

R E F E R E N C E S

1. G.A. Hagan, *Medical Clinics of North America*, 52, 417, (1968).

2. W.R. Greig, *British Journal of Surgery*, 60, 758 (1973).

3. W.D. Odell, J.F. Wilber and R.D. Utiger, *Recent Progress in Hormone Research*, 23, 47, (1967).

4. R. Hall, *Clinical Endocrinology*, 1, 115 (1972).

5. D.W. Slingerland, E.S. Dell and B.A. Burrows, *In* "6th International Thyroid Conference" (K. Fellinger and R. Hoefer, eds), Vienna 1970.

6. D.W. Slingerland, J.M. Hershman, E.S. Dell and B.A. Burrows, *J. Clin. Endocrinol. and Metab.* 35, 912 (1972).

7. A.D. Toft, E.W. Barnes, W.M. Hunter, J. Seth and W.J. Irvine, *Lancet* ii 644, (1973).

8. W.M.G. Tunbridge, P. Harsoulis and A.W.G. Goolden, *Brit. Med. J.* 3, 89 (1974).

9. A.D. Toft, W.J. Irvine, W.M. Hunter and J. Seth, *Brit. Med. J.* 3, 152 (1974).

10. A.D. Toft, W.M. Hunter, J. Seth and W.J. Irvine, *Lancet*, i, 704 (1974).

11. J. Seth, *Clin. Chim. Acta* 46, 43 (1973).

12. W.A. Ratcliffe, G.S. Challand and J.G. Ratcliffe, (in preparation).

13. W.J. Irvine, A.D. Toft, W.M. Hunter and K.E. Kirkham. *Clin. Endocrinology,* 2, 135 (1973).

14. K. Sterling, M.A. Brenner, E.S. Newman, W.D. Odell and D. Bellabarba, *J. Clin. Endocrinol. and Metab.* 33, 729 (1971).

15. D. Bellabarba, B. Bernard and M. Langlois, *Clin. Endocrinol.* 1, 345 (1972).

16. J.M. Hershman,C.L. Edwards, *J. Clin. Endocrinol. and Metab.* 34, 814 (1972).

17. J.L. Bakke, H. Kammer and L. Lawrence, *J. Clin. Endocrinol. and Metab.* 24, 281 (1964).

18. S. Murray and C. Ezrin, *J. Clin. Endocrinol. and Metab.* 26, 287 (1966).

19. F. Sanchez-Franco, M.D. Garcia, L. Cacicedo, A. Martin-Zurro, F. Escobar Del Rey and G. Morreale de Escobar, *J. Clin. Endocrinol. and Metab.* 38, 1098 (1974).

20. B.L.J. Treadwell, O. Savage, E.D. Sever and W.S.C. Copeman, *Lancet,* i, 355 (1963).

21. J. Landon, V. Wynn, V.H.T. James and J.B. Wood, *J. Clin. Endocrinol. and Metab.* 25, 602 (1965).

22. T. Livanou, D. Ferriman and V.H.T. James, *Lancet,* ii, 856 (1967).

23. M.K. Jasani, J.A. Boyle, W.R. Greig, T.G. Dalakos, M.C.K. Browning, A. Thompson and W.W. Buchanan, *Quart. J. Med.* 36, 261 (1967).

26. Evaluation of Serum T_3 Levels as a Routine Thyroid Test

D.R. HADDEN, ANNE McMASTER, T.K. BELL, J.A. WEAVER
AND D.A.D. MONTGOMERY.

Royal Victoria Hospital, Belfast.

INTRODUCTION

Measurement of serum triiodothyronine (T_3) is a pre-requisite for the diagnosis of T_3-toxicosis and its estimation may also be desirable in the differentiation of "hypothyroidism" from "compensated euthyroidism". Acute TRH and TSH tests have enhanced value by incorporation of serum T_3 responses. However, it is not clear whether measurement of serum T_3 has a major role in a routine thyroid clinic.

A priori, knowledge of a hormone that accounts for about 50% of thyroid metabolic activity seems desirable, but if T_3 simply reflected thyroxine (T_4) levels in most situations, its estimation might be an unnecessary laboratory task.

PATIENTS

In this study concomitant measurements of serum T_3 and T_4 have been undertaken in all patients attending a thyroid clinic to determine whether the knowledge of serum T_3 levels was helpful. Data from 549 patients, involving 1,470 T_3 and T_4 measurements are included representing clinic attendances from January 1973 to January 1974 (Table 1). In addition to

Table 1.   *Patients studied January 1973 - January 1974*

Hyperthyroid :	Untreated	90	
	Follow-up : Euthyroid	185	
	Relapsing	13	288
Hypothyroid :	Untreated	41	
	Follow-up	104	
	Hypopituitary	15	160
Euthyroid :	Simple goitre	61	
	Other thyroid states (cancer, thyroiditis, etc.)	8	
	Endocrine exophthalmos	6	
	Others	25	101
			549

serum T_3 and T_4, most patients had at various times radioiodine neck uptakes, protein bound iodine, serum TSH or thyroid antibody studies where appropriate. Data from 59 patients
without thyroid abnormality have been used for purposes of
comparison.

M E T H O D S

Serum thyroxine was estimated by competitive protein
binding using Thyopac-4 kits containing absorbent granules.
A free thyroxine index (FTI) was determined from these values
in association with a T_3-uptake ratio using Thyopac-3 kits
(with the Thyopac-3 test the uptake by the serum is measured
instead of the uptake by the secondary binder as in most other
techniques, consequently the FTI is calculated as $\frac{\text{Thyopac-4}}{\text{Thyopac-3}} \times 100$
A normal range for this FTI is 4.0 to 11.0 (1).

Serum T_3 was measured by specific radioimmune-assay
using sodium salicylate to block T_3 binding by serum proteins
(2). Figure 1 shows the standard curve for the assay. The
upper and lower limits of normality have been taken as 220
and 80 ng per 100ml, derived from a previous study of 170
control sera (mean 146 ng/100 ml, standard deviation 35 ng/100ml).

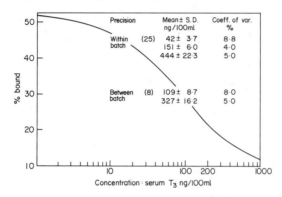

Figure 1. *The standard curve for the T₃-radioimmunoassay
(details of within-batch and between-batch precision are stated.*

HYPERTHYROIDISM

Ninety untreated hyperthyroid patients have been studied
(untreated implies no antithyroid treatment within the previous
12 months). This was the initial onset of hyperthyroidism in
69 of these patients. Figure 2 is a log/log scatter diagram
of serum T_3 and T_4 in 59 selected euthyroid subjects and the
90 hyperthyroid patients. Eighty-one of these patients showed
elevation of both serum T_3 and T_4 in keeping with the other
diagnostic findings of hyperthyroidism. Seven patients had T_3
above the normal range with normal T_4, and two patients had
high T_4 with normal T_3 values (although these were at the
upper range).

There were thus 7 patients in whom the diagnosis of T_3-

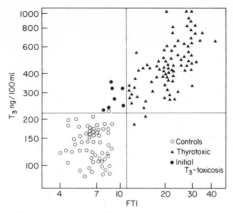

Figure 2. *Log/log scatter diagram of serum T3 and FTI in 59*
selected euthyroid subjects (controls), and 90 consecutive
hyperthyroid patients at the time of diagnosis. The inter-
secting lines at T3 220 ng per 100 ml and FTI 11.0 represent
the upper limits of the normal ranges. Eighty-three of the
hyperthyroid patients show elevated FTI values, 81 of which
are associated with an elevated T3. Seven patients represent
initial T3-toxicosis.

toxicosis was accepted on both clinical and laboratory evidence at their initial presentation. Six were female; their
mean age was 49 years (range 24 to 63). Five had vague and
indefinite symptoms of thyroid hormone excess including
sweating, palpitations, slow weight loss, tiredness and anxi-
ety: 2 presented for investigation of a goitre. Five had a
palpable thyroid gland (2 diffuse, 2 nodular and one a recurrent nodule after previous subtotal thyroidectomy). One had
minimal exophthalmos. The mean pulse rate (untreated) was 82
per minute. At the time the diagnosis was accepted the mean
free thyroxine index was 8.6 (range 7.0 to 10.7) and the mean
T_3 289 ng per 100ml (range 220 to 340). The mean serum T_3-
binding index (Thyopac-3) was 108% and the mean total T_4 8.8
μg per 100 ml (Thyopac-4).

Relative T_3 excess also occurred during the treatment of hyperthyroidism. Figure 3 shows 40 occasions where T_3 was elevated while T_4 was normal in the 90 patients. The 7 cases of initial T_3-toxicosis are contrasted with 33 episodes of similar T_3 and T_4 disparity developing during therapy. Two

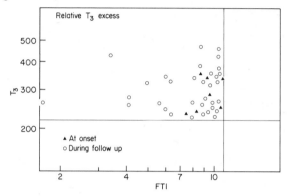

Fig. 3.*Relative T₃ excess (when FTI was normal) during treatment of hyperthyroidism. (Log/log scale with normal ranges as Fig. 2)*

values must represent overtreatment since the elevated T_3 is associated with an FTI level below 4.0. In 8 other instances FTI is at or below the mean FTI in controls (7.0) and the combined T_3 and T_4 levels probably represent euthyroidism. The remaining 23 seem acceptable as "episodic treatment phases of T_3-toxicosis".

A further 61 of the hyperthyroid patients were under active treatment at the time the T_3 assay became available to us and results from these patients have been combined with those from the 90 newly-diagnosed thyrotoxic patients. The total of 151 patients provided 281 tests at intervals during treatment for thyrotoxicosis, when T_3 and/or T_4 was elevated. Raised T_3 with normal T_4 was found in 87 instances, a pre-

valence of 31% of "biochemical T_3-toxicosis" as an isolated
phenomenon during treatment of hyperthyroidism. This state
was found particularly during treatment with carbimazole or
during a relapse of hyperthyroidism.

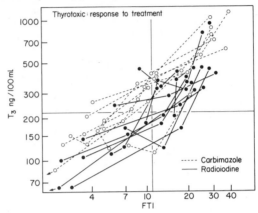

Fig. 4. *Response to treatment of hyperthyroidism by radioactive iodine or carbimazole. (log/log scale as Fig. 2). The
lines join observations in individual patients from the time
of diagnosis (upper right quadrant), at monthly intervals
during treatment for the first 3 months.*

Medical treatment of hyperthyroidism was either with a
low dose of radioactive iodine (usually 2.5 millicuries) and
propranolol (3) or with long-term carbimazole. Figure 4 con-
trasts the response to radioactive iodine with that to carbimazole. The pattern of response suggests a difference with
regard to serum T_3 and T_4 ratios during these treatments. A
consistent pattern of relative T_3 excess occurred with carbimazole treatment. This observation is confirmed in Table 2
which combines 45 episodes of relative T_3 excess and relative
T_4 excess among the 83 hyperthyroid patients during treatment
(7 initial T_3-toxicosis patients again excluded). The disparity
of T_4 and T_3 (high T_3 levels) during carbimazole is contrary

Table 2.   *T₃ or T₄ disparity during treatment of
hyperthyroidism*

	Carbimazole	Radioactive iodine	Total
High T_4 Normal T_3	2	14	16
High T_3 Normal T_4	20	9	29
	22	23	45

X^2 (with Yates' correction) = 10.99 : P < 0.001

to expectation. Other workers (4) have suggested that propyl-thiouracil may inhibit T_4 to T_3 conversion. It appears that carbimazole acts differently to propylthiouracil in this regard, and that intrathyroidal iodine deficiency is induced which favours higher T_3 production by the gland to a greater degree than any peripheral inhibition of T_4 to T_3 conversion. There is no explanation of relative T_4 preponderance after radioiodine treatment unless the intrathyroidal situation is envisaged as an iodine replete environment in terms of the functioning (non-damaged) thyroid cells, or that it is related to pro-pranolol therapy.

Figure 5 shows serum T_4 and T_3 levels at diagnosis in the 90 hyperthyroid patients displayed against an approximate index of the total serum binding capacity (thyopac-3). The lines represent the means of T_4 and T_3 values for each 10% change in binding. The similar slope of these lines shows there is as good a relationship for T_3 as for T_4 with the serum binding capacity: in both cases highest total hormone levels

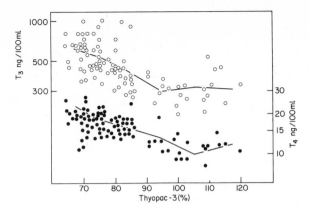

Fig. 5. T_3 and T_4 values (vertical log scales) in the 90 hyperthyroid patients at diagnosis plotted against the Thyopac-3 result. The lines represent means of T_3 and T_4 for each 10% change in binding.

are associated with lowest remaining binding capacity. The parallel nature of T_3 and T_4 levels to the binding measurement is to be expected since both hormones are practically all bound. Other relationships may exist in that total T_4 and degree of binding determines the free T_4 which must presumably be the precursor for T_3 derived by peripheral deiodination. It might be noted that the mean Thyopac-3 for the 7 cases of initial T_3-toxicosis in the present series was 108%. This might be the reason we have not found any of the very markedly raised T_3 levels in T_3-toxicosis described by some other workers, and that these must have been due to a primary abnormality of thyroid hormone production by the gland.

The maximum overall incidence of relative T_3 excess (T_3-toxicosis) in this large group of unselected consecutive patients with clinical hyperthyroidism was about 8% at the time of diagnosis: in hyperthyroid patients requiring treatment for thyrotoxicosis isolated episodes of relative T_3 excess can be demonstrated in 31%. The 8% incidence of T_3-toxicosis in this

unselected series is higher than the figure of 4% quoted by
Hollander *et al.* (5). Four of our 7 patients on repeated
testing before definitive antithyroid treatment were found
eventually to have a raised serum T_4 value and only 3 remained
persistently as T_3-toxicosis.

HYPOTHYROIDISM

Data from 36 of the untreated hypothyroid patients are
shown in Fig. 6 (22 primary, 8 post-radioiodine treatment, 6
post-thyroidectomy). The mean FTI in these patients was 1.4
(range <0.1 to 4.1). Thirty-seven patients with "compensated
euthyroidism" were selected for comparison from follow-up of
the radioiodine treated and post-thyroidectomy groups, and on
2 clinic visits had been accepted as euthyroid despite a low
free thyroxine index. Their mean FTI was 2.5 (range 0.3 to
3.9). All the patients in Fig. 6 therefore had an abnormally
low serum T_4. Inspection of serum T_3 and TSH levels shows that
the lowest T_3 levels were associated with the highest TSH res-

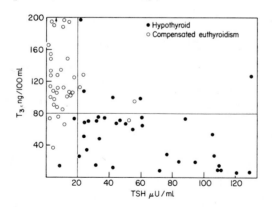

Fig. 6. *T_3 and TSH values (normal scales) in 36 untreated
clinically hypothyroid patients and 37 patients with compensated euthyroidism. All of these patients had FTI below 4.0.*

ponses (8 of 11 patients with T_3 below 20 ng per 100 ml had
a TSH level above 70 µU/ml). Five of the 34 clinically hypothyroid patients had serum T_3 levels within the normal range.
Four T_3 values in "compensated euthyroidism" were abnormally
low but no clinical evidence of hypothyroidism had been established. The borderline between the two states of clinical
hypothyroidism and "compensated euthyroidism" thus appears
indefinite but in this study most of the clinically hypothyroid patients had very low T_4 levels with serum T_3 below 80
ng per 100 ml and TSH elevated above 20 µU/ml. Compensated
cases had consistently slightly higher T_3 and T_4 levels and
lower TSH levels. These figures are conveniently compared as
a table (Table 3).

Table 3. *Comparison of the uncompensated and compensated*
states of subnormal serum thyroxine

	Uncompensated (clinically hypothyroid)	Compensated (clinically euthyroid)
T_4	0 - 2 µg per 100 ml	2 - 4 µg per 100 ml
T_3	Below 80 ng per 100 ml	Above 80 ng per 100 ml
TSH	Above 20 µU/ml	Below 20 µU/ml

T_4 and T_3 values in the hypothyroid patients already on
thyroxine therapy at various doses are shown as a log/log
scatter diagram in Fig. 7. This shows achievement of adequate
T_3 levels during T_4 therapy with a tendency for the results to
skew into the excess T_4 sector. The results confirm that many
cases are biochemically overtreated even with doses of thyroxine of 0.2 mg daily. Twenty-two patients had both T_4 and T_3
values above the normal range. Ten had high T_3 levels. In a
large number elevated T_4 values were found with T_3 levels in

the upper range of normal. Approximately one-third of the
patients appear biochemically overtreated although evidence of
clinical overtreatment in these patients is less certain.
Nevertheless, 7 out of 14 who were on 0.3 mg thyroxine daily
had T$_3$ and T$_4$ values within the normal range, indicating individual variation in the requirements of thyroxine dosage (these
figures are not corrected for body weight, age or sex).

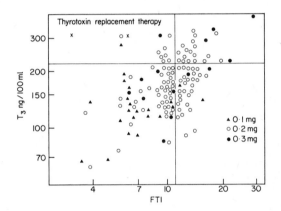

Fig. 7. *T$_3$ and FTI values (log/log scales as in Fig. 2) in
104 hypothyroid patients on treatment with various doses of
thyroxine. (The two cases labelled X were on treatment with
desiccated thyroid g 3, and triiodothyronine 80 ng daily).*

OPHTHALMIC GRAVES' DISEASE

Six euthyroid patients with endocrine exophthalmos were
studied: the mean T$_3$ value was 173 ng per 100 ml (range 145
to 210) and mean FTI 7.1 (range 4.5 to 9.4). In general these
patients tended to have higher T$_3$ values than euthyroid subjects and one patient is shown who progressed to frank T$_3$-
toxicosis (Fig. 8). It may be that measurement of serum T$_3$
will allow a further sensitive index of follow-up of these
patients.

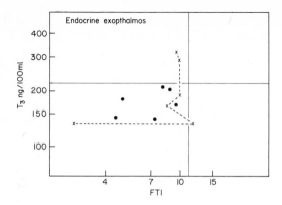

Fig. 8. *Endocrine exophthalmos : T₃ and T₄ values (log/log scales as Fig. 2) in 6 patients. Consecutive observations in one patient are joined by the dotted line.*

CONCLUSION

Routine knowledge of the T_3 level was useful in several clinical situations – the identification of T_3-toxicosis, early relapse of hyperthyroidism and in definition of the compensated euthyroid state. The occurrence of persistent elevation of T_3 without rise in T_4, with symptoms or signs of thyroid over-activity was relatively rare and in this clinic represented less than 5% of our hyperthyroid patients. We have found more frequently isolated episodes of relative T_3 excess, but these have not been associated with any recognisable new clinical features. We have not observed any instances of extremely high T_3 without T_4 also being very high and the clinical symptoms severe.

The patients we have described as T_3-toxicosis appear to represent merely one segment of that borderline area which includes the upper part of the normal range and the lower part of the hyperthyroid range. It appears that the same patient may

vary somewhat from time to time as to the segment of this
horderline area in which he falls.

Acknowledgements
We are grateful to Mrs. M. Burke for clerical assistance in
tracing the progress of these patients, and to Sister M. Murphy
at the Metabolic Outpatient Clinic who was responsible for
obtaining the blood specimens. Mr. D.W. Neill and his colleagues
in the Biochemistry Department also provided the routine bio-
chemical measurements.

R E F E R E N C E S

1.   T.K. Bell, D.A. Boyle, D.A.D. Montgomery and S.J. Todd,
     J. Clin. Path. <u>27</u>, 372-376 (1974).

2.   P.R. Larsen, *J. Clin. Invest.* <u>51</u>, 1939-1949 (1972).

3.   R.G. Shanks, D.R. Hadden, D.C. Lowe, D.G. McDevitt and
     D.A.D. Montgomery, *Lancet,* <u>1</u>, 993-995 (1969).

4.   L.S. Shenkman, T. Mitsuma and C.S. Hollander, *J. Clin.*
     Invest. <u>52</u>, 205-209 (1973).

5.   C.S. Hollander, C. Stevenson, T. Mitsuma, G. Pineda,
     L. Shenkman and E. Silva, *Lancet,* <u>2</u>, 1276-1278 (1972).

27. Thyroid Hormones during Treatment of Thyroid Cancer

C.J. EDMONDS, B.D. THOMPSON AND SUSAN HAYES

Medical Unit
MRC Department of Clinical Research,
University College Hospital Medical School, London, WC1
and Department of Chemical Pathology,
University College Hospital, London, WC1.

With the introduction of methods for measuring blood levels of thyroid hormones, it has become possible to follow the changes occurring during the course of treatment of functioning thyroid cancer and to relate these changes to the response to treatment and the degree of concentration of ^{131}I by the tumour. In the present account, we review some of our results obtained from studies on patients over several years and attempt to assess the value of the measurements in clinical situations.

METHODS USED

Measurements were made on blood samples obtained from patients with functioning thyroid carcinoma who were following our usual scheme of treatment, (Fig. 1), the general plan of which has been described by Pochin (1). No modifications of treatment were introduced for the present study, other than increased frequency of blood sampling; the patient's consent was always obtained after full explanation. Since there is often a significant remnant of normal thyroid tissue remaining

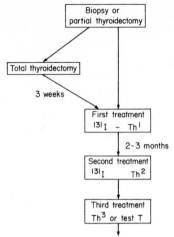

Fig. 1. *Treatment protocol that was followed in patients treated with ^{131}I.*

after total thyroidectomy, the first treatment dose (Th^1) at 80 mCi was smaller than subsequent ones at 150 mCi. Occasionally, the second treatment dose (ordinarily 150 mCi) was reduced where the tumour had a high production of organic iodine compounds which might give potentially dangerous whole body irradiation.

Plasma TSH was measured in 0.1 ml samples using the double antibody radioimmunoassay basically as described by Hall, Amas and Ormston (2). In normal individuals, the range was 0-4 μU/ml. Total plasma T_3 was measured by double antibody radioimmunoassay, the antisera to T_3 being raised in rabbits using T_3 conjugated to bovine serum albumin (3). Our normal range obtained from a large group of individuals is 0.8-2.0 ng/ml (conversion factor to nmol/l; multiply by 1.54). The lowest level that can be measured in the assay is 0.2 ng/ml. Total plasma T_4 was measured by competitive protein binding using the Amersham Thyopac μ kit method. The normal range is 4.0-

12.2 µg/100 ml (conversion factor to nmol/1 multiply by 12.9).

BEFORE TREATMENT

Rather few studies have been so far made on patients before treatment has begun since most patients have had extensive surgery before referral. The results (Table 1) are from patients who have had no or only minimal surgery where biopsy or local removal has been done when the surgeon had believed the condition benign. There has long been discussion as to the possibility that prolonged stimulation by elevated TSH levels might play a role in the genesis of thyroid cancer and there is evidence for this hypothesis from animal experiments. However, in none of our patients was there anything to support such a view, for, at least at the time they were first seen, plasma TSH was always within the normal range. For T_3, too, the mean values and ranges were similar to those obtained from the normal individuals. In the case of T_4, however, the mean value was relatively high, near the top limit of normal, accounted for by the fact that 4 patients had higher than normal values, ranging from 13.0 to 17.5 µg/100 ml. These patients had no signs of symptoms that could be associated with the T_4 elevation and its significance at present is obscure.

AFTER TOTAL THYROIDECTOMY

The measurements were made at about three weeks after total thyroidectomy in 38 patients (Table 2). In about 40% (14 patients), plasma TSH was within the normal range. In just over 40% (16 patients), plasma TSH was greater than 20 µU/ml while in the remaining 8 patients, it was in the range 4-20 µU/ml. Thus after total thyroidectomy alone, within three

P

Table 1. *Hormonal levels before*

	n	
(1) No surgery or biopsy only	8	(5F (3M
(2) After a localised removal	4	(3F (1M

weeks about half of the patients had little rise in TSH and
stimulation of the remaining tissue will have been slight.

The TSH elevation appeared to be closely related to the
reduction of plasma T_4 (Fig. 3) but with T_3, the relationship
was more variable, although on average being at its lowest
level in the patients with the highest TSH. The more variable
relationship between T_3 and TSH may be because the small remnant left after operation tends to produce T_3 in relatively
greater proportion when stimulated by high TSH levels.

AFTER THE FIRST TREATMENT DOSE OF ^{131}I

These measurements were derived from patients who had
received their first treatment dose two to three months previously. None of the patients had been receiving L-thyroxine
replacement. Only two of the 25 patients examined at this
stage had a plasma TSH level within the normal range (Table 2).
One of these two patients had had a low uptake of ^{131}I at the
first dose (less than 3.5% at 24 h) which appeared to be inadequate to destroy the thyroid remnant, for despite lack of
thyroxine supplement plasma T_4 was 8.4 µg/100 ml and T_3 1.5

treatment *(Mean and range).*

TSH μU/ml	T$_4$ (μg/100ml)	T$_3$ (ng/ml)
2.0	11.6	1.56
(< 1.0-3.9)	(4.6-17.5)	(1.0-2.1)
1.5	7.6	1.49
(< 1.0-2.1	(3.8-11.0)	(1.23-1.7)

ng/ml at the time of the second treatment dose. The results
obtained from the other patient are shown in Fig. 3. For the
second and third treatment doses, the ^{131}I uptakes were very
low and plasma TSH was also within the normal range for both
these doses. Unfortunately we have no certain explanation for
this anomaly as the full complement of hormonal studies was
not available at the time of the investigation. Presumably a
small remnant of normal tissue was producing just enough T$_4$
and T$_3$ to prevent increased TSH secretion. However that may be,
by the fourth treatment dose, considerable ^{131}I concentration
had appeared associated with an elevated TSH level. This concentration was almost certainly in tumour tissue being associated with the development of considerable blood activity
(organic iodine 0.84% dose/litre at 6 days after the dose)
more than 60% of which was due to iodoalbumin and other iodinated serum proteins.

In the remaining 23 patients, plasma TSH was elevated and
in nearly 90%, the values exceeded 20 μU/ml. Both plasma T$_4$
and T$_3$ were reduced in these patients well below the normal
level, T$_4$ averaging 1.9 ± 0.9 (S.D.) μg/100 ml and T$_3$ 0.44 ±

Table 2. TSH levels in patients with thyroid carcinoma after thyroidectomy and a single treatment dose of ^{131}I.

		TSH (μU/ml)					
		0-4	4-20	20-50	50-100	< 100	Total
3 weeks after thyroidectomy alone	Number of patients (n)	14	8	7	7	2	38
	% of total	38	21	18	18	5	
				41			
2-3 months after first ^{131}I therapy dose	Number of patients (n)	2	1	5	14	3	25
	% of total	8	4	20	56	12	
				88			

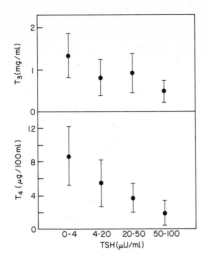

Fig. 2. *Relationship between plasma T_4, T_3 and TSH from meas-urements made on blood obtained two to three weeks after total thyroidectomy (mean ± S.D.).*

0.16 (S.D.) ng/ml. Thus after surgery and the first radio-iodine dose, there is in the great majority of patients con-siderable stimulation of any remaining normal or abnormal thy-roid tissue.

HORMONE LEVELS IN ATHYREOTIC PATIENTS

A number of measurements have been made in patients who have received several large doses of ^{131}I and have no detect-able residual tissue. The absence of functioning tissue was shown both by linear and two-dimensional scanning repeated over several days, to exclude the presence of any significant local concentration of ^{131}I. All these patients were maintained on 0.3 mg of thyroxine daily between treatment or test doses. The results of measurements made on a number of these patients while they were taking thyroxine are shown in Table 3. No detectable plasma TSH was present. The plasma T_4 was greater than normal while the T_3 level was within the normal range.

Table 3. *Hormonal levels in athyreotic patients maintained*
on thyroxine 0.3 mg daily (mean and range).

Patients	Time on T_4 (years)	TSH μU/ml	T_4 μg/100ml	T_3 ng/ml
M9			14.9	1.35
n=27	1-5	<1.0		
F18			(8.2-21.2)	(1.0-2.4)

Thus as has been shown by others (4) there is considerable
conversion of T_4 to T_3 in athyreotic individuals.

In eight patients, the effect of stopping thyroxine was
examined by obtaining blood samples at intervals over a period
of six weeks around the giving of a test dose (Fig. 4). TSH
was still undetectable in the blood one week after stopping
thyroxine administration but by two weeks was elevated above
the normal level in all patients and rose still further by
four weeks. It seems therefore that at least two weeks preceding the ^{131}I dose, any remaining tissue comes under continuous and considerable TSH stimulation.

When thyroxine 0.3 mg daily was restarted, three days
after the ^{131}I dose had been given, there was a rapid fall of
plasma TSH and rise of plasma T_4 so that within ten days these
had reached levels similar to those obtained during continuous
thyroxine administration.

Since the uptake of radioiodine by functioning tumour
tissue largely depends on the degree of TSH stimulation, it
is of some potential importance to know whether the TSH levels
reached after stopping thyroxine for four weeks are similar,
irrespective of the length of time thyroxine had been given
continuously. Because the length of time between doses was

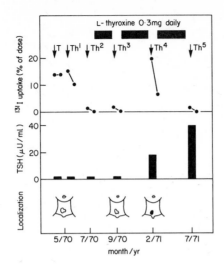

Fig. 3. *Radioiodine uptake measurements and localisation of concentration with plasma TSH measurements at various stages of treatment of thyroid carcinoma in a 46-year-old woman.*

variable, and dependent on the presence or absence of small residues, it was possible to examine the relationship between the TSH levels reached and the length of time that the patient had been receiving thyroxine without interruption. Although the data from this study are still rather limited, especially for those patients who have been maintained on thyroxine continuously for more than 3 years, the results (Fig. 5) nevertheless strongly suggest that the TSH response to four weeks' thyroxine withdrawal does progressively diminish as the time of continuous treatment increases. This is not due to any difference in plasma T_4 levels as these were of similar order in all the groups. The slightly higher average plasma T_4 in the patients treated continuously with thyroxine for one year or less, is probably accounted for by the presence of small functional remnants in some patients.

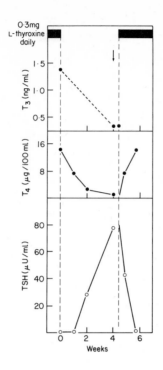

Fig. 4. *The effect on plasma T_4, T_3 and TSH of stopping and restarting thyroxine supplement in athyreotic patients (Mean values from eight patients).*

TSH AND TUMOUR ^{131}I UPTAKE

  In the patients studied so far, we have been unable to demonstrate a significant and unequivocal concentration of ^{131}I in tumour tissue unless the plasma TSH was elevated above the normal range. Undoubtedly there are occasional patients with an apparently autonomously functioning thyroid carcinoma not dependent on TSH stimulation or requiring very little (5, 6,7,8), but these seem to be rare and we have not found an example among about forty patients with functioning thyroid tumours seen during the last $3\frac{1}{2}$ years of the present study.

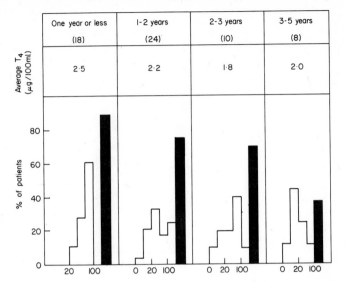

Fig. 5. *Rise of TSH at four weeks after stopping thyroxine supplement in relationship to the number of years of previous continuous treatment with thyroxine 0.3 mg daily. Open columns indicate % in ranges of TSH 0-4, 4-20, 20-50, 50-100 and > 100 μU/ml. The solid column in each group is the % of patients with TSH values > 20 μU/ml. The number of patients is given in parentheses.*

The level of TSH necessary to obtain a good ^{131}I uptake so as to give a satisfactory radiation dose to the tumour and metastases appears to vary from one individual to another. The patient illustrated in Fig. 3, for example, developed substantial tumour uptake when plasma TSH was less than 20 μU/ml. On the other hand, in another patient (Fig. 6), tumour uptake was absent when the TSH level was less than 20 μU/ml but developed strongly when it subsequently rose to over 60 μU/ml.

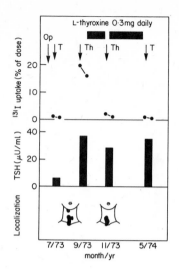

Fig. 6. *Radioiodine uptake measurements and localisation of concentration with plasma TSH measurements at various stages of treatment of thyroid carcinoma in a 35-year-old man. The initial arrow indicates the time of total thyroidectomy.*

VALUE OF HORMONE MEASUREMENTS

In most patients, an elevated level of TSH appears to be necessary to produce sufficient ^{131}I uptake for detection and treatment. Consequently if TSH levels at the time of a test or therapy dose of ^{131}I are normal or only mildly elevated, the failure of detectable concentration to develop may reflect inadequate TSH stimulation rather than the absence of tumour tissue or the presence of non-functioning tumour. Our measurements from patients after thyroidectomy showed that TSH levels in the majority were in the normal range or slightly elevated so that it is not surprising that ^{131}I concentration in tumour is not often detected with the first ^{131}I therapy, all the administered dose being concentrated in the normal thyroid remnant or excreted. The first dose does, however,

generally effect destruction of this remnant so that by the
time the second dose is given, the TSH levels are high in the
majority of patients and uptake in functioning tumour tissue
is generally demonstrable. Occasionally though, this does not
happen, and the availability of TSH measurements can then be
of considerable value in deciding whether to give the patient
further large doses of ^{131}I. In the patient illustrated in
Fig. 3, for example, the very small ^{131}I concentration found
at the second therapy dose, may have suggested that no further
therapy was needed. Because there was the additional information that TSH stimulation was low at the time of the second
dose, such a conclusion, based on ^{131}I uptakes, was not necessarily right. Further ^{131}I doses were given and subsequent
observations showed the correctness of this course.

Measurements of plasma TSH are also valuable at later
stages of treatment and follow-up (9). Thus plasma T_4 and TSH
values are useful in ensuring that the patient has properly
discontinued thyroxine. By the time the ^{131}I dose is given
four weeks after stopping thyroxine, the plasma T_4 should
be reduced to less than 2.5 µg/100ml. Having ensured that this
is so, the TSH value indicates the hypothalamic-pituitary response. If this is poor, with low TSH values, then it may be
necessary to give exogenous TSH in addition. Our observations
indicate that some patients maintained for long periods on
thyroxine seem to have impairment in the TSH response to its
withdrawal. This aspect calls for more detailed investigation;
such patients may need exogenous TSH or possibly a period of
TRH stimulation. The availability of hormonal measurements
is plainly going to be of considerable importance in the proper
evaluation of these new possibilities in treatment and as we

have tried to show in this preliminary account, has already
helped in the understanding and management of treatment of
patients with functioning thyroid cancer.

CONCLUSIONS

In none of the patients was the plasma TSH level found
to be elevated before surgery and T_4 and T_3 were also usually
within the normal range. Three weeks after total thyroidectomy, in only 40% of patients was plasma TSH much elevated.
Three months after a dose of 80 mCi of ^{131}I, however, plasma
TSH was considerably raised in 90% of patients and both T_4
and T_3 levels were low. With maintenance of patients on 0.3 mg
thyroxine daily, plasma TSH was undetectable and there seems,
therefore, no reason to use a higher dose to suppress TSH production. On stopping T_4 for four weeks preceding an [131]I
therapy or test dose, plasma TSH was elevated by two weeks
and rose progressively, while T_4 fell with a half-time of
7-8 days. In nearly all patients with functioning thyroid
cancer, elevation of plasma TSH appears to be necessary for
adequate ^{131}I uptake so that it is important to ensure that
plasma TSH is raised before concluding that ^{131}I uptake is
going to be inadequate for treatment. The combination of TSH,
T_4 and T_3 measurement is useful in ensuring that the hypothalamic-pituitary system is functioning properly, especially as
there is some evidence that with prolonged 0.3 mg daily L-thyroxine supplement, there may be impairment.

*Acknowledgement. We gratefully acknowledge the kindness of the
National Pituitary Agency (University of Maryland School of
Medicine U.S.A.) for providing human TSH for iodination and
rabbit anti-human HTSH, and of the Medical Research Council
for standard human TSH (MRC68/38) and rabbit anti-human TSH
serum.*

R E F E R E N C E S

1. E.E. Pochin, *In*"Modern Trends in Endocrinology"
    Ch. 5, Butterworths, London (1958).

2. R.A. Hall, J. Amos and B.J. Ormston, *Brit. Med. J.*
    1, 582 (1971).

3. J. Lieblich and R.D. Utiger, *J. Clin. Invest.* 51, 157
    (1972).

4. L.E. Braverman, S.H. Ingbar and K. Sterling, *J. Clin.
    Invest.* 49, 855 (1970).

5. D.D. Federman, *Medicine,* 43, 267 (1964).

6. E.E. Pochin, *Clin. Radiol.* 18, 113 (1967).

7. R.P. McLaughlin, D.A. Scholz, W.M. McConahey and D.S.
    Childs, *Mayo Clin. Proc.* 45, 328 (1970).

8. J.T. Dunn and S.C. Ray, *J. Clin. Endocr. Metab.* 36,
    1088 (1973).

9. T.J. Stahl and B. Shapiro, *J. Nucl. Med.* 14, 900, (1973).

28. Discussion of Thyroid Hormone Function in Clinical Investigation

Papers 17 and 18

Discussion of the paper by Drysdale, Ramsden and Hoffenberg on a routine method of estimation of thyroxine binding globulin in human serum started by consideration of the availability and desirability of absolute measurements of thyroxine binding globulin concentrations. Ramsden pointed out that to calibrate the described method it would be necessary to have a pure preparation of TBG. Oppenheimer suggested that in the clinical situation, a T_3 resin uptake was sufficient index of TBG binding capacity. Robbins agreed that knowledge of TBG binding capacity and the level of free T_4 would allow TBG concentration to be determined. He asked whether in the absence of TBG the technique presented would detect other transport proteins. Ramsden thought this was unlikely since TBPA was well separated from TBG in the method. In answer to a question from Hall, Ramsden said that his TBG levels in thyroid disorders compared well with most other reported values.

There followed a general discussion on variations in TBG metabolism in thyrotoxicosis, after oestrogen therapy and after surgery. Sterling raised the question, if alterations in T_3 resin tests in thyrotoxicosis might be due to alterations in TBG concentration rather than to saturation with thyroid hormone. There was also commentary on the dip in TBG concentration said to occur at the mid-point of the menstrual cycle

and the relationship to the observed five-day half life of
TBG. Rees asked if the antidiuresis after surgery could explain
the apparent diminution in concentration of TBG. Hoffenberg
did not consider this was a full explanation. He thought that
part of the problem was the increased catabolism of protein,
and also the sequestration of proteins in the region of the
wound in those patients who had major surgery. Sterling
agreed with this and pointed out that Gregerman had shown
that simple dilution could not explain the fall in TBG concentration.

The discussion ended on a number of technical points.
Sterling emphasised the importance of the position of the
antigen well in answer to a query from Nye. Ramsden indicated
that there was no interference from the agar in the TBG estimation. It was also stated that the method might be applied
to other proteins, such as transcortin, but because C-14 was
less suitable for autoradiography than I-125, it might prove
more technically difficult. This might be circumvented by the
use of fluorescent labels.

Discussion of the paper by Premachandra and Ibrahim was
opened by Wenzell who asked about the time necessary for
stripping. Premachandra said there was no simple answer. On
some occasions it might take 14 days, although many people used
only 24 hours. Larsen stated that his group had had similar
results. He stated that they used charcoal to obtain T_4-free
serum but that for T_3-free serum they used an ion exchange
resin. The latter method had the advantage that it did not
require a high-speed centrifuge to remove the particles as
required with charcoal.

The discussion ended with a consideration of the meaning

of the words "avidity" and "titre". Premachandra stated that
serum with high titre certainly takes longer to strip. Evered
said that his observations with T_4 and T_3 indicated that the
wide range of stripping times was related to titre but not to
avidity. Ekins asserted that stripping was determined by the
dissociation rate of the antibody and could have nothing to
do with either titre of affinity.

Papers 19, 20 and 21

Naegele showed slides of the plot of the Effective Thyroxine Ration (ETR) against the amount of serum added and
against the free-thyroxine concentration. He said that there
was a good correlation between the ETR and the clinically
evaluated thyroid status. All made a plea for the philosophy
of using the most sensitive available tests for screening
procedures rather than an initial simple test. He thought that
the logical thing would be to use TSH estimation for hypothyroidism and T_3 estimation or a TRH test for thyrotoxicosis.
Oppenheimer felt that the introduction of more tests tended
to lead to confusion and made a plea for a unified system of
nomenclature. Nicoloff felt that thyroid pathophysiology was
already almost unteachable to medical students. He said that
his laboratory had stopped reporting resin uptakes and instead
used them to adjust T_4 values. At this stage there was some
discussion of the importance of the free T_4 and free T_4 index.
Irvine (New Zealand) pointed out that caution was required
in ethanol extraction of serum since the process bringsdown
non-protein substances which bind T_4. Temperature variations
could also affect the various binding proteins differently,
and it was important to have a physiological buffer. He also
emphasised that free T_4 results are not necessarily related

to physiological activity.

Discussion of papers 20 and 21 were taken together. Oppenheimer enquired how Cavalieri visualised the molecular movement of T_3 from plasma into the kidney. He pointed out that the excretion of free hormone appeared to be higher than the free hormone flowing through the organ. Cavalieri replied that on the assumption of normal plasma flow, and of a uni-directional clearance of about 3% of the total T_3 entering the kidney, the results imply a debinding of T_3 during passage through the organ. He felt that the contribution of each specific binding protein could be derived from the total debinding rates. He also emphasised that the levels of free hormone estimated *in vitro* might not correspond to those found *in vivo* at the cellular level. In answer to a query from Burke, Cavalieri said that the renal uptake of T_3 correlated with the free T_3 levels in the plasma but not the total T_3 concentration. Ingbar enquired about the rising background counts, and Cavalieri confirmed his suspicion that this was due to rising activity in muscle, skin, etc. Robbins enquired if the limiting step in the transfer of T_3 was at the capillary wall or at the cell wall. Cavalieri said there was no direct information. In studies of the total T_3 uptake in the thigh there was no change in the pattern where the binding proteins in plasma were altered. He considered that the capillary barrier was perhaps the most important and pointed out that binding changes affect both sides of the capillary. Only if large doses of stable hormone are given could one cause a sudden disequilibrium. Irvine (New Zealand) found that the binding protein in renal lymph was about 60-70% of the binding protein concentration in the plasma and considered that the capillary

was not likely to be the barrier. He thought it more likely
that the barrier was at the cell wall in muscle and other
peripheral tissues. Rivlin noted the discrepancy between T_3
delivered to the kidney and the relatively small excretion.
He pointed to the evidence presented in his own paper that T_3
is transaminated in the kidney. Cavalieri, however, considered
that the time course of the experiment was too short to have
allowed for a major metabolic effect.

Hoffenberg asked why urinary thyroxine increased in the
presence of relatively trivial proteinuria. He also asked if
it would be more correct to express the clearances in terms
of creatinin clearance. Burke indicated that the creatinin
clearance, if used, does not alter the pattern of the data
but is potentially of use in neonates to enable a spot urine
to be used. He claimed that doubling the TBG concentration
would double or treble the total T_3 content in the urine.
In response to an enquiry from Ingbar, Burke said that triac
did not interfere with his estimations. Oppenheimer discussed
the problems of measuring free hormones both on technical
grounds and on a theoretical level, and enquired whether the
free hormone concentrations were the same at all sites of
the body. Ekins closed the discussion by indicating his experience of the estimation of free hormones by dialysis techniques, using a radioimmunoassay as the final estimation of
T_3 and T_4 concentrations. He claimed that these techniques
were not unduly difficult or time consuming.

Paper 22

There was a lengthy debate about the meaning of the
terms "subclinical hypothyroidism" and "compensated euthyroidism".
Following this, Evered made the point that T_4 might be important

in the feed back control of the thyroid while T_3 could be
considered more important in maintaining thyroid supply to the
tissues. There followed some discussion on the possibility
that TRH increases blood pressure. Oppenheimer stated that
his laboratory blood pressure readings were taken every minute
after the administration of TRH. Hall said that they had
observed no side effects from TRH in 2000 patients they studied
in Newcastle.

Paper 23

Hoffenberg raised the question of variable values for
T_3 in normal subjects. Sterling suggested that the differences
could result from the use of buffer alone as compared with
T_3-free serum diluted with buffer. Serum deprived of hormone
by passing it through charcoal had more unoccupied TBG sites.
Ingbar could not agree with Sterling's explanation. He had
tried T_3-free serum with low TBG. Ekins remarked that his
normal values were lower and he could not agree with Sterling's
higher values.

Paper 24

There was some discussion of what could be considered a
maintenance dose of T_3. Evered felt that 40 to 50 µg T_3 per
day could suppress thyroid function. Nicoloff agreed that
80 µg per day was high for a maintenance dose. He pointed out
that the existence of a normal level of T_4 in patients receiving T_3 reflects a higher than normal T_4 secretion since
T_3 increases the turnover of T_4. Evered said that the normal
response to T_3 was variable. Some patients responded to as
little as 10 µg per day whilst others required 16 µg per day
for a measurable response.

Papers 26 and 27

Discussion of the last two papers was taken together.
Ingbar stated that long-term follow-up of patients treated
with antithyroid drugs showed that hypothyroidism was very
common, sometimes developing as late as 20 years after treatment. McLarty said that in 50 clinically euthyroid thyrotoxic
cases two-thirds had flat TRH responses, 50% had raised T_3
levels, and the remainder had normal T_3 levels. There was
some discussion over the range of TSH concentrations found
in normal subjects, Ratcliffe believing that there was no
well defined normal range.

There was considerable discussion over the incidence
of "T_3 toxicosis". Larsen quoted a figure of 2-3%, Pochin
felt that T_3 toxicosis was not a separate form of thyroid
disease, but rather an extreme of the toxic range, a view
supported by Larsen.

There was also some discussion on the question of whether
TSH played a role in the development of thyroid cancer. Pochin
stated that TSH does increase the incidence of thyroid cancer
in animals, but that there was no evidence on this point in
humans. The use of bovine TSH to stimulate the uptake of
radioiodine for therapeutic purposes was considered. Pochin
pointed out that while TSH would be likely to increase the
thyroid uptake of radioiodine, the turnover of iodine within
the gland would also be greater than normal. TSH would
therefore have little effect on the radioactive dosage. The
discussion ended with a consideration of the decrease of
plasma T_3 concentrations with age.

Author Index

Abbreviations

cAMP, 3'5'cyclic adenosine monophosphate

ANS, 8-anilino-1-naphthalene sulfonic acid

CBP, Cytosol binding protein

DIT, 3,5-diiodo-L-tyrosine

$D-T_3$, 3,3',5-triiodo-D-thyronine

$D-T_4$, D-thyroxine

GPD or αGPD, α-glycerolphosphate dehydrogenase

K_α, Affinity constant

MBC, Maximal binding capacity

MIT, 3-iodo-L-tyrosine

PA, Thyroxine-binding prealbumin

PEG, Polyethylene glycol

PTU, 6-n-propylthiouracil

RBP, Retinol binding protein

SDS, Sodium dodecyl sulfate

STM, 0.25M sucrose, 20mM Tris-HCl, 1.1mM $MgCl_2$, pH 7.85

T_2, 3,5-diiodo-L-thyronine

T_3, 3,5,3'-triiodo-L-thyronine

T_4, L-thyroxine

TBG, Thyroxine binding globulin

TBPA, Thyroxine-binding prealbumin

TEM, 0.05M Tris-HCl, 2mM EDTA, 2mM 2-mercaptoethanol, pH 7.4

Tetrac, 3,3',5,5'-tetraiodothyroacetic acid

Tetraprop, 3,3',5,5'-tetraiodothyropropionic acid

Triac, 3,3',5-triiodothyroacetic acid

Triprop, 3,3',5-triiodothyropropionic acid

Subject Index*

A

Adenyl cyclase, 49, 201, 258

Athyreotic patients, 415

Aminotransferase ($L-T_3$), 213, 258

Analogues of thyroid hormones, 12, 40, 190, 223, 321

ANS, 14, 348

Antibodies, 148, 153, 281, 427

B

Biliary clearance, 69, 254

Bovine, 89

C

Cancer (thyroid), 409

Capillary, 428

Carbimazole, 368

Charcoal, 281

Cholesterol, 65, 150

Clofibrate, 65

Compartmental analysis, 163

Cyclic AMP, 49, 201, 258

Cytosol binding sites, 35, 47, 89, 105, 250, 253

D

Dolphin, 241

E

Effective thyroxine ratio, 427

Epinephrine, 202

Extraction, 293

F

Familial resistance, 139

G

Glucagon, 208, 258

Goitre, 142, 227, 341

GPD, 128, 195, 256

H

Hydroxyproline, 140, 255

Hyperthyroid, 151, 196, 201, 223, 259, 270, 299, 308, 322, 335, 367, 383, 397, 425, 427, 431

Hypothyroid, 151, 196, 201, 223, 259, 270, 299, 308, 322, 336, 383, 403, 427, 429, 431

I

^{131}I therapy, 383, 409

Subjects which occur throughout these proceedings (e.g. thyroxine) are not listed in the index. Where subjects occur throughout a chapter only the first page is given.